Anatomy
and
Physiology
for
Physiotherapists

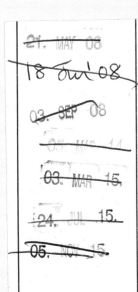

Anatomy
and
Physiology
for
Physiotherapists

Inderbir Singh
52, Sector One, Rohtak 124001

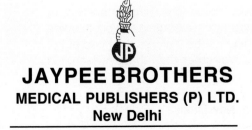

JAYPEE BROTHERS
MEDICAL PUBLISHERS (P) LTD.
New Delhi

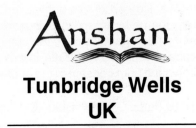

Tunbridge Wells
UK

First published in the UK by

Anshan Ltd
in 2006
6 Newlands Road
Tunbridge Wells
Kent TN4 9AT, UK

Tel/Fax: +44 (0)1892 557767
E-mail: info@anshan.co.uk
www.anshan.co.uk

ISBN 1 904798 594

British Library Cataloguing in Publication Data
A catalogue record for this book is available from the British Library

Printed in India by Paras Offset Pvt. Ltd., C-176, Naraina Indl. Area, New Delhi.

Preface

This book has been written to meet the requirements of students undergoing physiotherapy courses. Many of them are at present reading the subjects of Anatomy and Physiology from books meant for M.B.B.S students. It does not need to be emphasized that such books are not suited to the requirements of physiotherapy students. While the latter students require full details of some parts of the body, others can be dealt with briefly. The students also need guidance about what to read in detail, and what to omit.

The contents of the book have been framed keeping this in mind. The contents are also in keeping with the syllabi of various universities.

The language of the text has been kept simple. The book is illustrated with numerous diagrams in colour to make the subjects easy to comprehend.

Suggestions for improvement of the book will be welcomed.

Rohtak
January 2005

Inderbir Singh

Contents

PART ONE

INTRODUCTION
TO
THE HUMAN BODY

1

Learning the Language of Medicine

THE SUBJECT OF ANATOMY

Anatomy is the science that deals with the structure of the human body. Many features of structure can be seen by naked eye and such a study is called **gross anatomy** or **morphological anatomy**. Many other features can be observed only under a microscope, and a study of these features constitutes the science of **microscopic anatomy** or **histology**. Histology includes the study of details of the structure of cells (**cytology**), and of related chemical considerations (**histochemistry**). Many recent advances in our knowledge of the structure of the body have been made possible by the use of high magnifications available with an electron microscope, and such details are referred to as **ultrastructure**. The science of anatomy also includes the study of the development of tissues and organs before birth: this is called **embryology**. Aspects of anatomy that are of particular relevance to understanding of disease and its treatment are referred to as **applied anatomy** or **clinical anatomy**.

MAIN SUBDIVISIONS OF THE HUMAN BODY

For convenience of description the human body is divided into a number of major parts. Many of the parts bear names with which you will be already familiar, but even some of these may require more precise definition.

The uppermost part of the body is the **head**. The **face** is part of the head (and includes the region of the **forehead**, the **eyes**, the **nose**, the **cheeks** and the **chin**). Below the head there is the neck. Below the neck, there is the region that a layperson calls the chest. In anatomical terminology the chest is referred to as

the **thorax**. The thorax is in the form of a bony cage within which the heart and lungs lie. Below the thorax, there is the region commonly referred to as 'stomach' or 'belly'. Its proper name is **abdomen**. The abdomen contains several organs of vital importance to the body. Traced downwards, the abdomen extends to the hips. A part of the abdomen present in the region of the hips is called the **pelvis**.

The thorax and abdomen together form the **trunk**. Attached to the trunk there are the upper and lower **limbs**, or the upper and lower **extremities**. In relation to the upper limb the terms **shoulder**, **elbow**, **wrist**, **hand**, **palm**, **fingers** and **thumb** will be familiar. A layperson frequently refers to the entire upper limb as the **arm**, but in anatomy we use this term only for the region between the shoulder and elbow. The region between the elbow and wrist is the **forearm**. The fingers and thumb are also called **digits**.

In the lower limbs the terms **hip**, **knee**, **ankle**, **foot** and **toes** will be familiar. The region between the hip and the knee is the **thigh**, and that between the knee and the ankle is the **leg**. Like the fingers, the toes are also called **digits**. The innermost, and largest toe, is the **great toe**.

SOME COMMONLY USED DESCRIPTIVE TERMS

A student entering a hospital for the first time is very likely to find that doctors seem to use many strange sounding words. You will become familiar with them over the years. Many of these strange words are really terms used to describe different parts of the body, and they constitute the basis for the study of anatomy and physiology.

The learning of these terms is the basic foundation on which all subsequent studies of the human body depend. In short, the study of anatomy teaches us the language of medicine.

Of all the terms to be learnt the first, and most fundamental, are those used for precise description of the mutual relationships of various structures within the body. In describing such relationships the layperson uses terms like 'in front', 'behind', 'above', 'below' etc. However, in a study of anatomy, such terms are found to be inadequate; and the student's first task is to become familiar with the specialized terms used.

A major problem in describing anatomical relationships is that they keep changing with movement. For example, when a person stands upright the head is the uppermost part of the body and the feet the lowermost. However, on lying down the head and feet are at the same level. The problem is overcome by always describing relationships within the body presuming that the person is standing upright, looking directly forwards, with the arms held by the sides of the body, and with the palms facing forwards. (This posture is referred to as the **anatomical position**.) We will now consider some descriptive terms one by one.

(**1**) When structure **A** lies nearer the front of the body as compared to structure **B**, **A** is said to be **anterior** to **B** (Fig.1.1).

The opposite of anterior is **posterior**. In the above example, it follows that **B** is posterior to **A**. Using these terms we can say that the nose is anterior to the ears; and the ears are posterior to the nose.

(**2**) When structure **C** lies nearer the upper end of the body as compared to structure **D**, **C** is said to be **superior** to **D** (Fig. 1.1). The opposite of superior is **inferior**. In the above example **D** is inferior to **C**. (No difference in the quality of the structures is implied!). Using these terms we can say that the nose is superior to the mouth, but is inferior to the forehead.

(**3**) The body can be divided into two equal halves, right and left, by a plane passing vertically through it. (A plane is like a sheet of paper. It has length and breadth, but no thickness). The plane separating the right and left halves of the body is called the **median plane** (Fig. 1.2). When a structure lies in the median plane it is said to be **median** in position (e.g., G in Fig. 1.2). When structure **E** lies nearer the median plane than structure **F**, **E** is said to be **medial** to **F**. The opposite of medial is **lateral**. In the above example **F** is lateral to **E**.

In the anatomical position the palm faces forwards and the thumb lies along the outer side of the hand. Starting from the side of the thumb (or first digit) the

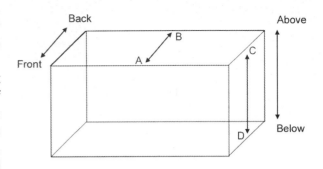

Fig. 1.1. Scheme to explain the terms anterior, posterior, superior, and inferior.

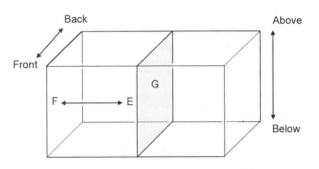

Fig. 1.2. Scheme to explain the terms medial, lateral and median.

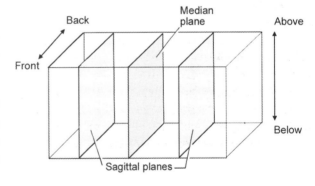

Fig. 1.3. Scheme showing median and paramedian planes.

fingers are named index finger (second digit), middle finger (third digit), ring finger (fourth digit) and little finger (fifth digit). To describe the medial-lateral relationships of the fingers we can say that the thumb lies lateral to the index finger. The index finger is medial to the thumb, but is lateral to the middle finger.

Various combinations of the descriptive terms mentioned above are frequently used. For example, each eye is anterior to the corresponding ear; and is also medial to it. Therefore, the eye can be said to be **anteromedial** to the ear. The tip of the nose is inferior and medial to each eye: we can say the nose is **inferomedial** to the eye.

We must now consider terms that are sometimes used as equivalent to some of the terms introduced above. The anterior aspect of the body corresponds to the ventral aspect of the body of four-footed animals. Hence the term **ventral** is often used as equivalent to anterior. (However, we shall see later that the two terms are not always equivalent, e.g., in the thigh). The opposite of ventral is **dorsal**. In the hand the palm is on the anterior or ventral aspect. This aspect of the hand is often called the **palmar** aspect. The back of the hand is the dorsal aspect, or simply the **dorsum**, of the hand. In the case of the foot the surface towards the sole is ventral: it is called the **plantar aspect**. The upper side of the foot is the **dorsum** of the foot.

While referring to structures in the trunk the term **cranial** (= towards the head) is sometimes used instead of superior; and **caudal** (= towards the tail) in place of inferior. In the limbs the term superior is sometimes replaced by **proximal** (= nearer) and inferior by **distal** (= more distant). Using this convention the phalanges of the hands are designated proximal, middle and distal. In the case of the forearm (or hand) the medial side is often referred to as the **ulnar** side, and the lateral side as the **radial** side. Similarly, in the leg (or foot) we can speak of the **tibial** (= medial) or **fibular** (= lateral) sides.

In addition to the terms described above there are some terms that are used to define planes passing through the body. (The concept of planes can be understood by reference to a cube. The angles of the cube are points: they have no length. The edges of the cube are lines: they have length but no width. The surfaces of the cube have length as well as breadth, but no thickness: these can be regarded as planes. (Remember than any flat surface is also called a plane surface: the essential thing about a plane is that it is absolutely flat).

We have already seen that a plane passing vertically through the midline of the body, so as to divide the body into right and left halves, is called the **median plane**. It is also called the **mid-sagittal plane**. Vertical planes to the right or left of the median plane, and parallel to the latter, are called **paramedian** or **sagittal planes** (Fig. 1.3). A vertical plane placed at right angles to the median plane (dividing the body into anterior and posterior parts) is called a **coronal plane** or a **frontal plane** (Fig. 1.4). Planes passing horizontally across the body (i.e., at right angles to both the sagittal and coronal planes) and dividing it into upper and lower parts, are called **transverse** or **horizontal planes** (Fig. 1.5). In addition there are innumerable oblique planes intermediate between those described above.

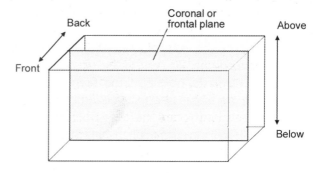

Fig. 1.4. Scheme showing a frontal or coronal plane.

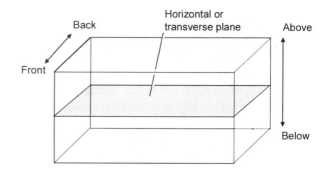

Fig. 1.5. Scheme showing a horizontal or transverse plane.

Sections through any part of the body in any of the planes mentioned above are given corresponding names. Thus we speak of median sections, sagittal sections, coronal or frontal sections, transverse sections and oblique sections.

STRUCTURES CONSTITUTING THE HUMAN BODY

The animal body is made up of various elements. The basic framework of the body is provided by a large number of **bones** that collectively form the **skeleton**. As bones are hard they not only maintain their own shape, but also provide shape to the part of the body within which they lie. In some situations (e.g., the nose or the ear) part of the skeleton is made up, not of bone but of, a firm but flexible tissue called **cartilage**. Bones meet each other at **joints**, many of which allow movements to be performed. At joints, fibrous bands called **ligaments** unite bones to one another. Overlying (and usually attached to) bones we see **muscles**. Muscles are what the layman refers to as flesh. In the limbs, muscles form the main bulk. Muscle tissue has the property of being able to shorten in length. In other words muscles can contract, and by contraction they provide power for movements. A typical muscle has two ends one (traditionally) called the *origin*, and the other called the *insertion*. Both ends are attached, typically, to bones. The attachment to bone may be a direct one, but quite often the muscle fibres end in cord like structures called *tendons*, which convey the pull of the muscle to bone. Tendons are very strong structures. Sometimes a muscle may end in a flat fibrous membrane. Such a membrane is called an *aponeurosis*.

Within a limb we find that the muscles are separated from skin, and from one another, by a tissue in which fibres are prominent. Such tissue is referred to as fascia. Immediately beneath the skin the fibres of the fascia are arranged loosely and this loose tissue is called *superficial fascia*. Over some parts of the body the superficial fascia may contain considerable amounts of fat. Deep to the superficial fascia the muscles are covered by a much better formed and stronger membrane. This membrane is the *deep fascia*. In the limbs, and in the neck, the deep fascia encloses deeper structures like a tight sleeve. Membranes similar to deep fascia may also intervene between adjacent muscles forming *intermuscular septa*. Such septa often give attachment to muscle fibres.

Running through the intervals between muscles (usually in relation to fascial septa) there are *blood vessels*, *lymphatic vessels*, and *nerves*.

Blood vessels are tubular structures through which blood circulates. The vessels that carry blood from the heart to various tissues are called *arteries*. Those vessels that return this blood to the heart are called *veins*. Within tissues plexuses of microscopic vessels called capillaries connect arteries and veins.

Lymphatic vessels are delicate, thin walled tubes. They are difficult to see. They often run alongside veins. Along the course of these lymphatic vessels small bean shaped structures are present in certain situations. These are *lymph nodes*. Lymphatic vessels and lymph nodes are part of a system that plays a prominent role in protecting the body in various ways that you will study later.

Running through tissues, often in the company of blood vessels, we have solid cord like structures called *nerves*. Each nerve is a bundle of a large number of *nerve fibres*. Each nerve fibre is a process arising from a *nerve cell* (or *neuron*). Most nerve cells are located in the brain and in the spinal cord. Nerves transmit impulses from the brain and spinal cord to various tissues. They also carry information from tissues to the brain. Impulses passing through nerves are responsible for contraction of muscle, and for secretions by glands. Sensations like touch, pain, sight and hearing are all dependent on nerve impulses traveling through nerve fibres.

Bones, muscles, blood vessels, nerves etc. that we have spoken of in the previous paragraphs are to be seen in all parts of the body. In addition to these many parts of the body have specialized *organs*, also commonly called *viscera*. Some of the viscera are solid (e.g., the liver, or the kidney), while others are tubular (e.g., the intestines) or sac like (e.g., the stomach). The viscera are grouped together in accordance with function to form various *organ systems*. Some examples of organ systems are the *respiratory system* responsible for providing the body with oxygen; the *alimentary* or *digestive system* responsible for the digestion and absorption of food; the *urinary system* responsible for removal of waste products from the body through urine; and the *genital system* which contains organs concerned with reproduction.

2

A Brief Introduction to Bones, Joints & Muscles of the Body

INTRODUCTION TO THE SKELETON

We have seen that the basic foundation of the body is provided by the skeleton. Although details of the features to be seen on individual bones are best studied along with the anatomy of the region concerned, any student embarking on a study of anatomy needs to have a general idea of the skeleton as a whole. The purpose of this section is to provide such information.

The human skeleton may be divided into:

(**a**) the **axial skeleton** consisting of the bones of the head, neck and trunk; and

(**b**) the **appendicular skeleton** consisting of the bones of the limbs.

A preliminary look at the skull

The skeleton of the head is called the skull. It is seen from the lateral side in Fig. 2.1 and from above in Fig. 2.2. The skull contains a large **cranial cavity** in which the brain is lodged. Just below the forehead the skull shows two large depressions, the right and left **orbits**, in which the eyes are lodged. In the region of the nose and mouth there are apertures that lead into the interior of the skull.

The skull is made up of a large number of bones that are firmly joined together. Some of these are as follows. In the region of the forehead there is the **frontal bone**. At the back of the head (also called the **occiput**) there is the **occipital bone**. The top of the skull, and parts of its side walls, are formed mainly by the right and left **parietal bones**. The region of the head just above the ears is referred to as the **temple**, and the bone here is the **temporal bone** (right or left). The bone that forms the upper jaw, and bears the upper teeth, is the **maxilla**. The prominence of the cheek is formed by the **zygomatic bone**. In the floor of the cranial cavity there is an unpaired bone called the **sphenoid bone**. The bone of the lower jaw is called

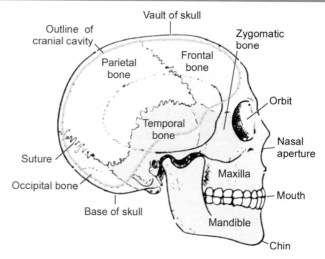

Fig. 2.1. Skull seen from the right side.

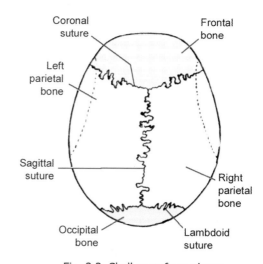

Fig. 2.2. Skull seen from above

the **mandible**. It is separate from the rest of the skull. In addition to these large bones there are several smaller ones that will be identified when we take up the study of the skull in detail.

The vertebral column

Below the skull the central axis of the body is formed by the backbone or **vertebral column** (Fig. 2.3). The vertebral column is made up of a large number of bones of irregular shape called **vertebrae**. There are seven *cervical vertebrae* in the neck. Below these there are twelve *thoracic vertebrae* that take part in forming the skeleton of the thorax. Still lower down there are five *lumbar vertebrae* that lie in the posterior wall of the abdomen. The lowest part of the vertebral column is made up of the *sacrum*, which consists of five sacral vertebrae that are fused together; and of a small bone called the *coccyx*. The coccyx is made up of four rudimentary vertebrae fused together. There are thus thirty three vertebrae in all. Taking the sacrum and coccyx as single bones the vertebral column has twenty six bones.

Skeleton of the thorax

The skeleton of the thorax forms a bony cage that protects the heart, the lungs, and some other organs (Fig. 2.4). Behind, it is made up of twelve thoracic vertebrae. In front, it is formed by a bone called the *sternum*. The sternum consists of an upper part, the *manubrium*; a middle part, the *body*; and a lower part, the *xiphoid process*. The side walls of the thorax are formed by twelve ribs on either side.

Each rib is a long curved bone that is attached posteriorly to the vertebral column. It curves round the sides of the thorax. Its anterior end is attached to a bar of cartilage (the *costal cartilage*) through which it gains attachment to the sternum. This arrangement is seen typically in the upper seven ribs (*true ribs*). The 8th, 9th and 10th costal cartilages do not reach the sternum, but end by getting attached to the next higher cartilage (*false ribs*). The anterior ends of the 11th and 12th ribs are free: they are, therefore, called *floating ribs*.

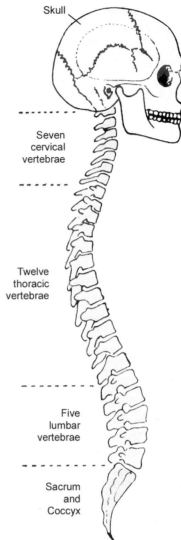

Fig. 2.3. Skull and vertebral column (side view).

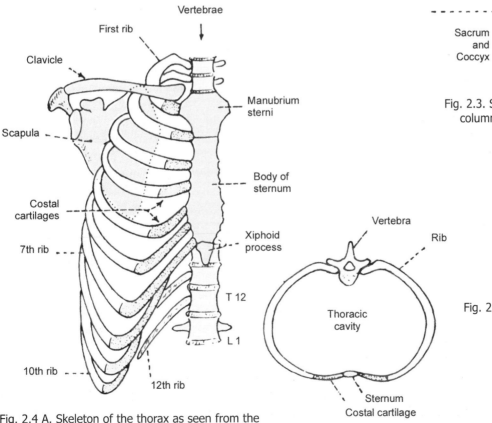

Fig. 2.4 A. Skeleton of the thorax as seen from the front. The bones of the shoulder girdle are also shown.

Fig. 2.4B. Section across thorax.

Skeleton of the Upper Limb

The skeleton of each upper limb (Fig. 2.5) consists of the bones of the **pectoral girdle** (or **shoulder girdle**) that lie in close relation to the upper part of the thorax (Fig. 2.4A), and those of the **free limb**.

The pectoral girdle consists of the collar bone or **clavicle**, and the **scapula**. The clavicle is a rod like bone placed in front of the upper part of the thorax. Medially, it is attached to the manubrium of the sternum, and laterally to the scapula. The scapula is a triangular plate of bone placed behind the upper part of the thorax.

The bone of the arm is called the **humerus**. There are two bones in the forearm: the bone that lies laterally (i.e., towards the thumb) is called the **radius**; and the bone that lies medially (i.e., towards the little finger) is called the **ulna**. The humerus, radius and ulna are long bones each having a cylindrical middle part called the **shaft**, and expanded upper and lower **ends**.

In the wrist there are eight small, roughly cuboidal, **carpal bones**. The skeleton of the palm is made up of five rod like **metacarpal bones**, while the skeleton of the fingers (or digits) is made up of the **phalanges**. There are three phalanges – **proximal, middle and distal** – in each digit except the thumb which has only two phalanges (proximal and distal).

The upper end of the humerus is joined to the scapula at the **shoulder joint**, and its lower end is joined to the upper ends of the radius and ulna to form the **elbow joint**. The **wrist joint** is formed where the lower ends of the radius and ulna meet the carpal bones. The upper and lower ends of the radius and ulna are united to one another at the **superior and inferior radioulnar joints**. There are numerous small joints in the hand: the **intercarpal** between the carpal bones themselves; the **carpometacarpal** between the carpal and metacarpal bones; the **metacarpophalangeal** between each metacarpal bone and the proximal phalanx; and the **interphalangeal** joints between the phalanges themselves.

Skeleton of the Lower Limb

The skeleton of the lower limb consists of the bones of the **pelvic girdle**, and those of the **free limb** (Fig. 2.6). The pelvic girdle is made up of one **hip bone** on either side. Each hip bone is made up of three parts that are fused together. The upper expanded part of the bone is called the **ilium**. A small part in front (shaded in the figure) is called the **pubis**. The lower part of the bone is called the **ischium**. Anteriorly, the two pubic bones meet in the midline to form a joint called the **pubic symphysis**. Posteriorly, the sacrum is wedged in between the two hip bones. The hip bones and sacrum (along with the coccyx) form the **bony pelvis**.

The bones of the free part of the limb are arranged in a pattern similar to that in the upper limb. The bone of the thigh is called the **femur**. There are two bones in the leg. The medial of the two (lying towards the great toe) is called the **tibia**, while the outer bone is called the **fibula**. The femur, tibia and fibula are long bones having cylindrical shafts with expanded upper and lower ends. In the region of the ankle, and the posterior part of the foot, there are seven roughly cuboidal **tarsal bones**. The largest of these is the **calcaneus**, which forms the heel. Next in size we have the **talus**. In the anterior part of the foot there are five **metatarsal bones**. Each digit (or toe) has three **phalanges** – proximal, middle and distal: however, the great toe has only

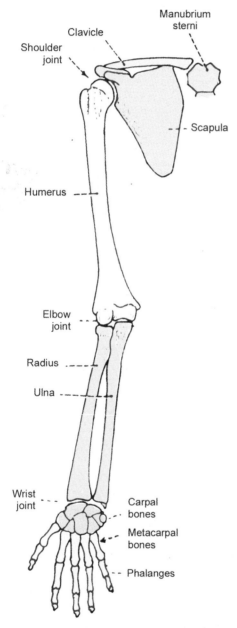

Fig. 2.5. Skeleton of the right upper limb. The manubrium sterni is included for orientation.

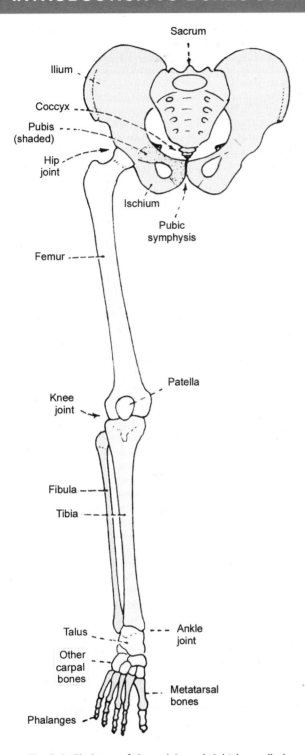

Fig. 2.6. Skeleton of the pelvis and right lower limb.

the **ankle joint**. Within the foot there are **intertarsal, tarsometatarsal, metatarsophalangeal and interphalangeal joints** on a pattern similar to those in the hand.

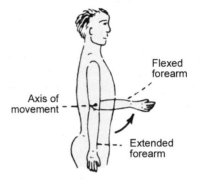

Fig. 2.7. Diagram to explain the movement of flexion of the forearm.

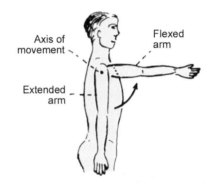

Fig. 2.8. Diagram to explain the movement of flexion of the arm.

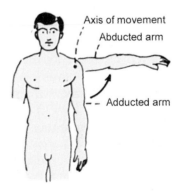

Fig. 2.9. Diagram to explain the movement of abduction of the arm.

two phalanges – proximal and distal.

The upper end of the femur fits into a deep socket in the hip bone (called the **acetabulum**) to form the **hip joint**. The lower end of the femur meets the tibia to form the **knee joint**. A small bone, the **patella**, is placed in front of the knee. The tibia and fibula are joined to each other at their upper and lower ends to form the superior and inferior **tibiofibular joints**. The lower ends of the tibia and fibula join the talus to form

SOME FEATURES OF JOINTS

We have seen that joints are formed where two (or more) bones meet. Some joints are merely bonds of union between different bones and do not allow movement. Joints of the skull (sutures) belong to this category. Some joints allow slight movement, while some (like the shoulder joint) allow great freedom of movement. In describing movements we use certain terms which the student must understand clearly.

In Chapter 1 we have introduced the concept of planes. Movements at any joint can take place in various planes. Movements taking place in a sagittal plane are referred to as *flexion* (= bending), and *extension* (= straightening). For example when we bend the upper limb at the elbow joint so that the front of the forearm tends to approach the front of the arm this movement is called flexion. Straightening the limb at the elbow is called extension. Bending the neck forwards is flexion of the neck, and straightening it is extension. Similarly, when we bow, the vertebral column is being flexed, and when the body is made upright the spine is being extended.

Movements in the coronal plane are referred to as *abduction* (= taking away) or *adduction* (= bringing near). When a limb is moved laterally so that it moves away from the trunk it is said to undergo abduction. For example, such a movement takes place at the shoulder joint when the upper limb is raised sideways. A similar movement takes place at the hip joint. Adduction and abduction can also take place at the wrist and at metacarpo-phalangeal joints.

Some joints allow *rotatory movements*. When the forearm is rotated so that the palm comes to face forwards, the movement is called *supination*. The opposite movement is called *pronation*. Side to side movements of the neck are also rotatory movements. The movement of the arm performed by a cricketer in bowling is a rotatory movement at the shoulder. Note that during this movement the hand moves in a circle. This movement is, therefore, called *circumduction*. When the foot is turned so that the sole looks somewhat inwards the movement is called *inversion*. The opposite movement is called *eversion*.

SOME FEATURES OF MUSCLES

Structure of Muscle

The power for movement is provided by muscle tissue. Muscle cells are specialized to shorten in length by contraction, and this shortening can pull two structures towards one another. That is how movements are produced. Three distinct types of muscle are recognized on the basis of their structure and function.

Large muscles are present in relation to the skeleton, specially in the limbs. These muscles constitute what a layperson describes as flesh. The contraction of these muscles is under our control i.e., it is voluntary. When examined through a microscope the muscle fibres show characteristic striations. Because of these reasons this kind of muscle is called *skeletal muscle*, *voluntary muscle* or *striated muscle*.

The walls of many hollow viscera contain a different kind of muscle that is not under our control, and does not show striations. This is called *smooth muscle*, or *involuntary muscle*.

A third kind of muscle forms the walls of the heart. This is called *cardiac muscle*.

The structure of muscle is considered in detail in Chapter 9.

How muscles are named

The human body contains a very large number of muscles, each of which bears a name. A muscle may be named on the basis of its action, its shape and size, and the region in which it lies. The name of a given muscle usually consists of two or more words based on these characteristics. How muscles are named will be clear from the following examples.

Some names based on region

1. The region on the front of the chest is called the *pectoral region*. There are two muscles in this region. The larger of the two is called the *pectoralis major*. The smaller one is called the *pectoralis minor*.

2. The region of the buttock is called the *gluteal region*. It contains three large muscles that are given the names *gluteus maximus* (largest), *gluteus medius* (intermediate in size) and *gluteus minimus* (smallest).

In each of the above examples note that the first word refers to the region concerned, and the second to relative size.

Some names based on shape

1. Muscles that are straight are given the name ***rectus*** (compare with 'erect'). One such muscle present in the wall of the abdomen is called the ***rectus abdominis***. Another in the thigh is called the ***rectus femoris***. (Femoris = thigh: that is why the bone of the thigh is the femur).

2. Over the shoulder there is a strong triangular muscle called the ***deltoid*** (after the Greek letter delta, which is shaped like a triangle).

3. A quadrilateral muscle present in the lumbar region is called the ***quadratus lumborum***.

4. Most muscles have a fusiform shape. The central thicker part is muscular and is called the ***belly***. The ends are usually tendinous, and gain attachment to bones.. Some muscles have two (or more) bellies each with a distinct origin (or head). A muscle having two heads is given the name ***biceps***. There is one such muscle in the arm and another in the thigh. The one in the arm is the ***biceps brachii*** (brachium = arm); and that in the thigh is the ***biceps femoris***. On the back of the arm there is a muscle that arises by three heads. It is called the ***triceps***. On the front of the thigh there is a muscle that has four heads. It is called the ***quadriceps femoris***. (Distinguish carefully between quadriceps and quadratus).

Some names based on action:

Muscles that produce flexion may be named ***flexors***, and those that cause extension may be called ***extensors***. Similarly, a muscle may be an ***abductor***, an ***adductor***, a ***supinator*** or a ***pronator***. In each case the word indicating action is followed by another word indicating the part on which the action is produced. For example, on the back of the forearm there is a muscle that is an extensor of the digits: it is called the ***extensor digitorum***. Sometimes we can have more than one muscle that qualifies for such a name. In that case we add a third word indicative of position. On the front of forearm there are two muscles that produce flexion at the wrist (or carpus). One of them, which lies towards the medial (or ulnar) side is called the ***flexor carpi ulnaris*** (= ulnar flexor of the carpus). The second muscle lies towards the lateral (or radial) side and is called the ***flexor carpi radialis***. Sometimes it is necessary to add a fourth word to the name. On the back of the forearm there are two radial extensors of the wrist: we call the longer one the ***extensor carpi radialis longus*** and the shorter one is named the ***extensor carpi radialis brevis***. On the medial side of the thigh there are three muscles that adduct it. Because of variations in size they are called the ***adductor longus***, the ***adductor brevis***, and the ***adductor magnus*** (magnus = largest).

Appreciation of these principles, used in naming muscles, can go a long way in easing the burden of remembering the names of muscles and their actions.

3

A Brief Introduction to
Organ Systems of the Body

We have seen that the body contains a number of organ systems that are essential to its working. We shall take a brief look at each system in the paragraphs that follow. Each of the organs mentioned will be studied in detail later.

INTRODUCTION TO THE RESPIRATORY SYSTEM

The respiratory system is meant, primarily, for the oxygenation of blood. The chief organs of the system are the right and left *lungs*. Oxygen contained in air reaches the lungs by passing through a series of respiratory passages, which also serve for removal of carbon dioxide released from the blood.

The respiratory passages are shown in Figs. 3.1 and 3.2. Air from the outside enters the body through the right and left *anterior nares* (or *external nares*) which open into the right and left *nasal cavities.* Apart from their respiratory function, the nasal cavities have olfactory areas that act as end organs for smell. At their posterior ends the nasal cavities have openings called the *posterior nares* (or *internal nares*) through which they open into the *pharynx.* The pharynx is a single cavity not divided into right and left halves. It is divisible, from above downwards, into an upper part the *nasopharynx* (into which the nasal cavities open); a middle part the *oropharynx* (which is continuous with the posterior end of the oral cavity); and a lower part the *laryngopharynx.* Air from the nose enters the nasopharynx and passes down through the oropharynx and laryngopharynx. Air can also pass through the mouth directly into the oropharynx and from there to the laryngopharynx. Air from the laryngopharynx enters a box-like structure called the *larynx.* The larynx is placed on the front of the upper part of the neck. Apart from being a respiratory passage it is the organ where voice is produced. It is, therefore, sometimes called the voice-box.

Inferiorly the larynx is continuous with a tube called the *trachea.* The trachea passes through the lower

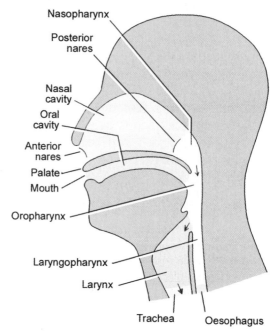

Fig. 3.1. Simplified diagram showing intercommunications between the nasal cavities, the mouth, the pharynx, the larynx and the oesophagus.

part of the neck into the upper part of the thorax. At the level of the lower border of the manubrium sterni the trachea bifurcates into the right and left *principal bronchi*, which carry air to the right and left lungs. Within the lung each principal bronchus divides, like the branches of a tree, into smaller and smaller *bronchi* that ultimately end in microscopic tubes that are called *bronchioles.* The bronchioles open into microscopic sac-like structures called *alveoli.* The walls of the alveoli contain a rich network of blood capillaries. Blood in these capillaries is separated from the air in the alveoli by a very thin membrane through which oxygen can pass into the blood and carbon dioxide can pass into the alveolar air.

The pumping of air in and out of the lungs is a result of respiratory movements performed by respiratory muscles. The most important of these is the *diaphragm*. The diaphragm is so called because it forms a partition between the thorax and the abdomen.

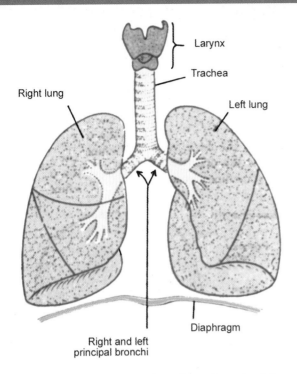

Fig. 3.2. Diagram to show the main parts of the respiratory system.

Another important set of respiratory muscles are the **intercostals muscles** that occupy the intercostal spaces (intervals between adjacent ribs).

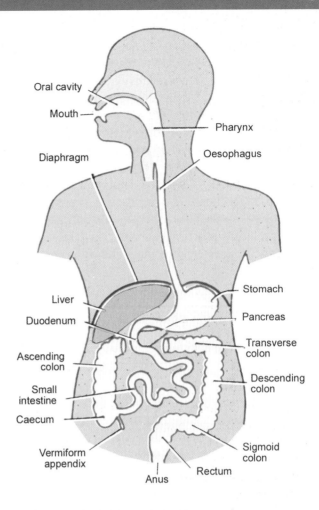

Fig. 3.3. Diagram to show the main parts of the digestive system.

INTRODUCTION TO THE ALIMENTARY SYSTEM

In ordinary English the word 'alimentary' means 'pertaining to nourishment'. The alimentary (or digestive) system includes all those structures that are concerned with eating, and with the digestion and absorption of food. The system consists of an alimentary canal which starts at the **mouth** and ends at the **anus**.

The external opening of the mouth is the **oral fissure** bounded by the upper and lower lips. Within the mouth cavity (or **oral cavity**) there are the **teeth** with which food is chewed; and the **tongue** which helps the processes of chewing and swallowing in addition to being an organ of taste. The roof of the mouth is formed by the **palate** (which separates the mouth from the nasal cavities). Posteriorly, the mouth opens into the **oral part of the pharynx**. We have already seen that this part of the pharynx is continuous, below, with the **laryngeal part of the pharynx**. The latter becomes

continuous with the **oesophagus**. The oesophagus is a tube that descends through the lower part of the neck, and then through the entire length of the thorax, to pierce the diaphragm and reach the abdomen (Fig. 3.3). Here the oesophagus ends by joining the **stomach**. The stomach is a large sac-like organ which acts as a store of swallowed food. After this food is partially digested in the stomach it passes into the **small intestine**. The small intestine is in the form of a tube about 5 meters long. It is divided, (rather arbitrarily) into three parts. These are the **duodenum**, the **jejunum** and the **ileum** (in that order). The small intestine is followed by the **large intestine**. The large intestine is about one and a half meters long. (It is described as large because it has a wider diameter). Its main subdivisions are the **caecum**, the **ascending colon**, the **transverse colon**, the **descending colon**, the **sigmoid** (or **pelvic**) **colon**, the **rectum** and the **anal canal**. These are shown in Fig. 3.3. The anal canal opens to the exterior at the **anus**.

After food has been digested and absorbed the useless remnants that remain are passed out to the exterior as faeces.

Closely related to the alimentary canal there are several accessory organs. In the region of the mouth there are three pairs of **salivary glands,** which produce a fluid the **saliva**, that helps to keep the oral cavity moist. In the abdomen we have two large glands: the **liver** and the **pancreas**. The liver occupies the upper right part of the abdomen. It is a very important organ having numerous functions. The pancreas lies transversely on the posterior wall of the abdomen. It produces digestive juices that are poured into the duodenum and help in digestion. It is also an important endocrine organ.

INTRODUCTION TO THE URINARY SYSTEM

The organs of the body that are concerned with the formation of urine and its elimination from the body are referred to as urinary organs. Urine is produced in the right and left **kidneys,** which lie on the posterior wall of the abdomen (Fig. 3.4). This urine passes through narrow tubes, the right and left **ureters**, to reach a sac-like reservoir called the **urinary bladder**. The urinary bladder lies in the true pelvis. It is connected to the exterior by a tube called the **urethra**.

INTRODUCTION TO THE REPRODUCTIVE SYSTEM

Both in the male and in the female the reproductive system consists of genital organs that are concerned with the function of reproduction. These organs may be divided into the **primary sex organs,** or **gonads,** which are responsible for the production of gametes; and the **accessory sex organs,** which play a supporting role. The genital organs are also divided into the **internal genital organs** (or **internal genitalia**) which include the gonads and those supporting organs that cannot be seen from the outside of the body; and the **external genital organs** (or **external genitalia**) which are visible on the outside. In

human beings (as in many other animal groups) fertilization takes place within the female body. This requires that male gametes be introduced into the female body through the process of **copulation** or **coitus** (commonly referred to as sexual intercourse). The male and female organs that are concerned with copulation are referred to as **copulatory organs**. The region of the body where the external genitalia (and anus) are located is referred to as the **perineum**.

Male Reproductive Organs

The male gonads are the right and left **testes** (singular = testis) (Fig. 3.5). They produce the male gametes, which are called **spermatozoa** (singular = **spermatozoon**). From each testis the spermatozoa pass through a complicated system of genital ducts. The most obvious of these are the **epididymis** and the **ductus deferens**. Near its termination, the ductus deferens is joined by the duct of the **seminal vesicle** (a sac-like structure), to form the **ejaculatory duct.** The right and left ejaculatory ducts open into the urethra.

The testis, epididymis and the initial part of the ductus deferens of both sides lie in a sac like structure covered by skin: this sac is called the **scrotum**. From here the ductus deferens passes upwards and

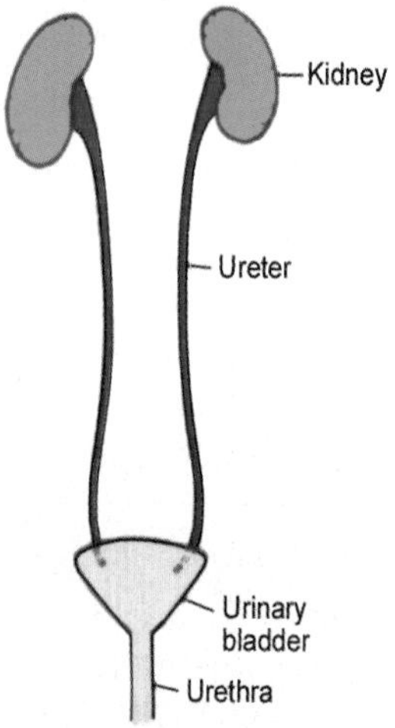

Fig. 3.4. Diagram to show the urinary organs.

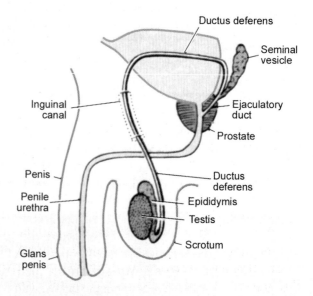

Fig. 3.5. Diagram to show the male reproductive organs.

enters the abdomen by passing through an oblique passage in the anterior abdominal wall: this passage is called the *inguinal canal*. Here the ductus deferens is surrounded by several structures that collectively form the *spermatic cord*.

As spermatozoa pass through the genital ducts, named above, they undergo maturation. They get mixed up with secretions produced by the seminal vesicle and the prostate to form the *seminal fluid* or *semen.* The process of ejection of semen from the body is called *ejaculation*. In this process semen is poured into the urethra and passes through it to the exterior. The male urethra is, therefore, both a urinary and a genital passage.

The *penis* is the male external genital organ. It is the organ of copulation. Because it is capable of becoming rigid it can be introduced into the vagina of the female, and semen can be injected into the vaginal cavity.

Female Reproductive Organs

The female reproductive organs are shown in Fig. 3.6. The female gonads are the right and left *ovaries*. The female internal genital organs are the *uterus*, the *uterine tubes* and the *vagina*. The vagina is the female organ of copulation. It opens to the exterior through a depression in the perineum called the *vestibule*. The female external genital organs are present around the vestibule. They are the *labia majora*, the *labia minora* and the *clitoris*; and some deeper structures that are associated with them. The *mammary glands* are accessory organs of reproduction.

In a mature female one ovum is produced every month (in the right or left ovary). It travels into the uterine tube towards the uterus. Spermatozoa introduced into the vagina can travel from the vagina into the uterus to reach the uterine tube. If a spermatozoon encounters an ovum fertilization can take place. (Fertilization normally takes place in the uterine tube). The fertilized ovum then travels to the uterus where it gets lodged and starts developing into a fetus (unborn child in the process of development).

The uterus provides the fetus with nutrition and with a suitable environment for its growth. The period during which a fetus is growing in the uterus is called *pregnancy*. During pregnancy a fetus receives nutrition and oxygen from the mothers' blood. Transfer of these from mother to fetus takes place through an organ called the *placenta*. The uterus enlarges greatly during pregnancy. At the end of pregnancy the fetus is expelled out of the uterus. It passes through the vagina

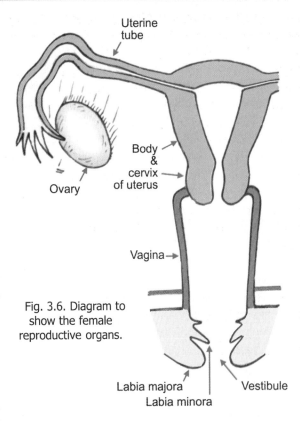

Fig. 3.6. Diagram to show the female reproductive organs.

to the exterior as a new-born infant. The process of childbirth is called *parturition*. The mammary glands provide the newborn baby with nourishment in the form of milk.

INTRODUCTION TO THE ENDOCRINE GLANDS

Some organs of the body produce secretions. Such organs are called *glands*. In the case of many glands the secretions produced by them pass through one or more ducts to be poured into a cavity. The salivary glands are of this type. Such glands are called *exocrine glands*. In contrast, there are other glands that have no duct. Their secretions are poured into blood. Such glands are called *endocrine glands*, and their secretions are called *hormones*. Hormones can travel through blood to distant organs and can influence their functions. One endocrine gland may produce more than one hormone. Some hormones influence only one organ, while some can have more widespread effects. Some endocrine glands constitute independent anatomical entities. These are the *hypophysis cerebri* (or *pituitary gland)* and the *pineal body* located within the cranial cavity; the *thyroid* and *parathyroid glands* located in the neck; and the *suprarenal glands* that lie in the abdomen just above the kidneys. Other endocrine glands are present in the form of histological elements embedded within organs having other functions. There are aggregations of cells having an endocrine function in the pancreas, the testes, and the ovaries. Some cells with endocrine functions are also present in the thymus, the kidney, the gastrointestinal tract, and the placenta.

THE LYMPHOID ORGANS

We have seen that tissues are permeated by lymph vessels, and that small rounded bodies called *lymph nodes* are associated with them. Within lymph nodes we find aggregations of large numbers of cells called *lymphocytes*. Similar aggregations of lymphocytes are also present in some other organs. All these are referred to as *lymphoid organs*.

The largest lymphoid organ is the *spleen*. It is located in the upper and left part of the abdomen, close to the stomach.

Another, very important, lymphoid organ is the *thymus*. It is located in the thorax just deep to the sternum.

In the lateral walls of the oropharynx we have small lymphoid organs called the *tonsils* (one right and one left). These are frequently inflamed (*tonsillitis*) resulting in sore throat.

Many aggregations of lymphocytes are also present in the walls of some organs including the intestines and the respiratory passages.

INTRODUCTION TO THE CARDIOVASCULAR SYSTEM

The cardiovascular system consists of the *heart* and *blood vessels*. The system is responsible for the circulation of blood through the tissues of the body. The heart acts as a pump and provides the force for this circulation. Blood vessels taking blood from the heart to the tissues are called *arteries*.

The largest artery in the body is called the *aorta*. Arising from the heart it divides, like the branches of a tree, into smaller and smaller branches. The smallest arteries are

called *arterioles*. The arterioles end in a plexus of thin-walled vessels that permeate the tissues. These thin walled vessels are called *capillaries*. Oxygen, nutrition, waste products etc., can pass through the walls of capillaries from blood to tissue cells and *vice versa*. In some organs these vessels are somewhat different in structure from capillaries and are called *sinusoids*. Blood from capillaries or sinusoids is collected by another set of vessels that carry it back to the heart: these are called *veins.* The veins adjoining the capillaries are very small and are called *venules.* Smaller veins join together (like tributaries of a river) to form larger and larger veins. Ultimately the blood reaches two large veins, the *superior vena cava* and the *inferior vena cava*, which pour it back into the heart. This blood reaching the heart through the veins has lost its oxygen. A special set of arteries and veins circulates this blood through the lungs where it is again oxygenated. This circulation through the lungs, for the purpose of oxygenation of blood, is called the *pulmonary circulation,* to distinguish it from the main or *systemic circulation.*

For further consideration of the cardiovascular system see Chapter 12.

INTRODUCTION TO THE NERVOUS SYSTEM

The nervous system may be divided into two parts.

(**a**) The *central nervous system* (CNS) is made up of the *brain* (lying in the cranial cavity) and the *spinal cord* (lying in the vertebral canal).

(**b**) The *peripheral nervous system* is made up nerves that arise from the brain and spinal cord.

The brain consists of the following parts (Fig. 3.7):

(**1**) The *cerebrum* made of two large *cerebral hemispheres*;

(**2**) the *cerebellum*,

(**3**) the *midbrain*,

(**4**) the *pons*, and

(**5**) the *medulla* oblongata.

The midbrain, pons and medulla together constitute the *brainstem*. The medulla is continuous, inferiorly, with the spinal cord.

Peripheral nerves attached to the brain are called *cranial nerves*; and those attached to the spinal cord are called *spinal nerves*.

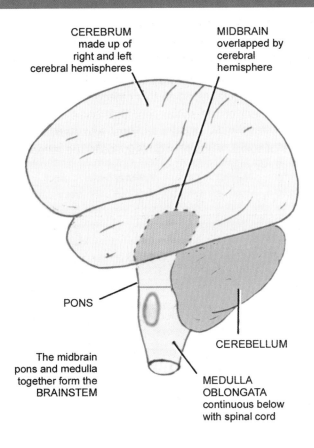

Fig. 3.7. Diagram to show the main parts of the brain.

The Cranial Nerves

There are twelve pairs of cranial nerves. They are identified by number and also bear names.

The **first** cranial nerve is called the **olfactory** nerve. It is the nerve of smell (olfaction = smell). It passes from the nose to the brain.

The **second** cranial nerve is called the **optic nerve**. It is the nerve of sight and passes from the eyeball to the brain.

The **third** cranial nerve is called the **oculomotor** nerve. It supplies several muscles that move the eyeball.

The **fourth** cranial nerve is called the **trochlear** nerve. It is so called because it supplies a muscle (superior oblique, of the eyeball) that passes through a pulley (trochlea = pulley).

The **fifth** cranial nerve is called the **trigeminal** nerve because it has three major divisions. These are the **ophthalmic division** to the orbit, the **maxillary division** to the upper jaw, and the **mandibular division** to the lower jaw.

The **sixth** cranial nerve is called the **abducent** nerve because it supplies a muscle (lateral rectus) which 'abducts' the eyeball.

The **seventh** cranial nerve is the **facial** nerve because it supplies the muscles of the face.

The **eighth** cranial nerve is called the **vestibulo-cochlear** nerve because it supplies structures in the vestibular and cochlear parts of the internal ear. It is sometimes called the **auditory nerve** (auditory = pertaining to hearing) or the **stato-acoustic** nerve (stato = pertaining to equilibrium; acoustic = pertaining to sound).

The **ninth** cranial nerve is called the **glossopharyngeal** nerve as it is distributed to the pharynx and to part of the tongue (glossal = pertaining to the tongue).

The **tenth** cranial nerve is called the **vagus**. It has an extensive course through the neck, the thorax and the abdomen. (The word vagus may be correlated with 'vagrant' = wandering from place to place).

The **eleventh** cranial nerve is called the **accessory** nerve because it appears to be a part of the vagus nerve (or 'accessory' to the vagus).

The **twelfth** cranial nerve is called the **hypoglossal** nerve (because it runs part of its course below the tongue before supplying the muscles in it (hypo = below; glossal = pertaining to tongue).

Spinal Nerves

We have seen that spinal nerves arise from the spinal cord. In the thoracic, lumbar and sacral regions the number of spinal nerves corresponds to that of the vertebrae. On each side (right or left) there are twelve thoracic nerves, five lumbar nerves, and five sacral nerves. In the cervical region there are eight cervical nerves (but only seven vertebrae). Below the sacral nerves there is one coccygeal nerve.

Each spinal nerve arises from the spinal cord by two roots, one dorsal and one ventral (Fig. 3.8). After a very short course the spinal nerve divides into a dorsal primary ramus (ramus = branch) and a ventral primary ramus.

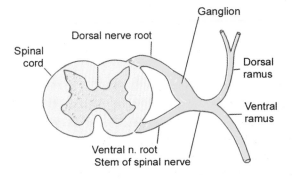

Fig. 3.8. Diagram to show the roots and main divisions of a typical spinal nerve.

As a rule the dorsal ramus is smaller than the ventral ramus. It passes backwards and divides into medial and lateral branches which supply the muscles and skin of the back. The ventral primary ramus passes forwards. In the thoracic region each ventral ramus remains distinct and forms an *intercostal nerve*. In the cervical, lumbar and sacral regions the ventral rami join those of neighbouring spinal nerves to form complicated plexuses.

Branches arising from these plexuses supply muscles and skin. In the upper cervical region we have a *cervical plexus*. In the lower cervical region there is the *brachial plexus* that gives origin to the nerves of the upper limb. In the lumbar region we have a *lumbar plexus*, and in the sacral region we have a *sacral plexus*. The lumbar and sacral plexuses send branches into the lower limb.

The cervical plexus gives off several branches to tissues in the head and neck. It also gives off the *phrenic nerve* which descends into the thorax to supply the diaphragm.

There are three prominent nerves in the upper limb. These are the *median, ulnar* and *radial* nerves. They are all branches of the brachial plexus and are so named because of their relative position in the forearm.

There are two main nerves in the lower limb. The *femoral nerve* is seen in the front of the thigh. It is a branch of the lumbar plexus. The *sciatic nerve* is seen on the back of the thigh. It is derived from the sacral plexus. It descends to the back of the knee where it divides into the *tibial nerve* (which supplies the back of the leg) and the *common peroneal nerve* (which supplies the front and lateral side of the leg. Branches of both these nerves descend into the foot.

Most of the nerves mentioned above supply tissues like skin and muscle. From the skin they carry impulses of touch, pain, temperature, etc. Such nerves are called *sensory nerves*. Nerves that supply muscles are called *motor nerves*. Nerves that contain both sensory and motor nerve fibres are *mixed nerves*, and the large majority of nerves belong to this category.

The segment of the spinal cord that gives origin to one spinal nerve is called a *spinal segment*. The number of spinal segments corresponds to the number of spinal nerves.

AUTONOMIC NERVOUS SYSTEM

Most internal organs of the body, (including the blood vessels), are supplied by nerves that belong to the autonomic nervous system. This system is divisible into two large subdivisions, *sympathetic* and *para-sympathetic*. Most autonomic nerves are very thin and difficult to see. They often form plexuses around blood vessels and in relation to viscera. The most prominent components of this system are the right and left *sympathetic trunks*. Each trunk extends vertically from the base of the skull (above) to the coccyx (below). The trunks lie along the sides of the vertebral column. Each trunk bears a large number of thickenings along its length. These thickenings are *sympathetic ganglia*.

The vagus nerve provides a parasympathetic supply to many organs of the body.

4

Introduction to Body Functions

External Environment

A living organism is in constant interaction with the external environment surrounding it. It is from this environment that the organism obtains food. This food provides energy required to perform various functions. Waste products left after utilisation of ingested food are thrown back into the external environment.

In addition to food, the animal body needs oxygen, and this is also obtained from the environment.

The body has to react to changes in the environment, for example changes in temperature. In mammals the body is maintained at a more or less constant temperature. When the environment is cold the body need mechanisms to provide it with heat. Conversely, when the environment is too warm, the body has to be cooled.

Internal Environment

The animal body is made up of very large numbers of cells. The cells are surrounded by intercellular fluid. The composition of this fluid is in constant change, but in a healthy person these changes are maintained within very narrow limits. The maintenance of the environment within these limits is called **homeostasis**. There are many mechanisms in the body for homeostasis.

Negative Feedback Mechanism

When the temperature of the body rises beyond normal, it triggers mechanisms that lower body temperature, e.g., by perspiration. In this example, the stimulus produces an effect (cooling) opposite to that of the stimulus. Such a mechanism is, therefore, called a negative feedback mechanism. Most central mechanisms of the body are of this variety.

Positive Feedback Mechanism

In such a mechanism the response is similar to the original stimulus and makes it stronger. For example, during childbirth (labour) the onset of uterine contractions acts as a stimulus for further strengthening of the contractions.

SOME ESSENTIAL BODY FUNCTIONS

Every animal body has to perform certain basic functions that are necessary for survival.

Procuring and Ingestion of Food

Every animal needs regular intake of nutrition. Substances that provide nutrition are called nutrients. The most important nutrients are water, carbohydrates, proteins, and fats. Small quantities of vitamins and mineral salts are also required. We obtain carbohydrates from sugar, and from food grains like wheat or rice. The richest sources of protein are the flesh of animals, and milk. Proteins are also available in some vegetarian foods specially in lentils (*daal*) and various kinds of beans (specially soya bean). Fats are present in milk (and milk products), in the flesh of animals, and in vegetable oils like mustard oil, groundnut oil and sunflower oil.

The nutrients taken into the body provide us with energy for various internal and external needs. Food is also necessary for growth in children, and for maintenance of tissues at all ages.

When ingested, food enters the alimentary canal. This is a long canal consisting of many parts. As food passes through the canal it undergoes a process of digestion. Sugar and carbohydrates are broken down into glucose. Proteins are broken down into amino acids; and fats are broken down into fatty acids and glycerol. It is in this form that food is absorbed from the intestine and is transported to various parts of the body for use.

Respiration

In addition to food, the body requires a constant supply of oxygen. This is obtained from the air we breathe. The parts of the body responsible for intake of air and absorption of oxygen into the blood constitute the respiratory system. The main organs of the system are the right and left lungs.

Excretion of Waste Products

1. After useful elements have been extracted from food, waste products are expelled from the body in the form of faeces.

2. When any fuel is burnt, oxygen is used and carbon dioxide is produced. This happens in the animal body too. Oxygen is necessary for "burning" food to create heat and energy. Carbon dioxide produced during this process has to be expelled from the body, and this is done through the lungs.

3. Many chemical reactions take places in various organs of the body and result in formation of chemicals (e.g., urea) that are harmful to the body. Most of these chemicals are excreted through urine. Urine is produced in the kidneys. It passes through a series of passages before being expelled to the exterior. The kidneys and the passages through which urine passes constitute the urinary system.

The Need for Movement

The capacity for movement is a fundamental characteristic of animals. Unicellular organisms (like amoeba) can move away from unpleasant stimuli. They can alter their shape in order to absorb particulate matter from the environment.

In the animal body the capacity for movement serves many functions that are essential to survival of the animal.

Movement in relation to the environment

1. Movement enables an animal to procure food.

2. Movement enables an animal to move away from danger. The same purpose is also served when animals come together to live in groups.

3. Movement is also essential for finding a mate. This is in turn, essential for preservation of the species.

Movement in relation the environment is made possible by:

(A). A skeleton made up of many bones. Movements occur at joints between the bones.

(B). The power for movement is provided by muscles.

The skeleton, joints and muscles collectively form the anatomical basis for production of movements in relation to the environment.

Movement within the body

1. Movement is necessary for eating food, and for its transport through the alimentary canal. This transport is dependent on muscle present in the walls of the canal.

2. The taking of air into the body (inspiration) and expelling it out of the body (expiration) is dependent on the action of muscles present in the walls of the thorax (chest) and abdomen.

3. Food absorbed from the intestines, and oxygen absorbed through the lungs, reach all parts of the body through blood. Blood is in constant circulation through all parts of the body. The power for this circulation is provided by the heart which is a pump made up mainly of muscle.

The circulation is also necessary for transporting waste products to excretory organs (e.g., kidneys, sweat glands) and for transporting numerous substances from one part of the body to another.

4. Movement is required for expelling faeces and urine from the body, and for childbirth.

From what has been said above it will be clear that movement is essential for life. Cessation of heart-beat, or of respiratory movements, results in death.

Modes of communication within the body

We have seen that substances can travel from one part of the body to another through circulating blood. This is one mode of communication. Apart from nutrients and oxygen, blood carries chemical messengers (called ***hormones***) through which one organ can have profound effect on the working of another.

The brain exerts a control on all parts of the body through nerves. Nerves can be compared to wires carrying an electric current. Contraction of muscles takes place through orders starting in the brain and travelling through nerves. The brain influences many other functions of the body in a similar manner.

The brain receives information about the external environment through sense organs like the eyes, the ears and the skin. Such information travels through nerves. Information is also received from various organs of the body. It provides the input on the basis of which the working of the organs is controlled.

In the chapters that follow we will consider the structure and functions of organs involved in the various functions very briefly introduced this chapter.

PART TWO

CELLS AND TISSUES
OF THE BODY

5

Cell Structure

CELL STRUCTURE

A cell is bounded by a *cell membrane* (or *plasma membrane*). This membrane encloses a complex material called *protoplasm*. The protoplasm consists of a central, more dense, part called the *nucleus*; and an outer less dense part called the *cytoplasm*. The nucleus is separated from the cytoplasm by a nuclear membrane. The cytoplasm has a fluid base (matrix) which is referred to as the *cytosol* or *hyaloplasm*. The cytosol contains a number of *organelles* which have distinctive structure and functions. Many of them are in the form of membranes that enclose spaces.

Basic Membrane Structure

When suitable preparations are examined by EM the cell membrane is seen to consist of two densely stained layers separated by a lighter zone, thus creating a trilaminar appearance (Fig. 5.1A).

It is now known that the trilaminar structure of membranes is produced by the arrangement of lipid molecules (predominantly phospholipids) that constitute the basic framework of the membrane (Fig. 5.1B).

Each phospholipid molecule consists of an enlarged head in which the phosphate portion is located; and of two thin tails. The head end is also called the *polar end* while the tail end is the *non-polar end*. The head end is soluble in water and is said to be hydrophilic. The tail end is insoluble and is said to be *hydrophobic*.

When such molecules are suspended in an aqueous medium they arrange themselves so that the hydrophilic ends are in contact with the medium; but the hydrophobic ends are not. They do so by forming a bilayer.

The dark staining parts of the membrane (seen by EM) are formed by the heads of the molecules, while the light staining intermediate zone is occupied by the tails, thus giving the membrane its trilaminar appearance.

THE CELL MEMBRANE

The membrane separating the cytoplasm of the cell from surrounding structures is called the *cell membrane* or the *plasma membrane*. It has the basic structure described above.

The cell membrane is of great importance in regulating the activities of the cell as follows.

(**a**) The membrane maintains the shape of the cell.

(**b**) It controls the passage of all substances into or out of the cell.

(**c**) The cell membrane forms a sensory surface. This function is most developed in nerve and muscle cells.

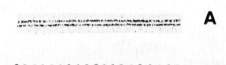

Fig. 5.1. A. Trilaminar structure of a cell membrane as revealed by EM.
B. Diagram showing the arrangement of phospholipid molecules forming a membrane.

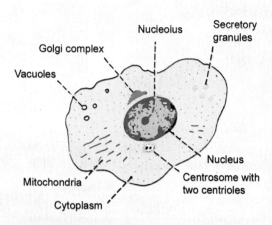

Fig. 5.2.Some features of a cell that can be seen with a light microscope.

The plasma membranes of such cells are normally polarized: the external surface bears a positive charge and the internal surface bears a negative charge. When suitably stimulated there is a selective passage of sodium and potassium ions across the membrane reversing the charge. This is called **depolarisation**: it results in contraction in the case of muscle, or in generation of a nerve impulse in the case of neurons.

(**d**) The surface of the cell membrane bears **receptors** that may be specific for particular molecules (e.g., hormones or enzymes). Stimulation of such receptors (e.g., by the specific hormone) can produce profound effects on the activity of the cell.

Role of cell membrane in transport of material into or out of the cell

Movement of various substances through cell membranes is an essential feature of cell function. Nutrients enter cells, and waste materials are expelled, in this way. The movement of some ions through cell membranes plays a very important role in functioning of nerve cells, muscle cells and others.

Transport through cell membrane can take place in two distinct ways:

(a) Transport can take place by diffusion or osmosis (from higher concentration to lower). For such transport the force required is provided by the concentration gradient, and no energy is used. It is, therefore, called **passive transport**.

(b) Sometimes substances have to be moved against the concentration gradient (from lower concentration to higher). For this to happen energy is required, and such transport is called **active transport**. Active transport is used for moving sodium and potassium ions across cell membranes (to neutralise their movement by diffusion).

Some molecules can enter cells by passing through channels in the cell membrane. Large molecules enter the cell by the process of **endocytosis**. In this process the molecule invaginates a part of the cell membrane, which first surrounds the molecule, and then separates (from the rest of the cell membrane) to form an **endocytic vesicle**. This vesicle can move through the cytosol to other parts of the cell.

The term **pinocytosis** is applied to a process similar to endocytosis when the vesicles (then called **pinocytotic vesicles**) formed are used for absorption of fluids into the cell.

Some cells use the process of endocytosis to engulf foreign matter (e.g., bacteria). The process is then referred to as **phagocytosis**.

Molecules produced within the cytoplasm (e.g., secretions) may be enclosed in membranes to form vesicles that approach the cell membrane and fuse with its internal surface. The vesicle then ruptures releasing the molecule to the exterior. The vesicles in question are called **exocytic vesicles**, and the process is called **exocytosis** or **reverse pinocytosis**.

CELL ORGANELLES

We have seen that (apart from the nucleus) the cytoplasm of a typical cell contains various structures that are referred to as organelles. They include the endoplasmic reticulum, ribosomes, mitochondria, the Golgi complex, and various types of vesicles (Fig. 5.2). The cytosol also contains a cytoskeleton made up of microtubules, microfilaments, and intermediate filaments. Centrioles are closely connected with microtubules.

Endoplasmic Reticulum and Ribosomes

The cytoplasm of most cells contains a system of membranes that constitute the endoplasmic reticulum (ER). The membranes form the boundaries of channels that may be arranged in the form of flattened sacs (or cisternae) or of tubules.

Because of the presence of the ER the cytoplasm is divided into two components, one within the channels and one outside them (Fig. 5.3). The cytoplasm within the channels is called the **vacuoplasm**, and that outside the channels is the **hyaloplasm** or **cytosol**.

In most places the membranes forming the ER are studded with minute particles of RNA called **ribosomes**. The presence of these ribosomes gives the membrane a rough appearance. Membranes of this type form what is called the rough (or granular) ER. In contrast some membranes are devoid of ribosomes and constitute the smooth or agranular ER (Fig. 5.3).

Rough ER represents the site at which proteins are synthesized. The attached ribosomes play an important role in this process.

Mitochondria

Mitochondria can be seen with the light microscope in specially stained preparations. They are so called because they appear either as granules or as rods (mitos = granule; chondrium = rod). The number of

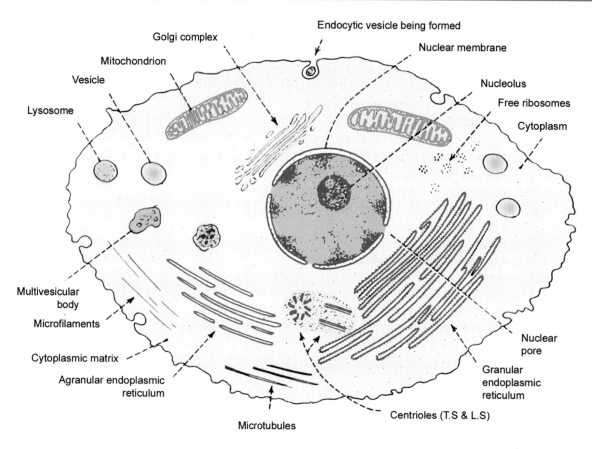

Fig. 5.3. Schematic diagram to show the various organelles to be found in a typical cell. The various structures shown are not drawn to scale.

mitochondria varies from cell to cell being greatest in cells with high metabolic activity (e.g., in secretory cells). Mitochondria vary in size and are large in cells with a high oxidative metabolism.

A schematic presentation of some details of the structure of a mitochondrion (as seen by EM) is shown in Fig. 5.4. The mitochondrion is bounded by a smooth *outer membrane* within which there is an *inner membrane*, the two being separated by an *intermembranous space*. The inner membrane is highly folded on itself forming incomplete partitions called *cristae*. The space bounded by the inner

membrane is filled by a granular material called the *matrix*. This matrix contains numerous enzymes. It also contains some RNA and DNA: these are believed to carry information that enables mitochondria to duplicate themselves during cell division.

Mitochondria are of great functional importance. They contain many enzymes including some that play an important part in Kreb's cycle (TCA cycle). ATP and GTP are formed in mitochondria from where they pass to other parts of the cell and provide energy for various cellular functions.

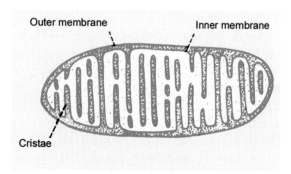

Fig. 5.4. Structure of a mitochondrion.

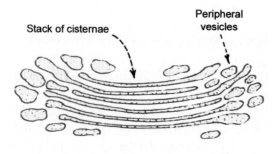

Fig. 5.5. Structure of the Golgi complex.

Golgi Complex

In light microscopic preparations suitably treated with silver salts the Golgi complex can be seen as a small structure of irregular shape, usually present near the nucleus (Fig. 5.2).

When examined by EM the complex is seen to be made up of membranes similar to those of smooth ER. The membranes form the walls of a number of flattened sacs that are stacked over one another. Towards their margins the sacs are continuous with small rounded vesicles (Fig. 5.5).

Membrane Bound Vesicles

The cytoplasm of a cell may contain several types of vesicles. The contents of any such vesicle are separated from the rest of the cytoplasm by a membrane which forms the wall of the vesicle.

Some vesicles serve to store material. Others transport material into or out of the cell, or from one part of a cell to another. Solid 'foreign' materials, including bacteria, may be engulfed by a cell by the process of **phagocytosis**. In this process the material is surrounded by a part of the cell membrane. This part of the cell membrane then separates from the rest of the plasma membrane and forms a free floating vesicle within the cytoplasm. Such membrane bound vesicles, containing solid ingested material are called **phagosomes**. Some fluid may also be taken into the cytoplasm by a process similar to phagocytosis. In the case of fluids the process is called **pinocytosis** and the vesicles formed are called **pinocytotic vesicles**. Just as material from outside the cell can be brought into the cytoplasm by phagocytosis or pinocytosis, materials from different parts of the cell can be transported to the outside by vesicles. Such vesicles are called **exocytic vesicles**, and the process of discharge of cell products in this way is referred to as **exocytosis** (or **reverse pinocytosis**).

The cytoplasm of secretory cells frequently contains what are called **secretory granules**. These can be seen with the light microscope. With the EM each 'granule' is seen to be a membrane bound vesicle containing secretion.

Lysosomes are vesicles which contain enzymes that can destroy unwanted material (e.g., bacteria) present within a cell.

Centrioles

All cells capable of division (and even some which do not divide) contain a pair of structures called centrioles. With the light microscope the two centrioles are seen as dots embedded in a region of dense cytoplasm which is called the **centrosome**. With the EM the centrioles are seen to be short cylinders that lie at right angles to each other. When we examine a transverse section across a centriole (by EM) it is seen to consist essentially of a series of microtubules arranged in a circle.

Centrioles play an important role in the formation of various cellular structures that are made up of microtubules. These include the mitotic spindles of dividing cells, cilia, flagella, and some projections of specialised cells (e.g., the axial filaments of spermatozoa).

PROJECTIONS FROM THE CELL SURFACE

Many cells show projections from the cell surface. The various types of projections are described below.

Cilia

These can be seen, with the light microscope, as minute hair-like projections from the free surfaces of some epithelial cells (Fig. 5.6). In the living animal cilia can be seen to be motile. Movements of cilia lining the respiratory epithelium help to move secretions in the trachea and bronchi towards the pharynx. Ciliary action helps in the movement of ova through the uterine tube, and of spermatozoa through the male genital tract.

Flagella

These are somewhat larger processes having the same basic structure as cilia. In the human body the best example of a flagellum is the tail of the spermatozoon.

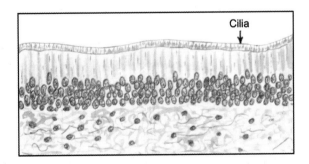

Fig. 5.6. Pseudostratified columnar epithelium showing cilia.

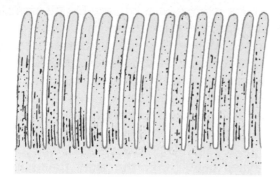

Fig. 5.7. Microvilli as seen in longitudinal section. The regular arrangement of microvilli is characteristic of the striated border of intestinal absorptive cells.

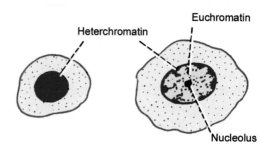

Fig. 5.8. Comparison of a heterochromatic nucleus (left), and a euchromatic nucleus (right).

Microvilli

Microvilli are finger-like projections from the cell surface that can be seen by EM (Fig. 5.7). With the light microscope the free borders of cells lining the small intestine appear to be thickened: the thickening has striations perpendicular to the surface. This *striated border* of light microscopy has been shown by EM to be made up of long microvilli arranged parallel to one another.

In some cells the microvilli are not arranged so regularly. With the light microscope the microvilli of such cells give the appearance of a *brush border*.

Microvilli greatly increase the surface area of the cell and are, therefore, seen most typically at sites of active absorption e.g., the intestine, and the proximal and distal convoluted tubules of the kidneys.

THE NUCLEUS

The nucleus constitutes the central, more dense, part of the cell. It is usually rounded or ellipsoid. Occasionally it may be elongated, indented or lobed. It is usually 4-10 μm in diameter. The nucleus contains inherited information which is necessary for directing the activities of the cell.

In usual class room slides stained with haematoxylin and eosin, the nucleus stains dark purple or blue while the cytoplasm is usually stained pink. In some cells the nuclei are relatively large and light staining. Such nuclei appear to be made up of a delicate network of fibres: the material making up the fibres of the network is called *chromatin* (because of its affinity for dyes). At some places (in the nucleus) the chromatin is seen in the form of irregular dark masses that are called *heterochromatin*. At other places the network is loose

and stains lightly: the chromatin of such areas is referred to as *euchromatin*. Nuclei which are large and in which relatively large areas of euchromatin can be seen are referred to as *open-face nuclei.* Nuclei which are made up mainly of heterochromatin are referred to as *closed-face nuclei* (Fig. 5.8).

Chromatin is made up of a substance called *deoxyribonucleic acid* (usually abbreviated to DNA); and of proteins.

During cell division the entire chromatin within the nucleus becomes very tightly coiled and takes on the appearance of a number of short, thick, rod-like structures called *chromosomes*. Chromosomes are made up of DNA and proteins.

In addition to the masses of heterochromatin (which are irregular in outline), the nucleus shows one or more rounded, dark staining bodies called *nucleoli.*

With the EM the nucleus is seen to be surrounded by a double layered *nuclear membrane* or *nuclear envelope*. At several points the inner and outer layers of the nuclear membrane fuse leaving gaps called *nuclear pores*. Nuclear pores represent sites at which substances can pass from the nucleus to the cytoplasm and vice versa (Fig. 5.3).

CHROMOSOMES

Haploid and Diploid Chromosomes

We have seen that during cell division the chromatin network in the nucleus becomes condensed into a number of thread-like or rod-like structures called chromosomes. The number of chromosomes in each cell is fixed for a given species, and in man it is 46. This is referred to as the *diploid number* (diploid = double). However, in spermatozoa and in ova the number is only half the diploid number i.e., 23: this is called the *haploid number* (haploid = half).

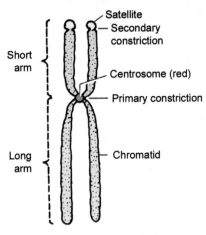

Fig. 5.9. Structure of a typical chromosome.

Autosomes and Sex Chromosomes

The 46 chromosomes in each cell can again be divided into 44 **autosomes** and two **sex chromosomes**. The sex chromosomes may be of two kinds, X or Y. In a man there are 44 autosomes, one X chromosome, and one Y chromosome; while in a woman there are 44 autosomes and two X chromosomes in each cell. When we study the 44 autosomes we find that they really consist of 22 pairs, the two chromosomes forming a pair being exactly alike (**homologous chromosomes**). In a woman the two X chromosomes form another such pair; but in a man this pair is represented by one X and one Y chromosome. We shall see later that one chromosome of each pair is obtained (by each individual) from the mother, and one from the father.

Significance of Chromosomes

Each cell of the body contains within itself a store of information that has been inherited from precursor cells. This information (which is necessary for the proper functioning of the cell) is stored in chromatin. Each chromosome bears on itself a very large number of functional segments that are called **genes**. Genes represent 'units' of stored information which guide the performance of particular cellular functions, which may in turn lead to the development of particular features of an individual or of a species.

The nature and functions of a cell depend on the proteins synthesized by it. Proteins are the most important constituents of our body. They make up the greater part of each cell and of intercellular substances. Enzymes, hormones, and antibodies are also proteins.

It is, therefore, not surprising that one cell differs from another because of the differences in the proteins that constitute it. We now know that chromosomes control the development and functioning of cells by determining what type of proteins will be synthesized within them.

Chromosomes are made up predominantly of a nucleic acid called **deoxyribonucleic acid** (or **DNA**), and all information is stored in molecules of this substance. When the need arises this information is used to direct the activities of the cell by synthesizing appropriate proteins.

One of the most remarkable properties of chromosomes is that they are able to duplicate themselves. Duplication of chromosomes involves the duplication (or replication) of DNA.

Structure of Fully Formed Chromosomes

Each chromosome consists of two parallel rod-like elements that are called **chromatids** (Fig. 5.9). The two chromatids are joined to each other at a narrow area which is light staining and is called the **centromere** (or **kinetochore**). Typically the centromere is not midway between the two ends of the chromatids, but somewhat towards one end. As a result each chromatid can be said to have a **long arm** and a **short arm**.

It is now possible to identify each chromosome individually and to map out the chromosomes of an individual. This procedure is called **karyotyping**.

CELL DIVISION

Multiplication of cells takes place by division of pre-existing cells. Such multiplication constitutes an essential feature of embryonic development. Cell multiplication is equally necessary after birth of the individual for growth and for replacement of dead cells.

We have seen that the chromosomes within the nuclei of cells carry genetic information that controls the development and functioning of various cells and tissues and, therefore, of the body as a whole. When a cell divides it is essential that the whole of the genetic information within it be passed on to both the daughter cells resulting from the division.

In other words the daughter cells must have chromosomes identical in number and in genetic content to those in the mother cell. This type of cell division is called **mitosis**.

A different kind of cell division called **meiosis** occurs during the formation of gametes. This consists of two successive divisions called the first and second meiotic divisions. The cells resulting from these divisions (i.e., the gametes) differ from other cells in the body in that:

(**a**) the number of chromosomes is reduced to half the normal number, and

(**b**) the genetic information in the various gametes produced is not identical.

Mitosis

Many cells of the body have a limited span of functional activity at the end of which they undergo division into two daughter cells. The daughter cells in turn have their own span of activity followed by another division. The period during which the cell is actively dividing is the phase of mitosis. The period between two successive divisions is called the *interphase*.

Mitosis is conventionally divided into a number of stages called *prophase, metaphase, anaphase* and *telophase*. For details of these phases consult a book on histology.

Meiosis

This type of division takes place only in the testis or ovary, for production of male and female gametes. Each ovum or spermatozoon contains only half the normal number of chromosomes i.e., 23.

At the time of fertilization the 23 chromosomes of the spermatozoon and the 23 chromosomes of the ovum together restore the number of chromosomes to 46.

The 46 chromosomes of a typical cell consist of 23 pairs, one chromosome of each pair being derived from the mother and one from the father.

We have seen that each cell of a human male has 44+X+Y chromosomes; and that each cell of a female has 44+X+X chromosomes. We have also seen that during the formation of gametes by meiosis the chromosome number is reduced to half. As a result all ova contain 22+X chromosomes. Spermatozoa are of two types. Some have the chromosomal constitution 22+X and the others have the constitution 22+Y. If an ovum is fertilised by a sperm bearing an X-chromosome the resulting child has (22+X)+(22+X) = 44+X+X chromosomes and is a girl. On the other hand if an ovum is fertilised by a sperm bearing a Y-chromosome the child has (22+X)+(22+Y) = 44+X +Y chromosomes and is a boy.

Abnormal Cell Growth and Tumours

Normally, cell multiplication is a controlled process and is just sufficient for replacing dead cells, for growth in children, or for repair of wounds and injuries.

Sometimes cell multiplication goes out of control and cells in an organ keep multiplying when more cells are not needed. These cells form an abnormal mass that is called a *tumour* or *neoplasm*.

In some tumours, growth is slow. The cells formed resemble normal cells of the tissue from which they originate (i.e., they are well differentiated). Surrounding connective tissue forms a capsule around the tumour. The tumour remains confined to one organ. Such tumours are said to be *benign*. They can cause problems by pressure on surrounding structures.

In other tumours the cells grow rapidly, and do not acquire characteristics of normal cells (i.e., they remain undifferentiated). Such tumours can invade adjoining structures. These are called *malignant* tumours. A malignant tumour arising from an epithelial cell is called a *carcinoma* (cancer). A malignant tumour arising from connective tissue cells is called a *sarcoma*. Some cells of the tumour can get detached and can travel to lymph nodes through lymphatic vessels. They can also spread to other organs, through blood, and can start growing there forming *secondary growths* or *metastases*.

In many cases there is no obvious cause for formation of a carcinoma. Some chemical substances can stimulate cancer formation and are called carcinogens. Other causes are exposure to some radiations (e.g., X-rays, and radiations from radioactive substances). Some viruses can also cause cancer.

6

Epithelia and Glands

The outer surface of the body and the luminal surfaces of cavities within it are lined by one or more layers of cells that completely cover them. Such layers of cells are called *epithelia* (singular=epithelium). Epithelia also line the ducts and secretory elements of glands.

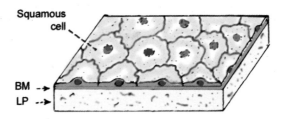

Fig. 6.1. Simple squamous epithelium (diagrammatic). BM= Basement membrane;

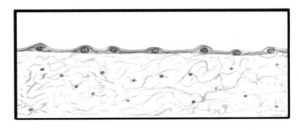

Fig. 6.2. Simple squamous epithelium as seen in a section.

CLASSIFICATION OF EPITHELIA

An epithelium may consist of only one layer of cells when it is called a *unilayered* or *simple* epithelium. Alternatively, it may be *multi-layered* or *stratified*.

Simple epithelia may be further classified according to the shape of the cells constituting them.

(1) In some epithelia the cells are flattened, their height being very little as compared to their width. Such an epithelium is called a *squamous epithelium* (Figs. 6.1, 6.2).

(2) When the height and width of the cells of the epithelium are more or less equal (i.e., they look like squares in section) it is described as a *cuboidal epithelium* (Fig. 6.6).

(3) When the height of the cells of the epithelium is distinctly greater than their width, it is described as a *columnar epithelium* (Figs. 6.3, 6.4).

Multi-layered epithelia are of two main types. In the most common type the deeper layers are columnar, but in proceeding towards the surface of the epithelium the cells become increasingly flattened (or squamous). Such an epithelium is described as *stratified squamous* (Fig. 6.10). It may be noted that all cells in this kind of epithelium are not squamous. In the second type of multi-layered epithelium all layers are made up of cuboidal, polygonal or rounded cells. The cells towards the surface of the epithelium are not flattened. This type of epithelium is called *transitional epithelium* (being transitional between unilayered epithelia and stratified squamous epithelium). As

transitional epithelium is confined to the urinary tract it is also called *urothelium*.

In some situations a columnar epithelium which is really single layered may give the appearance of a stratified epithelium. Such an epithelium is referred to as *pseudostratified columnar epithelium* (Figs. 6.8, 6.9).

The various types of epithelia named above are considered further below.

Squamous Epithelium

The cytoplasm of cells in this kind of epithelium forms only a thin layer. The nuclei produce bulgings of the cell surface (Fig. 6.1, 6.2). In surface view the cells have polygonal outlines that interlock with those of adjoining cells.

Squamous epithelium lines the alveoli of the lungs. It lines the free surface of the serous pericardium, of the pleura, and of the peritoneum: here it is called *mesothelium*. It lines the inside of the heart, where

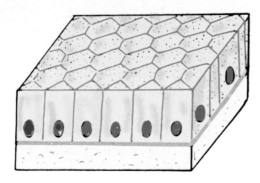

Fig. 6.3. Simple columnar epithelium (diagrammatic). Note the basally placed oval nuclei. The cells appear hexagonal in surface view.

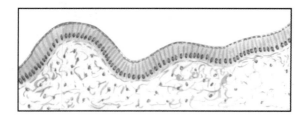

Fig. 6.4. Simple columnar epithelium as seen in a section.

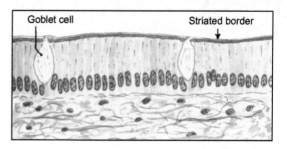

Fig. 6.5. Columnar epithelium with striated border as seen in a section.

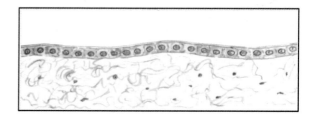

Fig. 6.6. Simple cuboidal epithelium as seen in a section.

it is called **endocardium**; and of blood vessels and lymphatics, where it is called **endothelium**.

Columnar Epithelium

Columnar epithelium (Figs. 6.3, 6.4) can be further classified according to the nature of the free surfaces of the cells as follows.

(**a**) In some situations the cell surface has no particular specialization: this is **simple columnar epithelium**.

(**b**) In some situations the cell surface bears cilia. This is **ciliated columnar epithelium**.

(**c**) In other situations the surface is covered with microvilli. Although the microvilli are visible only with the EM, with the light microscope the region of the microvilli is seen as a **striated border** (when the microvilli are arranged regularly) or as a **brush border** (when the microvilli are irregularly placed).

Some columnar cells have a secretory function. The apical parts of their cytoplasm contain secretory vacuoles.

Simple columnar epithelium (without cilia or microvilli) is present over the mucous membrane of the stomach and the large intestine.

Columnar epithelium with a striated border is seen most typically in the small intestine, and with a brush border in the gall bladder.

Ciliated columnar epithelium lines most of the respiratory tract, the uterus, and the uterine tubes. In the respiratory tract the cilia move mucous accumulating in the bronchi (and containing trapped dust particles) towards the larynx and pharynx. When excessive this mucous is brought out as sputum during coughing. In the uterine tubes the movements of the cilia help in the passage of ova towards the uterus.

Secretory columnar cells are scattered in the mucosa of the stomach and intestines. In the intestines many of them secrete mucous which accumulates in the apical part of the cell making it very light staining. These cells acquire a characteristic shape (Fig. 6.5) and are called **goblet cells**.

Cuboidal Epithelium

Cuboidal epithelium is similar to columnar epithelium, but for the fact that the height of the cells is about the same as their width. The nuclei are usually rounded (Fig. 6.6).

A typical cuboidal epithelium may be seen in the follicles of the thyroid gland, in the ducts of many glands, and on the surface of the ovary (where it is called **germinal epithelium**).

An epithelium that is basically cuboidal (or columnar) lines the secretory elements of many glands. In this situation, however, the parts of the cells nearest the lumen are more compressed (against neighbouring cells) than at their bases, giving them a triangular shape (Fig. 6.7).

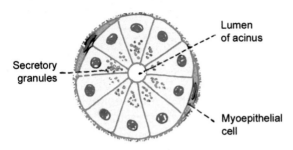

Fig. 6.7. Modified columnar cells in the wall of an acinus (of a gland) (diagrammatic). Note the triangular shape of the cells, the presence of secretory granules, and the myoepithelial cells lying between the gland cells and the basement membrane.

A cuboidal epithelium with a prominent brush border is seen in the proximal convoluted tubules of the kidneys.

Pseudostratified Columnar Epithelium

In usual class-room slides the boundaries between epithelial cells are often not clearly seen. In spite of this we can make out what type of epithelium it is. This is because the shape and spacing of the nuclei gives a good idea of where the cell boundaries must lie.

Normally, in columnar epithelium the nuclei lie in a row, towards the bases of the cells. Sometimes, however, the nuclei appear to be arranged in two or more layers giving the impression that the epithelium is more than one cell thick (Fig. 6.9). The reason for this will be understood easily from Fig. 6.8. It is seen that there is actually only one layer of cells, but some cells are broader near the base, and others near the

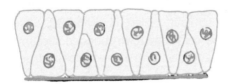

Fig. 6.8. Pseudostratified columnar epithelium (diagrammatic). This figure explains why the nuclei lie at various levels.

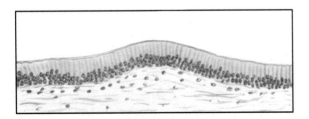

Fig. 6.9. Realistic appearance of pseudostratified columnar epithelium as seen in a section.

apex. The nuclei lie in the broader part of each cell and are, therefore, not in one layer. To distinguish this kind of epithelium from a true stratified epithelium, it is referred to as ***pseudostratified columnar epithelium***.

A pseudostratified columnar epithelium is found in some parts of the auditory tube, the ductus deferens, and the male urethra (membranous and penile parts). A ciliated pseudostratified columnar epithelium is seen in the trachea and in large bronchi.

Stratified Squamous Epithelium

This type of epithelium is made up of several layers of cells. The cells of the deepest (or basal) layer are usually columnar in shape. Lying over the columnar cells there are polyhedral or cuboidal cells. As we pass towards the surface of the epithelium these cells become progressively more flat, so that the most superficial cells consist of flattened squamous cells (Fig. 6.10).

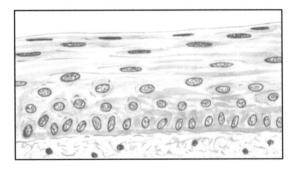

Fig. 6.10. Stratified squamous epithelium (non-keratinized) as seen in a section.

Stratified squamous epithelium can be divided into two types: ***non-keratinized*** and ***keratinized***. In situations where the surface of the epithelium remains moist, the most superficial cells are living and nuclei can be seen in them. This kind of epithelium is described as non-keratinized. In contrast, at places where the epithelial surface is dry (as in the skin) the most superficial cells die and lose their nuclei. These cells contain a substance called ***keratin***, which forms a non-living covering over the epithelium. This kind of epithelium constitutes keratinized stratified squamous epithelium.

Stratified squamous epithelium (both keratinized and non-keratinized) is found over those surfaces of the body that are subject to friction. As a result of friction the most superficial layers are constantly being removed and are replaced by proliferation of cells from the basal (or germinal) layer. This layer, therefore, shows frequent mitoses.

Keratinized stratified squamous epithelium covers the skin of the whole of the body and forms the epidermis. Non-keratinized stratified squamous epithelium is seen lining the mouth, the tongue, the pharynx, the oesophagus, the vagina and the cornea.

Transitional Epithelium

This is a multi-layered epithelium and is 4 to 6 cells thick. It differs from stratified squamous epithelium in that the cells at the surface are not squamous. The deepest cells are columnar or cuboidal. The middle layers are made up of polyhedral or pear-shaped cells. The cells of the surface layer are large and often shaped like an umbrella (Fig. 6.11).

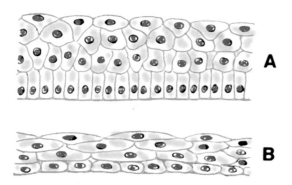

Fig. 6.11. Transitional epithelium (diagrammatic) in unstretched (A), and in stretched (B) conditions.

Transitional epithelium is found in the renal pelvis and calyces, the ureter, the urinary bladder, and part of the urethra. Because of this distribution it is also called *urothelium*.

Mucous Membranes

We have seen that epithelia line many tubular structures within the body. In such structures the epithelium rests on a layer of connective tissue called the *lamina propria* (or *corium*). The layer of epithelium along with its lamina propria is referred to as the *mucous membrane* or *mucosa* (as its surface is kept moist by secretions of mucous glands).

In the intestines the mucous membrane has a third layer formed by a thin stratum of smooth muscle. This smooth muscle is called the *muscularis mucosae* (= muscle of the mucous membrane).

GLANDS

We have seen that some epithelial cells may be specialised to perform a secretory function. Such cells, present singly or in groups, constitute glands.

From this it is obvious that some glands are *unicellular*. Unicellular glands are interspersed amongst other (non-secretory) epithelial cells. They can be found, for example, in the epithelium lining the intestines.

Most glands are, however, *multicellular*. Such glands develop as diverticula from epithelial surfaces. The 'distal' parts of the diverticula develop into secretory elements, while the 'proximal' parts form ducts through which secretions reach the epithelial surface.

Those glands that pour their secretions on to an epithelial surface, directly or through ducts are called *exocrine glands* (or *externally secreting glands*). Some glands lose all contact with the epithelial surface from which they develop: they pour their secretions into blood. Such glands are called *endocrine glands*, *internally secreting glands*, or *duct-less glands*.

When all the secretory cells of an exocrine gland discharge into one duct the gland is said to be a *simple gland*. Sometimes there are a number of groups of secretory cells, each group discharging into its own duct. These ducts unite to form larger ducts that ultimately drain on to an epithelial surface. Such a gland is said to be a *compound gland*.

Both in simple and in compound glands the secretory cells may be arranged in various ways.

(**a**) The secretory element may be *tubular*. The tube may be straight, coiled, or branched.

(**b**) The cells may form rounded sacs or *acini*.

(**c**) They may form flask-shaped structures called *alveoli*.

(**d**) Combinations of the above may be present in a single gland (Fig. 6.12).

Exocrine glands may also be classified on the basis of the nature of their secretions into *mucous glands* and *serous glands*. Unicellular cells secreting mucous are numerous in the intestines: they are called *goblet cells* because of their peculiar shape. (See Fig. 6.5 and Fig. 6.12). The secretions of serous glands are protein in nature.

The secretory elements of exocrine glands are held together by connective tissue. The connective tissue covering the entire gland forms a *capsule* for it.

The secretory cells of a gland constitute its **parenchyma**, while the connective tissue in which the former lie is called the **stroma**.

Endocrine glands are usually arranged in cords or in clumps that are intimately related to a rich network of blood capillaries or of sinusoids. In some cases (for example the thyroid gland) the cells may form rounded follicles.

Endocrine cells and their blood vessels are supported by delicate connective tissue, and are usually surrounded by a capsule.

Neoplasms can arise from the epithelium lining a gland. A benign growth arising in a gland is an **adenoma**; and a malignant growth is an **adenocarcinoma**.

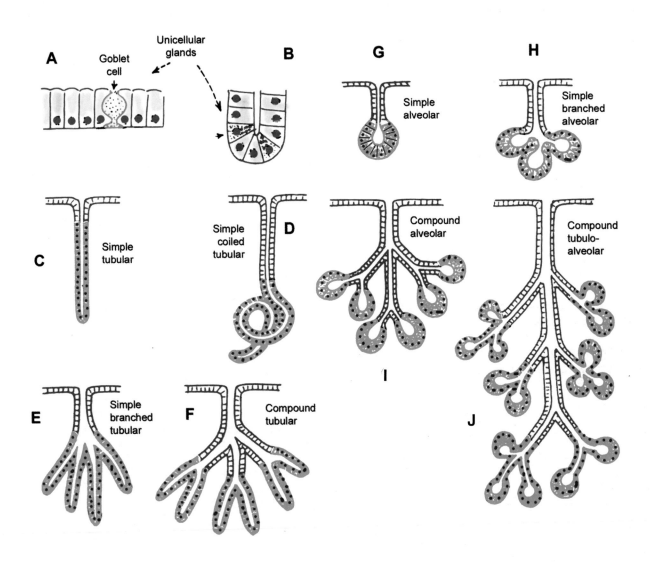

Fig. 6.12. Scheme to show various ways in which the secretory elements of a gland may be organized. A and B are examples of unicellular glands. All others are multicellular. Glands with a single duct are simple glands, while those with a branching duct system are compound glands.

7

Connective Tissue, Ligaments and Tendons

What is Connective Tissue?

The term **connective tissue** is applied to a tissue that fills the interstices between more specialized elements; and serves to hold them together and support them. Connective tissue serves to hold together, and to support, different elements within an organ. Such connective tissue is to be found in almost every part of the body. It is conspicuous in some regions and scanty in others. This kind of connective tissue is referred to as **general connective tissue** to distinguish it from more specialized connective tissues that we will consider separately. It is also called **fibro-collagenous tissue**.

Basic Components of General Connective Tissue

Many tissues and organs of the body are made up mainly of aggregations of closely packed cells e.g., epithelia, and solid organs like the liver. In contrast, cells are relatively few in connective tissue, and are widely separated by a prominent **intercellular substance**. The intercellular substance is in the form of a **ground substance** within which there are numerous **fibres** (Fig. 7.1). Connective tissue can assume various forms depending upon the nature of the ground substance, and of the type of fibres and cells present.

Fibres in connective tissue

The most conspicuous components of connective tissue are the fibres within it. These are of three main types.

(a) **Collagen fibres** are most numerous.

(b) **Reticular fibres** were once described as a distinct variety of fibres, but they are now regarded as one variety of collagen fibre.

(c) **Elastic fibres**.

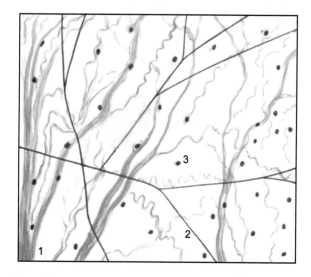

Fig. 7.1. Stretch preparation of omentum showing loose areolar tissue. 1- Collagen fibres. 2-Elastic fibres. 3-Nuclei of fibroblasts.

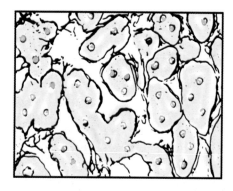

Fig. 7.2. Reticular fibres (black) forming a network in the liver. The white spaces represent sinusoids.

The three types of fibres mentioned above are embedded in an amorphous ground substance or **matrix**.

Cells in general connective tissue

Various types of cells are present in connective tissue. These can be classed into two distinct categories.

(a) Cells that are intrinsic components of connective tissue:

In typical connective tissue the most important cells are **fibroblasts**. Others present are **undifferentiated mesenchymal cells, pigment cells**, and **fat cells**. Other varieties of cells are present in more specialized forms of connective tissues.

(b) Cells that belong to the immune system and are identical or closely related with certain cells present in blood and in lymphoid tissues:

These include **macrophage cells** (or **histiocytes**), **mast cells, lymphocytes, plasma cells, monocytes** and **eosinophils**.

Different forms of Connective Tissue

Loose Connective Tissue

If we examine a small quantity of superficial fascia under a microscope, at low magnification, it is seen to be made up mainly of bundles of loosely arranged fibres that appear to enclose large spaces. This is **loose connective tissue**. Spaces are also called **areolae**, and such tissue is also referred to as **areolar tissue** (Fig. 7.1).

Fibrous Tissue

We have seen that in loose areolar tissue the fibre bundles are loosely arranged with wide spaces in between them. In many situations the fibre bundles are much more conspicuous, and form a dense mass. This kind of tissue is referred to as **fibrous tissue**. It appears white in colour and is sometimes called **white fibrous tissue**.

Elastic Tissue

We have seen that some elastic fibres can be seen in loose areolar tissue (Fig. 7.1). Some elastic fibres may also be present in any other variety of connective tissue. However, in some situations, most of the connective tissue is formed by elastic fibres: this is called **elastic tissue**. In contrast to white fibrous tissue, elastic tissue is yellow in colour. Some ligaments are made up of elastic tissue. These include the ligamentum nuchae (on the back of the neck). The vocal ligaments (of the larynx) are also made up of elastic fibres. Elastic fibres are numerous in membranes that are required to stretch periodically. For example the deeper layer of superficial fascia covering the anterior abdominal wall has a high proportion of elastic fibres to allow for distension of the abdomen.

Reticular Tissue

This is made up of reticular fibres. In many situations (e.g., lymph nodes, glands) these fibres form supporting networks for the cells (Fig. 7.2). In some situations (bone marrow, spleen, lymph nodes) the reticular network is closely associated with **reticular cells**. Most of these cells are fibroblasts, but some may be macrophages.

Other Connective Tissues

Bone and cartilage are regarded as forms of connective tissue as the cells in them are widely separated by intercellular substance. The firmness of cartilage, and the hardness of bone, are because of the nature of the ground substance in them. Cartilage and bone will be considered in Chapter 8. Blood is also included amongst connective tissues as the cells are widely dispersed in a fluid intercellular substance, the plasma. Blood is considered in Chapter 12. Connective tissue contain many fat cells is called adipose tissue.

FIBRES OF CONNECTIVE TISSUE

Collagen Fibres

With the light microscope collagen fibres are seen in bundles (Fig. 7.1). The bundles may be straight or wavy depending upon how much they are stretched. The bundles are made up of collections of individual collagen fibres. The bundles often branch, or anastomose with adjacent bundles, but the individual fibres do not branch.

Bundles of collagen fibres appear white with the naked eye. In sections stained with haematoxylin and eosin collagen fibres are stained light pink. With special methods they assume different colours depending upon the dye used.

Collagen fibres can resist considerable tensile forces (i.e., stretching) without significant increase in their length. At the same time they are pliable and can bend easily.

Reticular Fibres

These fibres are a variety of collagen fibre. They differ from typical collagen fibres as follows.

(**1**) They are much finer.

(2) They form a network (or reticulum) by branching, and by anastomosing with each other. They do not run in bundles (Fig. 7.2).

Reticular fibres provide a supporting network in many situations. These include the spleen, lymph nodes and bone marrow; most glands, including the liver; and the kidneys. Reticular fibres form an essential component of all basement membranes. They are also found in relation to smooth muscle and nerve fibres.

Elastic Fibres

In areolar tissue, elastic fibres are much fewer than those of collagen. They run singly (not in bundles), branch and anastomose with other fibres. Elastic fibres are thinner than those of collagen.

In some situations elastic fibres are thick (e.g., in the ligamenta flava). In other situations (as in walls of large arteries) they form fenestrated membranes.

As their name implies elastic fibres can be stretched (like a rubber band) and return to their original length when tension is released.

CELLS OF CONNECTIVE TISSUE

As mentioned earlier, the cells of connective tissue can be divided into those that are intrinsic components of the tissue, and those that belong to the immune system but are commonly seen in connective tissues. In the first group we include fibroblasts, undifferentiated mesenchymal cells, and pigment cells. Fat cells are commonly seen.

Cells of the immune system to be seen are some varieties of leucocytes and their derivatives. They include the following.

1. Lymphocytes, and plasma cells which are derived from lymphocytes.

2. Monocytes, and macrophages that are derived from monocytes.

3. Mast cells that are related to basophils.

4. Neutrophils and eosinophils are occasionally seen.

Fibroblasts

These are the most numerous cells of connective tissue. They are called fibroblasts because they are concerned with the production of collagen fibres. They also produce reticular and elastic fibres. Where associated with reticular fibres they are usually called **reticular cells**.

Fibroblasts are present in close relationship to collagen fibres. In tissue sections these cells appear to be spindle shaped, and the nucleus appears to be

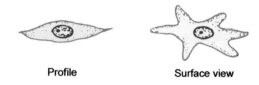

Profile   Surface view

Fig. 7.3. Structure of a fibroblast.

flattened. When seen from the surface the cells show branching processes (Fig. 7.3).

Fibroblasts become very active when there is need to lay down collagen fibres. This occurs, for example, in wound repair. When the need arises fibroblasts can give rise, by division, to more fibroblasts.

Undifferentiated Mesenchymal Cells

Embryonic connective tissue is called **mesenchyme**. It is made up of small cells with slender branching processes that join to form a fine network.

Pigment cells

Pigment cells are easily distinguished as they contain brown pigment (melanin) in their cytoplasm. They are most abundant in connective tissue of the skin, and in the choroid and iris of the eyeball. Along with pigment containing epithelial cells they give the skin, the iris, and the choroid their dark colour. Variations in the number of pigment cells, and in the amount of pigment in them accounts for differences in skin colour of different races, and in different individuals.

Pigment cells prevent light from reaching other cells. The importance of this function in relation to the eyeball is obvious. Pigment cells in the skin protect deeper tissues from the effects of light (specially ultraviolet light). The darker skin of races living in tropical climates is an obvious adaptation for this purpose.

Fat Cells (Adipocytes)

Although some amount of fat (lipids) may be present in the cytoplasm of many cells, including fibroblasts, some cells store fat in large amounts and become distended with it. These are called **fat cells**, **adipocytes**, or **lipocytes**. Aggregations of fat cells constitute **adipose tissue** .

Macrophage Cells

Macrophage cells of connective tissue are part of a large series of cells present in the body that have similar functions. These collectively form the **mononuclear phagocyte system**.

Macrophage cells of connective tissue are also called **histiocytes** or **clasmatocytes** (Fig. 7.4). They have

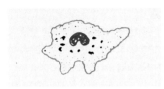

Fig. 7.4. Macrophage cell (histiocyte)

the ability to phagocytose (eat up) unwanted material like bacteria.

Mast Cells

These are small round or oval cells. They are also called **mastocytes**, or **histaminocytes** (Fig. 7.5). The nucleus is small and centrally placed. The distinguishing feature of these cells is the presence of numerous granules in the cytoplasm. The granules can be demonstrated by special stains.

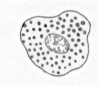

Fig. 7.5. Mast cell.

Mast cells release histamine when a tissue is exposed to an antigen to which it is sensitive (because of previous exposure). The release of histamine leads to local reactions like urticaria, or to severe general reactions like anaphylactic shock.

Lymphocytes

Lymphocytes represent one variety of leucocytes (white blood cells) present in blood. Large aggregations of lymphocytes are present in lymphoid tissues. They reach connective tissue from these sources, and are specially numerous when the tissue undergoes inflammation. Lymphocytes play an important role in defence of the body against invasion by bacteria and other organisms.

Plasma Cells or Plasmatocytes

Very few plasma cells can be seen in normal connective tissue. Their number increases in the presence of certain types of inflammation. It is believed that plasma cells represent B-lymphocytes that have matured and have lost their power of further division. Plasma cells produce antibodies.

LIGAMENTS

Ligaments are very important structures responsible for maintaining the integrity of joints. They are made up of bundles of collagen fibres. In other they consist of fibrous tissue. We have seen that collagen fibres are flexible, but they cannot be stretched. This is true of ligaments as well.

We will try and understand some aspects of ligaments by taking the example of the elbow joint. This joint is surrounded all round by a capsular ligament (often simply called the capsule). The capsule is thickened at some places to form ligaments. When the elbow is flexed the ligaments on the anterior (or ventral) aspect of the joint are relaxed, while those on the posterior aspect are stretched. The opposite happens in extension. When a ligament is fully stretched further movement in that direction is not possible. In other words **ligaments limit the range of movement** at a joint. The ligaments around a joint **hold the articulating bones together** and prevent their separation. The fibres in a ligament can run in different directions, depending upon the direction of pull exerted on them. The ligament is thickest where the fibres are stretched most often, and with greatest force.

In some injuries a joint may be forcefully twisted. The ligaments that resist the movement can get strained, or even torn. This is one of the commonest causes of pain for which a person may come to a physiotherapist.

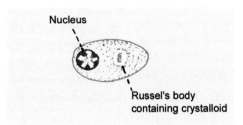

Fig. 7.6. Plasma cell.

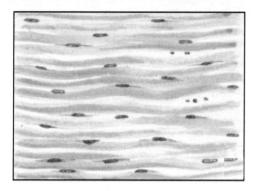

Fig. 7.7. Longitudinal section through a tendon. Note the collagen fibres running parallel to one another. Fibroblasts are present in intervals between the fibres.

TENDONS

Tendons are cord like bands attached to the ends of muscles. Like ligaments, tendons are made up of bundles of collagen fibres. The difference is that the fibres in a tendon are arranged very regularly and run parallel to each other (Fig. 7.7). Tendons have a smooth surface so that friction with other structures is minimal. For this purpose many tendons are covered with double layered synovial sheaths. The two layers are separated by a thin layer of fluid.

The functions performed by tendons are as follows.

1. At one end the tendon receives the attachment of a large number of muscle fibres. At its other end the tendon is attached to a narrow area of bone. In this way a tendon serves to concentrate the pull of a muscle on a narrow area, making precise movements possible.

2. Many large muscles that are responsible for movements of the fingers are placed in the forearm. The pull of these muscles reaches the phalanges of the fingers through long tendons. Tendons allow the main muscle mass to be placed at a convenient distance away from the point where pull is to be exerted.

3. Many long tendons curve around bony prominences that serve as pulleys. This changes the direction of pull of the muscle. It is only because of the presence of tendons that a muscle can be placed in a direction different from that in which its pull is to be exerted.

RETINACULA

In the region of the wrist, and at the ankle, the deep fascia is thickened to form strong ribbon like bands called retinacula. Retinacula are composed of fibrous tissue. Their function is to keep tendons in place during movements. One retinaculum placed on the front of the wrist is called the flexor retinaculum. The tendons that pass from the front of the forearm into the hand pass deep to this retinaculum. The presence of the retinaculum prevents the tendons from bulging forwards when the wrist is flexed. The retinaculum also acts as a pulley allowing the tendons to change direction as they pass from the forearm into the palm. This example illustrates the usefulness of retinacula. Many other retinacula are present around the wrist and ankle.

SUMMARY OF THE FUNCTIONS OF CONNECTIVE TISSUES

Mechanical Functions

1. In the form of loose connective tissue, it holds together structures like skin, muscles, blood vessels, etc. It binds together various layers of hollow viscera. In the form of areolar tissue and reticular tissue it forms a framework that supports the cellular elements of various organs like the spleen, lymph nodes, and glands, and provides capsules for them.

2. The looseness of areolar tissue facilitates movement between structures connected by it. The looseness of superficial fascia enables the movement of skin over deep fascia. In hollow organs this allows for mobility and stretching.

3. In the form of deep fascia connective tissue provides a tight covering for deeper structures (specially in the limbs and neck) and helps to maintain the shape of these regions.

4. In the form of ligaments it holds bone ends together at joints.

5. In the form of deep fascia, intermuscular septa and aponeuroses, connective tissue provides attachment for the origins and insertions of many muscles.

6. In the form of tendons it transmits the pull of muscles to their insertion.

7. Thickened areas of deep fascia form retinacula that hold tendons in place at the wrist and ankle.

8. Both areolar tissue and fascial membranes provide planes along which blood vessels, lymphatics, and nerves travel. The superficial fascia provides passage to vessels and nerves going to the skin, and supports them.

9. In the form of dura mater it provides support to the brain and spinal cord.

Other Functions

(**a**) In the form of adipose tissue it provides a store of nutrition. In cold weather the fat provides insulation and helps to generate heat.

(**b**) Because of the presence of cells of the immune system (macrophages and plasma cells), connective tissue helps the body to fight against invading foreign substances (including bacteria) by destroying them, or by producing antibodies against them.

8

Cartilage, Bone and Joints

CARTILAGE

Cartilage is a tissue that forms the 'skeletal' basis of some parts of the body e.g., the auricle of the ear, or the lower part of the nose. Feeling these parts readily demonstrates that while cartilage is sufficiently firm to maintain its form, it is not rigid like bone. It can be bent, returning to its original form when the bending force is removed.

Cartilage is considered to be a modified connective tissue. It resembles ordinary connective tissue in that the cells in it are widely separated by a considerable amount of intercellular material or *matrix*. The latter consists of a homogeneous *ground substance* within which fibres are embedded. Cartilage differs from typical connective tissue mainly in the nature of the ground substance: this is firm and gives cartilage its characteristic consistency. Three main types of cartilage can be recognised depending on the number and variety of fibres in the matrix. These are *hyaline cartilage*, *fibrocartilage*, and *elastic cartilage*.

As a rule, the free surfaces of hyaline cartilage are covered by a fibrous membrane called the *perichondrium*, but fibrocartilage is not.

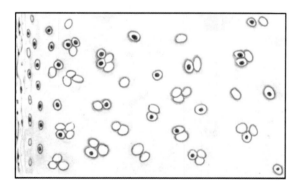

Fig. 8.1. Hyaline cartilage. Note groups of chondrocytes surrounded by homogenous matrix. Perichondrium is seen at the left end of the figure.

Cartilage Cells

The cells of cartilage are called *chondrocytes*. They lie in spaces (or *lacunae*) present in the matrix. At first the cells are small. As the cartilage cells mature they enlarge considerably.

Ground Substance

The ground substance of cartilage is made up of complex molecules containing proteins and carbohydrates (proteoglycans). These molecules form a meshwork that is filled by water and dissolved salts.

HYALINE CARTILAGE

Hyaline cartilage is so called because it is transparent (hyalos = glass). Its intercellular substance appears to be homogeneous, but using special techniques it can be shown that many collagen fibres are present in the matrix.

Towards the centre of a mass of hyaline cartilage the chondrocytes are large and are usually present in groups (of two or more) (Fig. 8.1). Groups of cartilage cells are called *cell-nests* (or *isogenous cell groups*). Immediately around lacunae housing individual chondrocytes, and around cell nests the matrix stains deeper than elsewhere giving the appearance of a capsule. Towards the periphery of the cartilage the cells are small, and elongated in a direction parallel to the surface. Just under the perichondrium the cells become indistinguishable from fibroblasts.

Embedded in the ground substance of hyaline cartilage, there are numerous collagen fibres. The fibres are arranged so that they resist tensional forces. Hyaline cartilage has been compared to a tyre. The ground substance (corresponding to the rubber of the tyre) resists compressive forces, while the fibres (corresponding to the treads of the tyre) resist tensional forces.

Distribution of Hyaline Cartilage

Hyaline cartilage is widely distributed in the body as follows.

(1) Costal Cartilages

These are bars of hyaline cartilage that connect the ventral ends of the ribs to the sternum, or to adjoining costal cartilages. They show the typical structure of hyaline cartilage described above.

(2) Articular Cartilage

The articular surfaces of most synovial joints are lined by hyaline cartilage. These articular cartilages provide the bone ends with smooth surfaces between which there is very little friction. They also act as shock absorbers. Articular cartilages are not covered by perichondrium. Their surface is kept moist by synovial fluid that also provides nutrition to them.

(3) Other sites where Hyaline Cartilage is found

(**a**) The skeletal framework of the larynx is formed by a number of cartilages and most of these are composed of hyaline cartilage.

(**b**) Hyaline cartilage is also present in the walls of the trachea and bronchi, and in parts of the nose.

(**c**) In growing children long bones consist of a bony *diaphysis* (corresponding to the shaft) and of one or more bony *epiphyses* (corresponding to bone ends or projections). Each epiphysis is connected to the diaphysis by a plate of hyaline cartilage called the *epiphyseal plate*. This plate is essential for bone growth.

FIBROCARTILAGE

On superficial examination this type of cartilage (also called *white fibrocartilage*) looks very much like dense fibrous tissue (Fig. 8.2). However, in sections it is seen to be cartilage because it contains typical cartilage cells surrounded by capsules. The matrix is pervaded by numerous collagen bundles amongst which there are some fibroblasts. The fibres merge with those of surrounding connective tissue, there being no perichondrium over the cartilage. This kind of cartilage has great tensile strength combined with considerable elasticity.

White fibrocartilage is found at the following sites.

(**1**) Fibrocartilage is most conspicuous in secondary cartilaginous joints or *symphyses*. These include the joints between bodies of vertebrae (where the cartilage

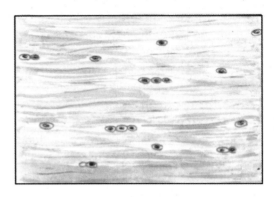

Fig. 8.2. Fibrocartilage. Cartilage cells are embedded amongst thick bundles of collagen fibres.

forms intervertebral discs); the pubic symphysis; and the manubriosternal joint.

(**2**) In some synovial joints the joint cavity is partially or completely subdivided by an articular disc. These discs are made up of fibrocartilage. (Examples are discs of the temporo-mandibular and sternoclavicular joints, and menisci of the knee joint).

(**3**) The glenoidal labrum of the shoulder joint and the acetabular labrum of the hip joint are made of fibrocartilage.

ELASTIC CARTILAGE

Elastic cartilage (or yellow fibrocartilage) is similar in many ways to hyaline cartilage. The main difference is that instead of collagen fibres, the matrix contains numerous elastic fibres which form a network (Fig. 8.3). The surface of elastic cartilage is covered by perichondrium.

Elastic cartilage possesses greater flexibility than hyaline cartilage, and readily recovers its shape after being deformed.

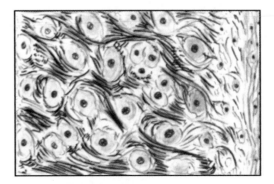

Fig. 8.3. Elastic cartilage. Note chondrocytes surrounded by bundles of elastic fibres. The section has been stained by Verheoff's method in which elastic fibres are stained bluish black.

Elastic cartilage is found in the auricle (or pinna) of the ear, and in some internal parts of the ear. It is found in the epiglottis and in some other parts of the larynx.

During fetal life cartilage is much more widely distributed than in the adult. The greater part of the skeleton is cartilaginous in early fetal life. The ends of most long bones are cartilaginous at the time of birth, and are gradually replaced by bone. The replacement is completed only after full growth of the individual (i.e., by about 18 years of age).

Replacement of cartilage by bone is called *ossification*. Ossification of cartilage has to be carefully distinguished from *calcification* in which the matrix hardens because of the deposition in it of calcium salts, but true bone is not formed. Calcification of hyaline cartilage is often seen in old people.

BONE

Some Features of Gross Structure

If we examine a longitudinal section across a bone (such as the humerus) we see that the wall of the shaft is tubular and encloses a large *marrow cavity* (Fig. 8.4). The wall of the tube is made up of a hard dense material that appears, on naked eye examination, to have a uniform smooth texture with no obvious spaces in it. This kind of bone is called *compact bone*. It is seen further, that compact bone is thickest midway

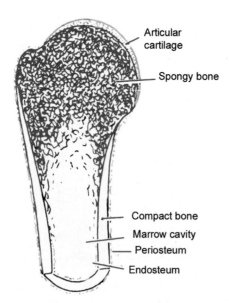

Fig. 8.4. Some features of bone structure as seen in a longitudinal section through one end of a long bone.

between the two ends of the bone and gradually tapers towards the ends.

When we examine the bone ends we find that the marrow cavity does not extend into them. They are filled by a meshwork of tiny rods or plates of bone and contain numerous spaces, the whole appearance resembling that of a sponge. This kind of bone is called *spongy* or *cancellous bone* (cancel= cavity).

Where the bone ends take part in forming joints they are covered by a layer of articular cartilage. With the exception of the areas covered by articular cartilage, the entire outer surface of bone is covered by a membrane called the *periosteum*. The wall of the marrow cavity is lined by a membrane called the *endosteum*.

The marrow cavity and the spaces of spongy bone (present at the bone ends) are filled by a highly vascular tissue called *bone marrow*. At the bone ends the marrow is red in colour. Apart from blood vessels this *red marrow* contains numerous masses of blood forming cells (*haemopoietic tissue*). In the shaft of the bone of an adult, the marrow is yellow. This *yellow marrow* is made up predominantly of fat cells. In bones of a fetus, or of a young child, the entire bone marrow is red. The marrow in the shaft is gradually replaced by yellow marrow with increasing age.

BASIC FACTS ABOUT BONE STRUCTURE

Elements Comprising Bone Tissue

Like cartilage, bone is a modified connective tissue. It consists of bone cells or *osteocytes* that are widely separated from one another by a considerable amount of intercellular substance. The latter consists of a homogeneous ground substance or matrix in which collagen fibres and mineral salts (mainly calcium and phosphorus) are deposited.

In addition to mature bone cells (osteocytes) two additional types of cells are seen in developing bone. These are bone producing cells or *osteoblasts*, and bone removing cells or *osteoclasts* (Fig. 8.9). Other cells present include *osteoprogenitor cells* from which osteoblasts and osteocytes are derived.

Lamellar Bone

When we examine the structure of any bone of an adult, we find that it is made up of layers or *lamellae* (Fig. 8.5). This kind of bone is called *lamellar bone*. Each lamellus is a thin plate of bone consisting of collagen fibres and mineral salts that are deposited in a gelatinous ground substance. Even the smallest piece

The unit of bone structure is called a lamellus

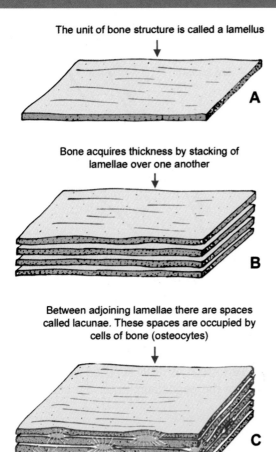

Bone acquires thickness by stacking of lamellae over one another

Between adjoining lamellae there are spaces called lacunae. These spaces are occupied by cells of bone (osteocytes)

Fig. 8.5. Scheme to show how lamellae constitute bone.

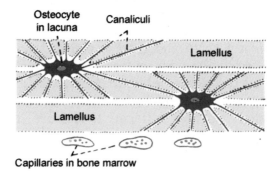

Fig. 8.6. Diagram to show the relationship of osteocytes to bone lamellae.

of bone is made up of several lamellae placed over one another.

Between adjoining lamellae we see small, flattened spaces or *lacunae*.

Each lacuna contains one osteocyte (Fig. 8.6). Spreading out from each lacuna there are fine canals or *canaliculi* that communicate with those from other lacunae. The canaliculi are occupied by delicate cytoplasmic processes of osteocytes.

Woven Bone

In contrast to mature bone, newly formed bone does not have a lamellar structure. The collagen fibres are present in bundles that appear to run randomly in different directions, interlacing with each other. Because of the interlacing of fibre bundles, this kind of bone is called *woven bone*. All newly formed bone is woven bone. It is later replaced by lamellar bone.

We have seen that bone may be classified as compact or cancellous, and as lamellar or woven. On the basis of the manner of its development, bone can also be classified as *cartilage bone* or as *membrane bone.*

Structure of Cancellous Bone

The bony plates or rods that form the meshwork of cancellous bone are called *trabeculae*. Each trabeculus is made up of a number of lamellae (described above) between which there are lacunae containing osteocytes. Canaliculi, containing the processes of osteocytes, radiate from the lacunae.

The trabeculae enclose wide spaces which are filled in by bone marrow. They receive nutrition from blood vessels in the bone marrow (Fig. 8.7).

Structure of Compact Bone

When we examine a section of compact bone we find that this type of bone is also made up of lamellae, and is pervaded by lacunae (containing osteocytes), and by canaliculi (Fig. 8.8). Most of the lamellae are arranged in the form of concentric rings that surround a narrow *Haversian canal* present at the centre of each ring. The Haversian canal is occupied by blood vessels, nerve fibres, and some cells. One Haversian

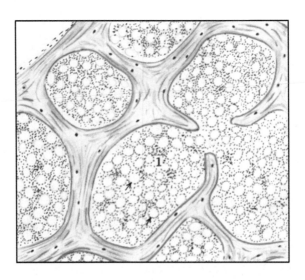

Fig. 8.7. Structure of cancellous bone as seen in a section. 1-Bone marrow.

canal and the lamellae around it constitute a *Haversian system* or *osteon*.

Compact bone consists of several such osteons. Between adjoining osteons there are angular intervals that are occupied by *interstitial lamellae*. Near the surface of compact bone the lamellae are arranged parallel to the surface: these are called *circumferential lamellae*.

From what has been said above it will be appreciated that there is an essential similarity in the structure of cancellous and compact bone. Both are made up of lamellae. The difference lies in the relative volume occupied by bony lamellae and by the spaces. In compact bone the spaces are small and the solid bone is abundant; whereas in cancellous bone the spaces are large and actual bone tissue is sparse.

THE PERIOSTEUM

We have seen that the external surface of any bone is, as a rule, covered by a membrane called periosteum. (The only parts of the bone surface devoid of periosteum are those that are covered with articular cartilage). The periosteum consists of two layers, outer and inner. The outer layer is a fibrous membrane. The inner layer is cellular. In young bones the inner layer contains numerous osteoblasts, and is called the *osteogenetic layer*. In the periosteum covering the bones of an adult osteoblasts are not conspicuous, but osteoprogenitor cells present here can form osteoblasts when need arises e.g., in the event of a

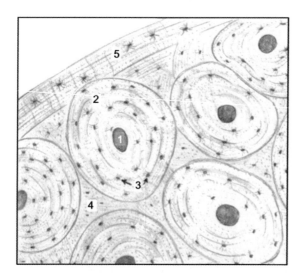

Fig. 8.8. Structure of compact bone as seen in a ground section. 1. Haversian canal. 2.Concentric lamellae forming Haversian system. 3. Lacunae. 4. Interstitial lamellae. 5. Circumferential lamellae.

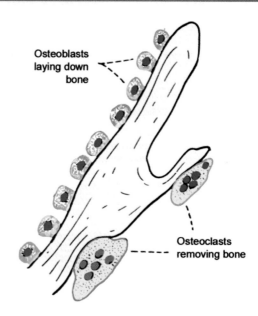

Fig. 8.9. Relationship of osteoblasts and osteoclasts to developing bone.

fracture. Periosteum is richly supplied with blood. Many vessels from the periosteum enter the bone and help to supply it.

FORMATION OF BONE

The process of bone formation is called *ossification*. Formation of most bones is preceded by the formation of a cartilaginous model, which is subsequently replaced by bone. This kind of ossification is called *endochondral ossification*; and bones formed in this way are called *cartilage bones*. In some situations (e.g., the vault of the skull) formation of bone is not preceded by formation of a cartilaginous model. Instead bone is laid down directly in a fibrous membrane. This process is called *intramembranous ossification*; and bones formed in this way are called *membrane bones*. The bones of the vault of the skull, the mandible, and the clavicle are membrane bones.

Development of a Typical Long Bone

In the region where a long bone is to be formed mesenchymal cells get converted to cartilage producing chondroblasts. These cells produce a cartilaginous model of the bone. This cartilage is covered by perichondrium. Endochondral ossification starts in the central part of the cartilaginous model (i.e., at the centre of the future shaft).

This area is called the *primary centre of ossification*. Gradually, bone formation extends from the primary centre towards the ends of shaft. This is

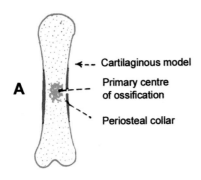

A

Cartilaginous model

Primary centre
of ossification

Periosteal collar

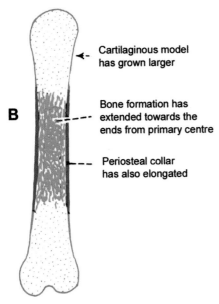

B

Cartilaginous model
has grown larger

Bone formation has
extended towards the
ends from primary centre

Periosteal collar
has also elongated

Fig. 8.10. Formation of a typical long
bone: primary centre of ossification and
periosteal collar.

accompanied by progressive enlargement of the cartilaginous model.

Soon after the appearance of the primary centre, and the onset of endochondral ossification in it, the perichondrium (which may now be called periosteum) becomes active. The osteoprogenitor cells in its deeper layer lay down bone on the surface of the cartilaginous model by **intramembranous ossification**. This periosteal bone completely surrounds the cartilaginous shaft and is, therefore, called the **periosteal collar** (Fig. 8.10).

At about the time of birth the developing bone consists of (a) a part called the **diaphysis** (or shaft), that is bony, and has been formed by extension of the primary centre of ossification, and (b) ends that are cartilaginous (Fig. 8.11). At varying times after birth **secondary centres** of ossification appear in the cartilages forming the ends of the bone (Fig. 8.11B). These centres enlarge until the ends become bony (Fig. 8.12). More than one secondary centre of ossification may appear at either end. The portion of bone formed from one secondary centre is called an **epiphysis**.

For a considerable time after birth the bone of the diaphysis and the bone of any epiphysis are separated by a plate of cartilage called the **epiphyseal cartilage**, or **epiphyseal plate**. This is formed by cartilage into which ossification has not extended either from the diaphysis or from the epiphysis. This plate plays a vital role in growth of the bone.

Metaphysis

The portion of the diaphysis adjoining the epiphyseal plate is called the metaphysis (Fig. 8.12). It is a region of active bone formation and, for this reason, it is highly vascular. The metaphysis is frequently the site of infection.

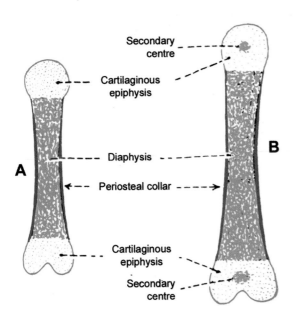

Secondary
centre

Cartilaginous
epiphysis

Diaphysis

A

Periosteal collar

B

Cartilaginous
epiphysis

Secondary
centre

Fig. 8.11. Formation of a typical long bone:
secondary centres of ossification.

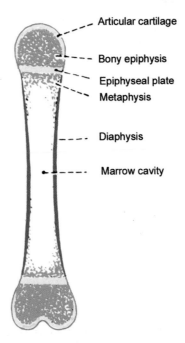

Articular cartilage

Bony epiphysis

Epiphyseal plate

Metaphysis

Diaphysis

Marrow cavity

Fig. 8.12. Formation of a typical long bone:
bony epiphyses and epiphyseal plates.

SOME DISORDERS OF BONE

Fractures

The most common condition affecting a bone is fracture. Nature tries to rejoin the broken ends. The process of fracture healing is described below.

Fracture Healing

1. When a bone fractures, there is bleeding at the site, and a haematoma forms between the two bone ends.

2. An inflammatory reaction sets in. Macrophages collect in the region and gradually remove clotted blood and bone fragments. Granulation tissue consisting of new capillaries and fibroblasts is formed.

3. Osteoblasts (present in periosteum) multiply and lay down new bone, that joins the bone ends. This new bone is temporary and is called *callus*. The union is at first weak but gradually increases in strength.

4. Activity of osteoblasts and osteoclasts gradually replaces the callus with normal bone.

Fracture healing is best if the two bone ends are brought close together (= reduction of fracture); and maintained in that position (= immobilisation). Regions of bone that have a rich blood supply heal better than areas with scanty supply. Healing is best in children and young adults, and is often delayed in the elderly.

Osteoporosis

Reduced density of bone is called osteoporosis. It is common in old persons, and in those in whom mobility is restricted for any reason. Calcium content of bone decreases so that bones break easily. Vertebrae can undergo compression. Osteoporosis can be prevented or cured by sufficient intake of calcium and vitamin D.

Rickets

Deficiency of vitamin D in children leads to rickets. Bones are weak, and growth of the body is not normal. Bones of the legs can get bent (bowed legs).

Osteomalacia

Deficiency of vitamin D in adults leads to osteomalacia. The bones become soft and can be deformed. Such deformity of the pelvis, in women, causes difficulty during childbirth.

Osteomyelitis

Infection in bone is called osteomyelitis. It is difficult to treat and easily becomes chronic. Sinuses discharging pus may form, and spicules of bone may come out through the sinus.

Tumours

Both benign and malignant tumours can arise in bone. A benign tumour arising from osteoblasts is called an *osteoma*. A malignant tumour arising from the same cells is called an *osteosarcoma*. Osteosarcomas are most commonly seen in bones adjoining the knee joint. They can spread to distant sites in the body through the blood stream.

CLASSIFICATION OF JOINTS

Some facts about joints and related movements have been considered in Chapter 2. In this section we will see how joints can be classified. Joints can be divided into three main types on the basis of structure.

Fibrous joints

The two bone ends are connected directly by fibrous tissue. Examples of such joints areas follows.

(a) Joints between flat bones of the skull (called *sutures*) (Fig. 8.13).

(b) Joints between teeth and jaw (*peg and socket joints*).

(c) Joint between lower ends of tibia and fibula (*syndesmosis*) (Fig. 8.14).

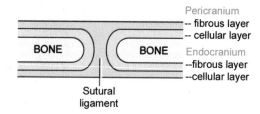

Fig. 8.13. Section across a suture between two bones of the skull.

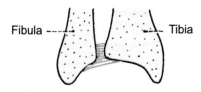

Fig. 8.14. Diagram showing the lower ends of the tibia and fibula united by fibrous tissue. Such a joint is classified as a syndesmosis.

Cartilaginous joints

The two bones are joined by cartilage. Such joints are of two types.

(a) We have seen that in growing individuals the shaft (diaphysis) of a long bone is united to the bone end (epiphysis) by the epiphyseal plate (Fig. 8.12). This plate is made of hyaline cartilage, and this kind of joint is called a **synchondrosis**. As explained above these joints serve as areas of growth and disappear after growth is completed.

(b) Some cartilaginous joints are permanent. These are secondary cartilaginous joints or **symphyses**. The structure is such a joint is shown in Fig. 8.15. The bone ends forming the joint are covered by a thin layer of hyaline cartilage. The two layers of hyaline cartilage are united by an intervening plate of fibrocartilage. Examples of this type of joint are the pubic symphysis, and joints between bodies of vertebrae.

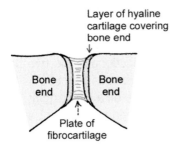

Fig. 8.15. Structure of the pubic symphysis, which is an example of a secondary cartilaginous joint, also called a symphysis.

Synovial joints

Most of the joints of the body are of this type. The articulating surfaces are not directly connected to each other, by any tissue. They are covered by a layer of hyaline cartilage (called **articular cartilage**). This makes the surfaces smooth and helps them to glide over each other (Fig. 8.16).

The two bone ends are held together by a **capsule** made up of fibrous tissue. The capsule encloses the articular surfaces within a cavity.

The inside of the capsule is lined by a **synovial membrane** which secretes synovial fluid. This fluid has a lubricating and nutritive function.

Synovial joints are of various types as follows.

1. In many small joints the articulating surfaces are flat. These are **plane joints**.

2. In several joints, a convex articular surface on one bone fits into a concavity on the other (as shown in Fig. 8.16). When the convex surface is rounded (like part of a sphere) and the concave surface is cup-shaped, the joint is said to be of the **ball and socket**

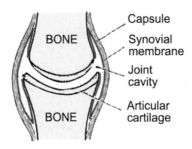

Fig. 8.16. Structure of a typical synovial joint.

variety. The shoulder joint and the hip joint are of this type. They allow the maximum movement.

3. In some joints the convex surface is elliptical rather than rounded. These are **ellipsoid joints**, and the wrist joint is of this type.

4. In some cases one bone end may have two convex surfaces (or condyles) that fit into two cavities on the opposite bone. Such joints are **condylar joints**. The knee joint is of this type (Fig. 8.17).

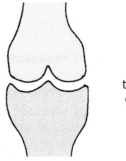

Fig. 8.17. Scheme to show the shape of bone ends in a condylar joint.

5. In some cases one bone end may be convex in one direction and concave in another. The opposite bone shows a reciprocal curvature. Such joints are called **saddle joints**. The carpometacarpal joint of the thumb is of this type.

6. In a **pivot joint** one bone end is rod shaped. It fits into a ring made up partly of bone and partly of a ligament. Two examples are shown in Fig. 8.18.

CLASSIFICATION OF JOINTS ON BASIS OF MOVEMENTS

I. Immovable Joints:

These are synchondroses and sutures. About sutures it may be noted that at the time of birth the fibrous tissue of the sutural ligaments is sufficiently lax to permit over-riding of skull bones on one another. This 'moulding' allows the head to pass easily through the mother's pelvis. In later life sutures permit no movement. Syndesmoses and gomphoses are usually

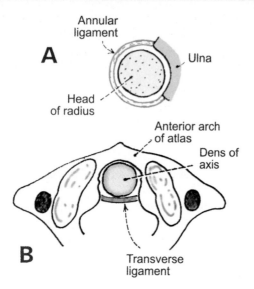

Fig. 8.18. Two examples of pivot joints. A. Superior radioulnar joint. B. Joint between the first cervical vertebra (atlas) and the second cervical vertebra (axis).

included among immovable joints, but they do allow slight movement that affords resilience to these joints.

II. Joints permitting slight movement

Slight movement is possible at secondary cartilaginous joints. In the case of the vertebral column the movements between succeeding vertebrae get added together so that the total movement becomes considerable. Synovial joints of the plane variety also permit slight gliding movements only. These joints provide resilience to regions like the wrist and ankle, and increase the total range of movement in these regions.

III. Joints Allowing Free Movement:

Free movement is possible only at synovial joints, but within these there is considerable variability in the type and range of movement permitted.

(**a**) If we study the movements of the arm at the shoulder joint we find that the arm can be moved forwards and backwards; from side to side; and can also be rotated on itself. In other words it can be moved in almost any direction. This is possible only when the joint is of the ball and socket variety. Apart from the shoulder the only other joint of this variety is the hip joint.

(**b**) Next, if we consider the movements at the wrist we find that the hand can be moved forwards and backwards, and from side to side, but cannot be rotated (independently of the forearm). In other words movement is permitted only on two axes (at right angles to each other), whereas a ball and socket joint permits

movement in intermediate axes also. Rotation is not possible at the wrist because this joint is of the ellipsoid variety. The metacarpophalangeal joints are also examples of ellipsoid joints.

(**c**) The movements permitted at a saddle joint are like those of an ellipsoid joint except that forward and backward movement, or side to side movement are accompanied by a certain amount of rotation. The rotation is automatic and is produced because of the shape of the articular surfaces: it cannot be performed independently.

(**d**) In some joints the movements are like those of a door on a hinge: forward and backward movement is permitted, but side to side movement or rotation is not possible. These are called ***hinge joints***. Typically a hinge joint is of the condylar variety which is seen in its pure form in the interphalangeal joints. The knee is also a hinge joint of the condylar variety, but because of differences in the size and shape of the medial and lateral femoral condyles the movements of the knee are associated with some rotation. The elbow is a hinge joint, but here instead of two condyles we have a pulley shaped trochlea. Functionally the two halves (medial and lateral) of the trochlea function as two condyles. Yet another example of a hinge joint is seen at the ankle where side to side movement and rotation are prevented partly by the pulley like shape of the upper surface of the talus and partly by the presence of the medial and lateral malleoli on either side of the talus. From the above it may be noted that the term hinge joint refers to a functional entity and not to a structural one.

(**e**) From what has been said above it will be clear that ball and socket joints are ***multiaxial***, ellipsoid and saddle joints are ***biaxial***, and hinge joints are ***uniaxial***. The pivot joint is another joint of the uniaxial type. A pivot is a rod around which something else rotates. At the median atlantoaxial joint the dens of the axis vertebra represents the pivot around which the atlas vertebra rotates. The movement is reversed in the superior radioulnar joint: the ring formed by the radial notch of the ulna and the annular ligament remains fixed, while the head of the radius (i.e., the pivot itself) moves within the ring.

Compound And Complex Joints

When more than two bone ends are enclosed within a single capsule the joint is said to be ***compound***. For example, in the elbow we really have three separate joints within one capsule: the humeroulnar, the humeroradial, and the superior radioulnar.

A complex joint is one in which the cavity is divided completely or incompletely into two parts by an ***intra-articular disc*** of fibrocartilage.

Examples are the ***temporomandibular joint***, the ***sternoclavicular joint***, and the ***knee joint***. The intra-articular disc may perform various functions. It may help to provide better adaptation of articular surfaces to each other. The two halves of the joint may permit different types of movements. For example, the upper part of the temporomandibular joint permits forward and backward gliding; and its lower part acts like a hinge joint. The intra-articular disc may facilitate lubrication, and may act as a shock absorber. The discs of the sternoclavicular and inferior radioulnar joints act as important bonds of union between the bones concerned.

9

Muscle

Introductory Remarks

Muscle tissue is composed predominantly of cells that are specialized to shorten in length by contraction. This contraction results in movement. It is in this way that virtually all movements within the body, or of the body in relation to the environment, are ultimately produced.

Muscle tissue is made up basically of cells that are called *myocytes*. Myocytes are elongated in one direction and are, therefore, often referred to as *muscle fibres*. We shall see, however, that in some cases muscle fibres are made up of several myocytes joined to each other; or of greatly elongated myocytes containing multiple nuclei.

The force generated by contraction of a muscle fibre is transmitted to other structures through connective tissue. Each muscle fibre is closely invested by connective tissue which is continuous with that around other muscle fibres. Because of this fact the force generated by different muscle fibres gets added together. In some cases a movement may be the result of simultaneous contraction of thousands of muscle fibres.

The connective tissue framework of muscle also provides pathways along which blood vessels and nerves reach muscle fibres.

From the point of view of its histological structure muscle is of three types.

(1) The first variety of muscle tissue is present mainly in the limbs and in relation to the body wall. Because of its close relationship to the bony skeleton, this variety is called **skeletal muscle**. When examined under a microscope fibres of skeletal muscle show prominent transverse striations. Skeletal muscle is, therefore, also called **striated muscle**. Skeletal muscle can normally be made to contract under our will (to perform movements we desire). It is, therefore, also called **voluntary muscle**. Skeletal muscle is supplied by somatic motor nerves.

(2) The second variety of muscle is present mainly in relation to viscera. It is seen most typically in the walls of hollow viscera. As fibres of this variety do not show transverse striations it is called **smooth muscle**, or **nonstriated muscle**. As a rule, contraction of smooth muscle is not under our control; and smooth muscle is, therefore, also called **involuntary muscle**. It is supplied by autonomic nerves.

(3) The third variety of muscle is present exclusively in the heart and is called **cardiac muscle**. It resembles smooth muscle in being involuntary; but it resembles striated muscle in that the fibres of cardiac muscle also show transverse striations. Cardiac muscle has an inherent rhythmic contractility the rate of which can be modified by autonomic nerves that supply it.

SKELETAL MUSCLE

Elementary Facts about Skeletal Muscle

Skeletal muscle is made up essentially of long, cylindrical 'fibres'. The length of the fibres is highly variable, the longest being as much as 30 cm in length. The diameter of the fibres also varies considerably (10 to 60 μm: usually 50-60 μm). Each 'fibre' is really a syncytium with hundreds of nuclei along its length.

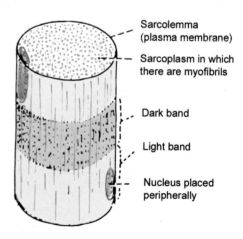

- Sarcolemma (plasma membrane)
- Sarcoplasm in which there are myofibrils
- Dark band
- Light band
- Nucleus placed peripherally

Fig. 9.1. Scheme to show the structure of a muscle fibre.

(The 'fibre' is formed, during development, by fusion of numerous myoblasts). The nuclei are elongated and lie along the periphery of the fibre, just under the cell membrane (which is called the **sarcolemma**). The cytoplasm (or **sarcoplasm**) is filled with numerous longitudinal fibrils that are called **myofibrils.**

The most striking feature of skeletal muscle fibres is the presence of transverse striations in them. After staining with haematoxylin the striations are seen as alternate dark and light bands that stretch across the muscle fibre. The dark bands are called **A-bands**, while the light bands are called **I-bands**. (As an aid to memory note that 'A' and 'I' correspond to the second letters in the words d**a**rk and l**i**ght.

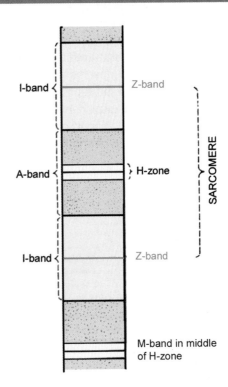

Fig. 9.4. Scheme to show the terminology of transverse bands in a myofibril. Note that the A-band is confined to one sarcomere, but the I-band is made up of parts of two sarcomeres that meet at the Z-band.

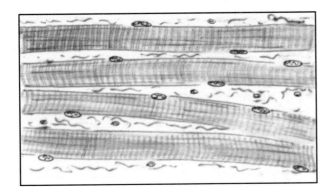

Fig. 9.2. Skeletal muscle seen in longitudinal section.

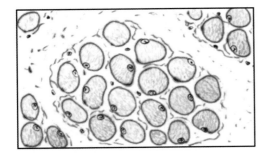

Fig. 9.3. Skeletal muscle seen in transverse section.

Running across the middle of each I-band there is a thin dark line called the **Z-band**. The centre of the A-band is traversed by a lighter band called the **H-band** (or **H-zone**). Running through the centre of the H-band a thin dark line can be made out. This is the **M-band.** The various bands described are really present in myofibrils. They appear to run transversely across the whole muscle fibre because corresponding bands in adjoining myofibrils lie exactly opposite one another.

The part of a myofibril situated between two consecutive Z-bands is called a **sarcomere**. The significance of the striations of myofibrils has to be understood in terms of their ultrastructure which is described later in this chapter.

In addition to myofibrils the sarcoplasm of a muscle fibre contains the usual cell organelles which tend to aggregate near the nuclei. Mitochondria are numerous. Substantial amounts of glycogen are also present. Glycogen provides energy for contraction of muscle.

Organisation of Muscle Fibres in Muscles

Within a muscle, the muscle fibres are arranged in the form of bundles or fasciculi. The number of fasciculi in a muscle, and the number of fibres in each fasciculus, are both highly variable. In small muscles concerned with fine movements (like those of the eyeball, or those of the vocal folds) the fasciculi are delicate and their number small. In large muscles (in which strength of contraction is the main consideration) fasciculi are coarse and numerous.

Muscles differ in the way their fasciculi are arranged. Some muscles (e.g., the sartorius) are strap-like, the fasciculi running the whole length of the muscle. Other muscles are fusiform, the fasciculi being attached at one or both ends to tendons. In still other muscles, the fasciculi are much shorter than the total length of the muscle, and gain attachment to tendinous intersections within the muscle. Some variations in fascicular architecture are illustrated in Figs. 9.5 A to F.

Variations in the fascicular architecture are to be correlated with the kind of movements performed by a muscle. A muscle fibre can shorten to about two-thirds of its full length. The total displacement that a muscle can produce is, therefore, proportional to the length of its fibres. In contrast the strength of contraction of

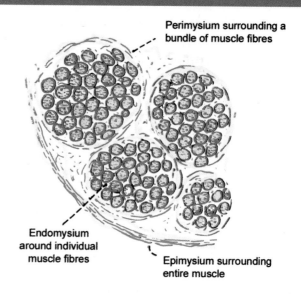

Fig. 9.6. Diagram to show the connective tissue present in skeletal muscle.

a muscle depends on the number of fibres in a muscle (irrespective of their length). In some muscles a large number of short fasciculi are packed into a relatively small total volume (e.g., in a multipennate muscle like the deltoid: Fig. 9.5F). Such a muscle can exert much greater force than a long strap muscle having the same total volume.

Connective Tissue Framework of Muscles

Muscles are pervaded by a network of connective tissue fibres that support muscle fibres and unite them to each other. Individual muscle fibres are surrounded by delicate connective tissue that is called the **endomysium**. Individual fasciculi are surrounded by a stronger sheath of connective tissue called the **perimysium**. Connective tissue that surrounds the entire muscle is called the **epimysium**. At the junction of a muscle with a tendon the fibres of the endomysium, the perimysium and the epimysium become continuous with the fibres of the tendon.

Innervation of Skeletal Muscle

The nerve supplying a muscle enters it (along with the main blood vessels) at an area called the **neurovascular hilus**. This hilus is usually situated nearer the origin of the muscle than the insertion. After entering the muscle the nerve breaks up into many branches that run through the connective tissue of the perimysium and endomysium to reach each muscle fibre. The nerve fibres supplying skeletal muscle are axons arising from large neurons in the anterior (or ventral) grey columns of the spinal cord (or of corresponding nuclei in the brain stem). These **alpha-efferents** have a large diameter and are myelinated.

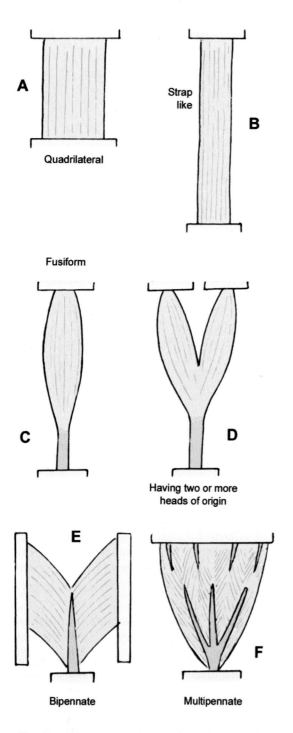

Fig. 9.5. Scheme to show some ways in which the fasciculi of a skeletal muscle may be arranged.

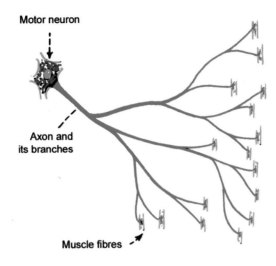

Fig. 9.7. Scheme to illustrate the concept of a motor unit.

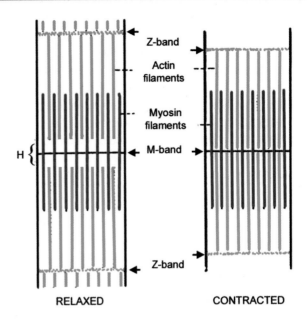

Fig. 9.8. Scheme to show how a myofibril shortens by sliding of actin filaments into the intervals between the myosin filaments. Note that the width of the I-band becomes less, and that the H-zone disappears when the myofibril contracts.

Because of repeated branching of its axon, one anterior grey column neuron may supply many muscle fibres all of which contract when this neuron 'fires'. One anterior grey column neuron and the muscle fibres supplied by it constitute one ***motor unit***. The number of muscle fibres in one motor unit is variable. The units are smaller where precise control of muscular action is required (as in ocular muscles), and much larger in limb muscles where force of contraction is more important. The strength with which a muscle contracts at a particular moment depends on the number of motor units that are activated.

The junction between a muscle fibre and the nerve terminal that supplies it is highly specialized and is called a ***motor end plate***. The structure of a motor end plate is described in Chapter 10.

Apart from the alpha efferents described above every muscle receives smaller myelinated ***gamma-efferents*** that arise from gamma neurons in the ventral grey column of the spinal cord. These fibres supply special muscle fibres that are present within sensory receptors called ***muscle spindles*** (see Chapter 10). These special muscle fibres are called ***intrafusal fibres***. Nerves to muscles also carry autonomic fibres that supply smooth muscle present in the walls of blood vessels.

Ultrastructure of Striated Muscle

Each muscle fibre is covered by a plasma membrane that is called the ***sarcolemma***. The sarcolemma is covered on the outside by a ***basement membrane*** (also called the ***external lamina***) which establishes an intimate connection between the muscle fibre and the fibres (collagen, reticular) of the endomysium.

The cytoplasm (***sarcoplasm***) is permeated with myofibrils which push the elongated nuclei to a peripheral position. Between the myofibrils there is an elaborate system of membrane lined tubes called the ***sarcoplasmic reticulum***. Elongated mitochondria (***sarcosomes***) and clusters of glycogen are also scattered amongst the myofibrils. Perinuclear Golgi bodies, ribosomes, lysosomes, and lipid vacuoles are also present.

Structure of Myofibrils

When examined by EM each myofibril is seen to be made of fine myofilaments. These are of two types: ***actin*** and ***myosin***, made up of molecules of corresponding proteins. (Each myosin filament is about 12 nm in diameter, while an actin filament is about 8 nm in diameter. They are therefore referred to as thick and thin filaments respectively). The arrangement of actin and myosin filaments within a sarcomere is shown in Fig. 9.8. It will be seen that myosin filaments are confined to the A-band, the width of the band being equal to the length of the myosin filaments. The actin filaments are attached at one end to the Z-band. From here they pass through the I-band and extend into the 'outer' parts of the A-band, where they interdigitate with the myosin filaments. Note that the I-band is made up of actin filaments alone. The H-band represents the part of the A-band into which actin filaments do not extend. The Z-band is really a complicated network at which the actin filaments of adjoining sarcomeres meet. The M-band is produced by fine interconnections between adjacent myosin filaments.

In an uncontracted myofibril, overlap between actin and myosin filaments is minimal. During contraction the fibril shortens by sliding in of actin filaments more and more into the intervals between the myosin filaments. As a result the width of the I-band decreases, but that of the A-band is unchanged. The H-bands are obliterated in a contracted fibril.

Sarcoplasmic Reticulum

In the intervals between myofibrils, the sarcoplasm contains an elaborate system of tubules called the sarcoplasmic reticulum (Fig. 9.9). The larger elements of this reticulum run in planes at right angles to the long axes of the myofibrils, and form rings around each myofibril. At the level of every junction between an A and I band the myofibril is encircled by a set of three closely connected tubules which constitute a *muscle triad*. For purposes of description each such triad can be said to be composed of an upper, a middle, and a lower tubule (Fig. 9.9). The upper and lower tubules of the triad are connected to the tubules of adjoining triads through a network of smaller tubules. There is one such network opposite each A-band, and another opposite each I-band. These networks, along with the upper and lower tubules of the triad, constitute the sarcoplasmic reticulum. This reticulum is a closed system of tubes.

The middle tube of the triad is an entity independent of the sarcoplasmic reticulum. It is called a *centrotubule* and belongs to what is called the *T-system* of membranes. The centrotubules are really formed by invagination of the sarcolemma into the sarcoplasm. Their lumina are, therefore, in communication with the exterior of the muscle fibre. As already noted the centrotubules permeate the entire muscle fibre as they form networks around myofibrils as part of the muscle triads.

Contraction of muscle is dependent on release of calcium ions into myofibrils. In a relaxed muscle these ions are strongly bound to the membranes of the sarcoplasmic reticulum. When a nerve stimulus reaches a motor end plate the sarcolemma is depolarized. The wave of depolarization is transmitted to the interior of the muscle fibre through the centrotubules. As a result of this wave calcium ions are released from the sarcoplasmic reticulum into the myofibrils causing their contraction.

Red (or Slow Twitch) & White (or Fast Twitch) Muscle

It has been known since long that some skeletal muscle fibres are reddish in colour while others are whitish. As compared to white fibres the contraction of red fibres is relatively slow. Hence red fibres are also called *slow twitch fibres*, or *type I fibres*; while white fibres are also called *fast twitch fibres* or *type II fibres*.

The colour of red fibres is due to the presence (in the sarcoplasm) of a pigment called *myoglobin*. This pigment is similar (but not identical with) haemoglobin. It is present also in white fibres, but in much lesser quantity.

In addition to colour and speed of contraction there are several other differences between red and white fibres. In comparison to white fibres red fibres differ as follows.

Red fibres are narrower than white fibres. Relative to the volume of the myofibrils the sarcoplasm is more abundant. Probably because of this fact the myofibrils, and striations, are less well defined; and the nuclei are not always at the periphery, but may extend deeper into the fibre. Mitochondria are more numerous in red fibres, but the sarcoplasmic reticulum is less extensive. The sarcoplasm

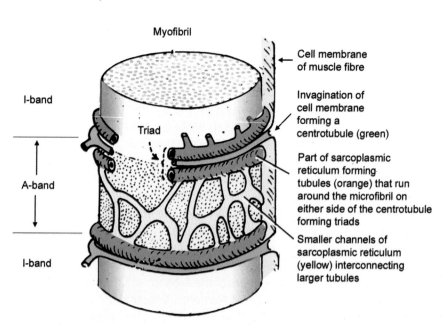

Myofibril

Cell membrane of muscle fibre

Invagination of cell membrane forming a centrotubule (green)

Part of sarcoplasmic reticulum forming tubules (orange) that run around the microfibril on either side of the centrotubule forming triads

Smaller channels of sarcoplasmic reticulum (yellow) interconnecting larger tubules

I-band

Triad

A-band

I-band

Fig. 9.9. Diagram to show relationship of the sarcoplasmic reticulum, an the T-tubes to a myofibril.

contains more glycogen. The capillary bed around red fibres is richer than around white fibres. Differences have also been described in enzyme systems and the respiratory mechanisms in the two types of fibres. Fibres intermediate between red and white fibres have also been described.

In some animals complete muscles may consist exclusively of red or white fibres, but in most mammals, including man, muscles contain an admixture of both types. Although red fibres contract slowly their contraction is more sustained, and they fatigue less easily. They predominate in the so called postural muscles (which have to remain contracted over long periods), while white fibres predominate in muscles responsible for sharp active movements.

Blood Vessels and Lymphatics of Skeletal Muscle

Skeletal muscle is richly supplied with blood vessels. The arteries form a plexus in the epimysium and in the perimysium, and end in a network of capillaries that surrounds each muscle fibre. This network is richer in red muscle than in white muscle.

Veins leaving the muscle accompany the arteries. A lymphatic plexus extends into the epimysium and the perimysium, but not into the endomysium.

CARDIAC MUSCLE

The structure of cardiac muscle has many similarities to that of skeletal muscle; but there are important differences as well.

Similarities between Cardiac & Skeletal Muscle

These are as follows. Like skeletal muscle, cardiac muscle is made up of elongated 'fibres' within which there are numerous myofibrils. The myofibrils (and, therefore, the fibres) show transverse striations similar to those of skeletal muscle. A, I, Z and H bands can be made out in the striations. The connective tissue framework, and the capillary network around cardiac muscle fibres are similar to those in skeletal muscle.

With the EM it is seen that myofibrils of cardiac muscle have the same structure as those of skeletal muscle and are made up of actin and myosin filaments. A sarcoplasmic reticulum, T-system of centrotubules, numerous mitochondria and other organelles are present.

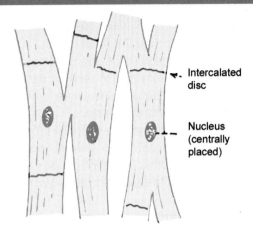

Fig. 9.10. Cardiac muscle (diagrammatic).

Intercalated disc

Nucleus (centrally placed)

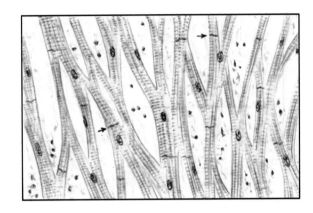

Fig. 9.11. Cardiac muscle as seen in a section.

Differences between Cardiac & Skeletal Muscle

These are as follows.

1. The fibres of cardiac muscle do not run in strict parallel formation, but branch and anastomose with other fibres to form a network.

2. Each fibre of cardiac muscle is not a multinucleated syncytium as in skeletal muscle, but is a chain of cardiac muscle cells (or **cardiac myocytes**) each having its own nucleus. Each myocyte is about 80 μm long and about 15 μm broad.

3. The nucleus of each myocyte is located centrally (and not peripherally as in skeletal muscle).

4. The sarcoplasm of cardiac myocytes is abundant and contains numerous large mitochondria. The myofibrils are relatively few. At places, the myofibrils merge with each other. As a result of these factors, the myofibrils and striations of cardiac muscle are not as distinct as those of skeletal muscle. In this respect cardiac muscle is closer to the red variety of skeletal muscle than to the white variety. Other similarities with red muscle are the presence of significant amounts of

glycogen and of myoglobin, and the rich density of the capillary network around the fibres.

5. With the light microscope the junctions between adjoining cardiac myocytes are seen as dark staining transverse lines running across the muscle fibre. These lines are called ***intercalated discs***.

6. Cardiac muscle is involuntary and is innervated by autonomic fibres (in contrast to skeletal muscle that is innervated by cerebrospinal nerves). Nerve endings terminate near the cardiac myocytes, but motor end plates are not seen.

Isolated cardiac myocytes contract spontaneously in a rhythmic manner. In the intact heart the rhythm of contraction is determined by a pace maker located in the sinuatrial node. From here the impulse spreads to the entire heart through a conducting system made up of a special kind of cardiac muscle. From the above it will be appreciated that a nerve supply is not necessary for contraction of cardiac muscle. Nervous influences do, however, influence the strength and rate of contraction of the heart.

SMOOTH MUSCLE

Basic Facts About Smooth Muscle

Smooth muscle (also called ***non-striated, involuntary*** or ***plain muscle***) is made up of long spindle shaped cells (myocytes) having a broad central part and tapering ends. The nucleus, which is oval or elongated, lies in the central part of the cell. The length

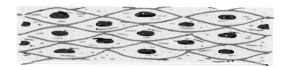

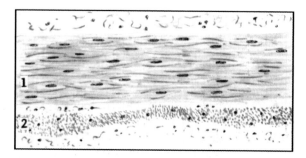

Fig. 9.12. Smooth muscle cells (diagrammatic).

Fig. 9.13. Smooth muscle as seen in section. 1 – L.S. 2 – T.S.

of smooth muscle cells (often called fibres) is highly variable (15 μm to 500 μm).

With the light microscope the sarcoplasm appears to have indistinct longitudinal striations, but there are no transverse striations.

Smooth muscle cells are usually aggregated to form bundles, or fasciculi, that are further aggregated to form layers of variable thickness. In such a layer the cells are so arranged that the thick central part of one cell is opposite the thin tapering ends of adjoining cells. Aggregations of smooth muscle cells into fasciculi and layers is facilitated by the fact that each myocyte is surrounded by a network of delicate fibres (collagen, reticular, elastic) that holds the myocytes together. The fibres between individual myocytes become continuous with the more abundant connective tissue that separates fasciculi or layers of smooth muscle.

Distribution of Smooth Muscle

(a) Smooth muscle is seen most typically in the walls of hollow viscera including the stomach, the intestines, the urinary bladder and the uterus.

(b) It is present in the walls of several structures that are in the form of narrow tubes e.g., arteries, veins, bronchi, ureters, deferent ducts, uterine tubes, and the ducts of several glands.

(c) The muscles that constrict and dilate the pupil are made up of smooth muscle.

(d) Some smooth muscle is present in the orbit (orbitalis); in the upper eyelid (Muller's muscle); in the prostate; in the skin of the scrotum (Dartos muscle). In the skin delicate bundles of smooth muscle are present in relation to hair follicles. These bundles are called the *arrector pili* muscles.

Variations in Arrangement of Smooth Muscle

Smooth muscle fibres may be arranged in a variety of ways depending on functional requirements.

(a) In some organs (e.g., the gut) smooth muscle is arranged in the form of two distinct layers: an inner circular and an outer longitudinal. Within each layer the fasciculi lie parallel to each other. Such an arrangement allows peristaltic movements to take place for propulsion of contents along the tube.

In some organs (e.g., the ureter) the arrangement of layers may be reversed, the longitudinal layer being internal to the circular one. In yet other situations there may be three layers: inner and outer longitudinal with a circular layer in between.

(b) In some regions (e.g., urinary bladder, uterus) the smooth muscle is arranged in layers, but the layers are not distinctly demarcated from each other. Even within layers the fasciculi tend to run in various directions and may form a network. In these organs contraction of muscle reduces the size of the lumen of the organ and pushes out its contents.

(c) In some tubes (e.g., the bile duct) a thick layer of circular muscle may surround a segment of the tube forming a *sphincter*. Contraction of the sphincter occludes the tube.

(d) In the skin, and in some other situations, smooth muscle occurs in the form of narrow bands.

Innervation of Smooth Muscle

Smooth muscle is innervated by autonomic nerves, both sympathetic and parasympathetic. The two have opposite effects. For example, in the iris, parasympathetic stimulation causes constriction of the pupil, and sympathetic stimulation causes dilatation. It may be noted that sympathetic or parasympathetic nerves may cause contraction of muscle at some sites, and relaxation at other sites.

PHYSIOLOGY OF SKELETAL MUSCLE

Muscle is an excitable tissue. The exciting stimulus can be chemical, mechanical or electrical. The muscle responds to the stimulus by contraction. Within the body, a muscle contracts on receiving a nerve impulse.

Electrical phenomena in muscle

A muscle fibre is covered by a cell membrane, the sarcolemma. In the resting fibre the membrane is polarised. Its internal surface (towards sarcoplasm) has a negative charge, while its outer surface (towards extracellular fluid) as a positive charge. The difference in potential on the two sides of the membrane is the resting membrane potential. By convention, it is expressed in terms of the voltage inside the muscle cell, and is about −90 millivolts.

When a stimulus is applied to the muscle, the membrane undergoes polarisation. This means that voltage on the two sides of the membrane becomes equal. This is the action potential. The action potential lasts only for 2-4 ms (milliseconds) at a given site. Depolarisation begins at the motor end plate. It spreads through the sarcolemma like a wave, succeeding segments being depolarised followed by repolarisation. In this way the entire muscle fibre is stimulated to contract.

Ionic basis of resting membrane potential

Positively charged sodium and potassium ions and negatively charged ions are present on both sides of the membrane. However, there are more positively charged ions on the external surface than inside the cell. This is the reason for the resting membrane potential. This potential is kept constant by movement of ions as described below.

Ions can move across a cell membrane, by passive transport, in two ways. When the concentration of ions is greater on one side of the membrane than on the other, this concentration gradient tends to move ions from region of higher concentration to lower. Similarly an electric gradient can move positive ions towards the side having a lower potential, and negative ions towards the side of higher potential. These two forces may act in the same direction or in opposing directions. In the first instance the two reinforce one another, and in the second instance the two forces oppose one another.

Chloride ions (Cl⁻)are present in higher concentration outside the cell, than inside it. Hence the concentration gradient tends to move chloride ions into the cell (Fig. 9.14). On the other hand the electric gradient tends to move negatively charged Cl⁻ ions out of the cell and equilibrium is reached when the two forces are equal. In the case of potassium (K^+) ions, the concentration gradient pushes the ions out of the cell, but the electric gradient tends to move K^+ ions into the cell. In the case of sodium (Na^+) both the concentration gradient and the electric gradient tend to move ions inwards. Such passive movement of ions would have the effect of changing the resting membrane potential. However, this is not allowed to happen. Sodium ions are moved

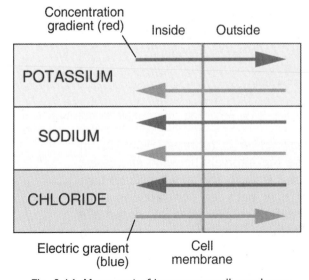

Fig. 9.14. Movement of ions across cell membrane.

out of the cell by active transport (using Na$^+$-K$^+$ATPase).

CONTRACTION OF MUSCLE

Some features of muscle contraction can be studied experimentally using isolated muscle and its nerve.

Muscle twitch

(1) When the nerve supplying a muscle is stimulated using a single brief electric current the muscle contracts once and then relaxes. This is called a muscle twitch (Fig. 9.15).

(2) If a second stimulus is given before relaxation sets in, a second contraction gets added to the first one, resulting in a higher curve. The adding together of two or more contractions is called **summation of contractions**.

Two types of summation are recognized. When the two stimuli produce a single curve that is higher than that produced by a single stimulus, it is called **quantal summation** (Fig. 9.16). When the stimuli produce two curves that overlap it is called **wave summation** (Fig. 9.17).

(3) If repeated stimuli are given, the muscle shows a prolonged response. This is called a **tetanic**

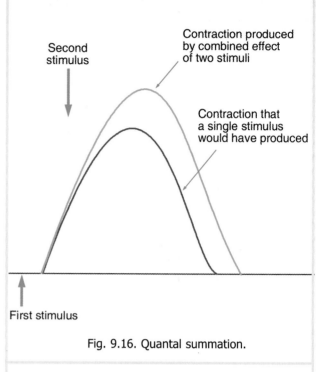

Fig. 9.16. Quantal summation.

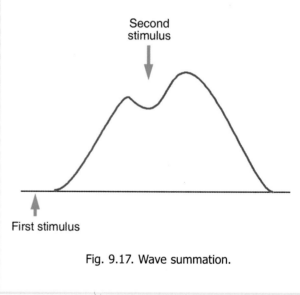

Fig. 9.17. Wave summation.

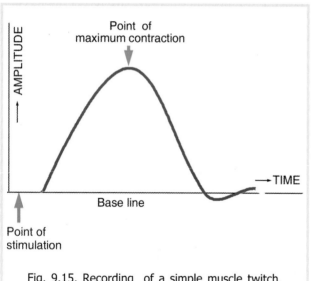

Fig. 9.15. Recording of a simple muscle twitch.

contraction (or **tetanus**) (Fig. 9.18). In case the intervals between successive stimuli is short, the muscle gets no time to relax between contractions. This condition is described as **complete tetanus**. When the interval between stimuli is slightly more prolonged, the muscle may undergo partial relaxation between stimuli. This is **incomplete tetanus**.

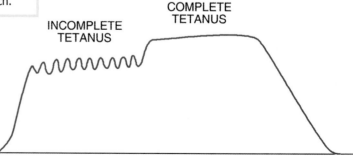

Fig. 9.18. Complete and incomplete tetanus.

(4) There is a limit to the number of times a muscle can keep contracting in response to stimuli. After the first few contractions, the force of each contraction gradually decreases. Finally the muscle stops responding. This is called *fatigue*. Fatigue is caused by exhaustion of acetyl choline in the motor end plate, lack of oxygen and nutrients, and accumulation of lactic acid.

(5) If one end of a muscle is fixed, and the other end is free to move, contraction leads to shortening. Because of shortening, tension on the muscle fibres remains more or less constant. This kind of contraction is called *isotonic contraction*.

(6) If both ends of a muscle are fixed, and such a muscle is made to contract, tension develops within the muscle, but there is no shortening. This kind of contraction is called *isometric contraction*.

(7) Using a suitable machine a muscle can be made to contract in such a way that speed of movement remains constant through the full range of contraction. This is called *isokinetic contraction*.

From paragraphs 4 to 6 note that muscle exercise can be isotonic, isometric or isokinetic.

All or none law

When a single muscle fibre is subjected to stimuli of increasing intensity we observe the following.

1. A specific strength of stimulus is necessary for contraction of the muscle fibre. This is the *threshold intensity* of stimulus required. Stimuli of lesser intensity cannot produce any response.

2. Any stimulus above the threshold intensity produces a maximal response. Increasing strength of stimulus beyond the threshold does not increase strength of contraction. In other words if a stimulus is strong enough to produce a response the fibre contracts with its full strength. This is called the *all or none law*. However, note that this law applies only a single muscle fibre, and not to the muscle as a whole. The strength of contraction of a muscle depends on the total number of fibres that contract at a given time.

Effect of temperature

The strength of muscle contraction is increased by moderate increase in temperature (to about 40ºC). The increase is due to increased excitability of muscle, to accleration of chemical processes, and reduced viscosity of muscle. Cooling the muscle (to about 10ºC) has the opposite effect. Exposure to very high temperatures (60ºC) leads to coagulation of muscle proteins, which in turn leads to stiffness and shortening of the muscle. This is called *rigor*.

CHEMICAL PROCESSES INVOLVED IN MUSCLE CONTRACTION

Muscle contraction requires a large amount of energy, in the form of ATP (adenosine triphosphate). The structure of ATP is explained in Fig. 9.19. The storage and release of energy from ATP is shown in Fig. 9.20.

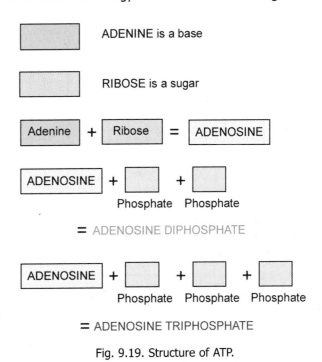

Fig. 9.19. Structure of ATP.

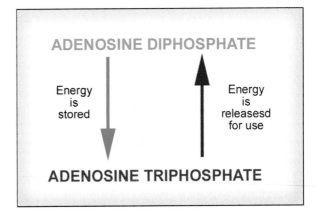

Fig. 9.20. Role of ATP in metabolism.

Muscle fibres store large quantities of glycogen. Glycogen is readily converted to glucose. ATP is obtained by metabolism of glucose as shown in Fig. 9.21. The process is efficient when oxygen is available in adequate quantity. Utilization of glucose in the presence of oxygen is called aerobic catabolism. Some utilization of glucose can also take place in the absence of oxygen (anaerobic catabolism) but this process is not efficient. The steps involved in utilization of glucose are summarised below.

A large quantity of energy is locked up in one molecule of glucose. However, a series of chemical reactions are required to release this energy, which is then stored in the form of ATP

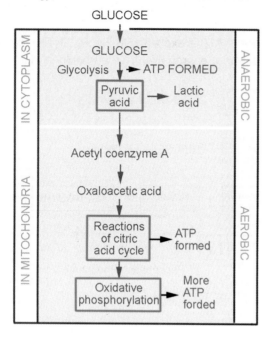

Fig. 9.21. Deriving energy from glucose.

Remember that energy released is stored in the form of ATP.

Glycolysis

Step 1. Glucose (from the circulation) enters the cytoplasm of a cell. Each molecule of glucose forms two molecules of pyruvic acid. Energy is released in the form of two molecules of ATP. Glucolysis is an anaerobic process (Fig. 9.21).

Step 2. The two molecules of pyruvic acid enter mitochondria and undergo a series of reactions that are known as the citric acid cycle or Krebs' cycle. In this process two more molecules of ATP are generated. Oxygen is required for this reaction.

Step 3. Some substances produced in the citric acid cycle undergo oxidative phosphorylation to produce several more molecules of ATP. This takes place within mitochrondria and requires adequate supply of oxygen.

Step 4. When adequate supply of oxygen is not available (e.g., during heavy exercise) the two molecules of pyruvic acid formed by glycolysis (see step 1 above) remain in the cytoplasm and are converted to lactic acid. Accumulation of lactic acid in muscles, leads to pain and cramps (that athletes often complain of). Later when adequate blood supply (oxygen supply) is restored accumulated lactic acid is removed as follows.

Some of it is reconverted into pyruvic acid. Pyruvic acid is oxidized to form CO_2 and water. CO_2 enters blood and is removed through the lungs. Water (if in excess) is removed from the body through urine.

Muscle contains the compound phosphorylcreatine. This compound can be hydrolyzed to creatine and phosphate. This reaction releases considerable energy which can be stored as ATP. This is an alternative source of energy available in muscle. A third source of energy are free fatty acids present in blood. They are oxidised to CO_2 and H_2O releasing energy in the form of ATP.

Oxygen debt

When a muscle is at rest the oxygen used by it is the **basal consumption**.

During exertion the oxygen consumption becomes much higher, as oxygen is needed for aerobic metabolism of glucose using the pathway shown in Fig. 9.21. As intensity of exercise increases, oxygen supply falls short of demand. When this happens the muscle uses anaerobic pathways for production of ATP. These are

1. Anaerobic conversion of glucose to pyruvate, and of pyruvate to lactic acid.

2. Hydrolysis of phosphorylcreatine.

The availability of these anaerobic pathways enables muscle contraction to continue for a longer period. When activity of muscle has ceased, for some time the muscle continues to use a higher quantity of oxygen than in the resting state. This oxygen is needed for:

a). Replenishing exhausted stores of ATP.

b). Replenishing exhausted stores of phosphorylcreatine.

c). Reconverting some accumulated lactate to pyruvate.

d). Removal of excessive lactate.

The extra oxygen used to bring the muscle back to the state that existed before beginning of exercise is called the **oxygen debt**.

Strength, power and endurance of muscle

The term **strength** is applied to the maximum force that can be generated by a muscle. It is about 3 to 4 kg per square centimeter of cross sectional area of the muscle. Hence the thicker the muscle, the more its strength. The force generated by shortening of the muscle is called **contractile strength**. The force required to stretch a contracted muscle is called **holding strength**.

Power is a measure of work done by a muscle (expressed in kg per minute). Power depends on strength, its force of contraction and frequency of contraction.

The capacity of a muscle to maintain activity over a period of time is called *endurance*. This depends mainly on availability of glycogen in the muscle. It is increased by training in athletes, and by a high carbohydrate diet.

GENERAL AND CARDIORESPIRATORY ENDURANCE

Endurance of muscular activity is only possible by adequate supply of blood and oxygen.

The factors that increase blood supply are as follows.

1. *Increase in heart rate*: This is produced by increased sympathetic tone and reduced vagal tone. Factors affecting these include proprioceptive impulses from muscle, increased carbon oxide tension, raised body temperature, and increased secretion of catecholamines.

2. *Increase in cardiac output*: This is produced by increased heart rate and increased stroke volume.

3. *Increased venous return*: This is a result of the pumping action of muscle, greater activity of respiratory pump and reduced blood supply to viscera.

4. *Increased blood pressure*: In isotonic exercise systolic blood pressure rises, but the diastolic pressure remains normal, or less than normal. Diastolic pressure increases in isometric exercise.

The factors that increase oxygen supply to muscle are as follows.

1. *Increased pulmonary ventilation*: This is a result of increase in rate and depth of respiration. These are produced through stimulation of the respiratory centre, by stimulation of chemoreceptors by hypoxia, by increase of body temperature, and by acidosis.

2. *Increased blood flow* through pulmonary capillaries increases diffusion capacity for oxygen.

3. *Increased consumption of oxygen*. The oxygen consumed by tissues, specially by muscle, greatly increases during exercise. This is possible because of increased availability of oxygen through blood.

4. See oxygen debt (page 60) and respiratory quotient (page 103).

Comparison of aerobic and anaerobic work

1. Aerobic work (or exercise) can be done over a long period of time (e.g., walking a long distance). Anaerobic work can be done for a limited time only, as exhaustion sets in fast (e.g., after running at high speed).

2. A healthy person may not experience fatigue after aerobic work. In contrast a period of rest is essential after anaerobic work.

3. Greater speeds can be attained only with anaerobic work, but they cannot be maintained for long.

4. Anaerobic utilization of glycogen stores (in muscle) takes place at the beginning of exercise. All the glycogen available in muscle is consumed within a few minutes. After this the source of energy is glucose obtained through blood (from glycogen stored in the liver). This is also used up in about 20 minutes. After this, fat stored in the body is used as a source of energy.

It follows that if a person wants to lose fat, the exercise must last beyond 20 minutes. This is possible only if the exercise is aerobic. In contrast anaerobic exercise calls for a diet rich in carbohydrate, so that adequate stores of glycogen are available in muscle.

The various factors described above become more efficient with training and are responsible for development of endurance in trained athletes.

EFFECTS OF AGEING ON ACTIVITY

Muscle mass and strength increase as a child grows, reaching a maximum at about the age of 20 years. A person's physical efficiency is at its peak between 20-30 years of age. In most persons physical and muscle strength gradually declines after the age of 50. Endurance is reduced and fatigue sets in faster.

Decrease in activity with age is to be correlated with reduced efficiency of the cardiovascular and respiratory systems. Narrowing of arteries, due to atherosclerosis begins as early as the age of 20 and pregressively increases thereafter. This progressively reduces blood and oxygen supply to all parts of the body. Narrowing of arteries leads to increased peripheral resistance, with reduced arterial compliance. Increased resistance leads to elevation of systolic blood pressure and ultimately to some degree of left ventricular hypertrophy. The cardiac output falls and the body is less able to adjust to a rise in heart rate, to dehydration, or to postural changes.

The respiratory system becomes less efficient as lung elasticity decreases, and chest wall stiffness increases.

Changes also take place in the nervous system. Atrophy of brain tissue has been observed. Reflexes become slower. The gait becomes stiff. Orientation of time and space many be impaired. Impairment of vision and hearing are contributory causes. However, many old persons remain mentally sharp till a late age.

10

Nervous Tissue

The nervous system is made up, predominantly, of tissue that has the special property of being able to conduct impulses rapidly from one part of the body to another. The specialized cells that constitute the functional units of the nervous system are called **neurons**. Within the brain and spinal cord neurons are supported by a special kind of connective tissue that is called **neuroglia.** Nervous tissue, composed of neurons and neuroglia, is richly supplied with blood.

The nervous system of man is made up of innumerable neurons. The neurons are linked together in a highly intricate manner. It is through these connections that the body is made aware of changes in the environment, or of those within itself; and appropriate responses to such changes are produced e.g., in the form of movement or in the modified working of some organ of the body. There is no doubt that higher functions of the brain, like those of memory and intelligence, are also to be explained on the basis of connections between neurons, but as yet little is known about the mechanisms involved. Neurons are, therefore, to be regarded not merely as simple conductors, but as cells that are specialized for the reception, integration, interpretation and transmission of information.

NEURON STRUCTURE

Elementary Structure of a Typical Neuron

Neurons vary considerably in size, shape and other features. However, most of them have some major features in common and these are described below (Figs. 10.1 to 10.16).

A neuron consists of a **cell body** which gives off a variable number of **processes** (Fig. 10.1). Like a typical cell it consists of a mass of cytoplasm surrounded by a cell membrane. The cytoplasm contains a large central nucleus (usually with a prominent nucleolus), numerous mitochondria, lysosomes and a Golgi complex (Fig. 10.2). In addition to these features, the cytoplasm of a neuron has some distinctive characteristics not seen

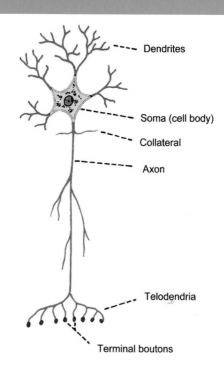

Fig. 10.1. Scheme to show some parts of a neuron.

in other cells. The cytoplasm shows the presence of a granular material that stains intensely with basic dyes; this material is the **Nissl substance** (Fig. 10.3). When examined by EM, these bodies are seen to be composed of rough surfaced endoplasmic reticulum (Fig. 10.2). The presence of abundant granular endoplasmic reticulum is an indication of the high level of protein synthesis in neurons. The proteins are needed for maintenance and repair, and for production of neurotransmitters and enzymes.

Another distinctive feature of neurons is the presence of a network of fibrils permeating the cytoplasm (Fig. 10.5). These **neurofibrils** are seen, with the EM, to consist of microfilaments and microtubules. Some neurons contain pigment granules.

The processes arising from the cell body of a neuron are called **neurites.** These are of two kinds. Most neurons give off a number of short branching processes called **dendrites** and one longer process called an **axon.**

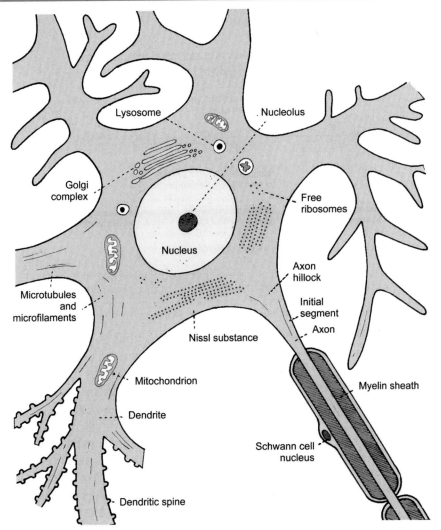

Fig. 10.2. Schematic presentation of some features of the structure of a neuron as seen by EM.

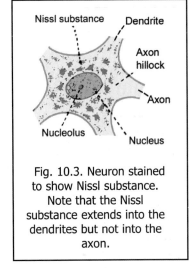

Fig. 10.3. Neuron stained to show Nissl substance. Note that the Nissl substance extends into the dendrites but not into the axon.

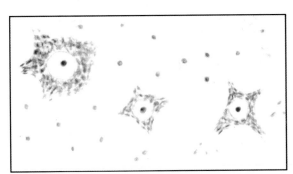

Fig. 10.4. Section of spinal cord showing large neurons in the ventral grey column.

The dendrites are characterized by the fact that they terminate near the cell body. They are irregular in thickness, and Nissl granules extend into them. They bear numerous small spines which are of variable shape.

The axon may extend for a considerable distance away from the cell body. The longest axons may be as much as a metre long. Each axon has a uniform diameter, and is devoid of Nissl substance.

In addition to these differences in structure, there is a fundamental functional difference between dendrites and axons. In a dendrite, the nerve impulse travels **towards the cell body** whereas in an axon the impulse travels **away from the cell body.**

We have seen above that the axon is free of Nissl granules. The Nissl-free zone extends for a short distance into the cell body: this part of the cell body is called the **axon hillock.** The part of the axon just beyond the axon hillock is called the **initial segment** (Fig. 10.2).

Some axons are surrounded by a **myelin sheath**. In peripheral nerves, the myelin sheath is formed by **Schwann cells**. A thin layer of Schwann cell cytoplasm persists outside the myelin sheath, to form an additional sheath which is called the **neurilemma** (also called the neurilemmal sheath or Schwann cell sheath). Axons lying within the central nervous system are provided a myelin sheath by a kind of neuroglial cell called an **oligodendrocyte.**

Axons having a myelin sheath are called **myelinated axons**. The presence of a myelin sheath increases the

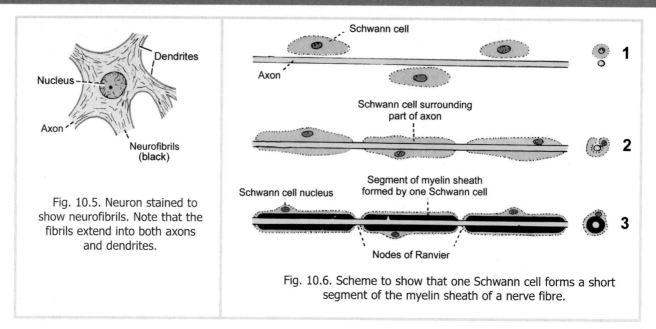

Fig. 10.5. Neuron stained to show neurofibrils. Note that the fibrils extend into both axons and dendrites.

Fig. 10.6. Scheme to show that one Schwann cell forms a short segment of the myelin sheath of a nerve fibre.

velocity of conduction (for a nerve fibre of the same diameter). It also reduces the energy expended in the process of conduction.

An axon is related to a large number of Schwann cells over its length. Each Schwann cell provides the myelin sheath for a short segment of the axon. At the junction of any two such segments there is a short gap in the myelin sheath. These gaps are called the *nodes of Ranvier* (Fig. 10.6).

There are some axons that are devoid of myelin sheaths. These are *unmyelinated axons*.

An axon may give off a variable number of branches (Fig. 10.1). Some branches, that arise near the cell body and lie at right angles to the axon are called *collaterals*. At its termination the axon breaks up into a number of fine branches called *telodendria* which may end in small swellings (*terminal boutons* or *bouton terminaux*).

An axon (or its branches) can terminate in two ways. Within the central nervous system, it always terminates by coming in intimate relationship with another neuron, the junction between the two neurons being called a *synapse*. Outside the central nervous system, the axon may end in relation to an effector organ (e.g., muscle or gland), or may end by synapsing with neurons in a peripheral ganglion.

Axons (and some dendrites that resemble axons in structure: see below) constitute what are commonly called *nerve fibres.*

Variability in Neuron Structure

Neurons vary considerably in the size and shape of their cell bodies (somata) and in the length and manner of branching of their processes. The shape of the cell body is dependent on the number of processes arising from it. The most common type of neuron gives off several processes and the cell body is, therefore, *multipolar* (Fig. 10.7). Some neurons have only one axon and one dendrite and are *bipolar.*

Another type of neuron has a single process. This process divides into two. One of the divisions represents the axon; the other is functionally a dendrite, but its structure is indistinguishable from that of an axon. This neuron is described as *unipolar*, but from a functional point of view it is to be regarded as bipolar. Depending on the shapes of their cell bodies some neurons are referred to as *stellate* (star shaped) or *pyramidal.*

In addition to the variations in size and shape, the cell bodies of neurons may show striking variations in the appearance of the Nissl substance. In some neurons, the Nissl substance is very prominent and is in the form of large clumps. In some others, the granules are fine and uniformly distributed in the cytoplasm, while yet other neurons show gradations between these extremes. These differences are correlated with function.

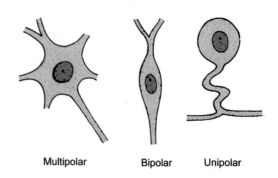

Fig. 10.7. Diagram showing three types of neurons.

SOME PHYSIOLOGICAL PROPERTIES OF NEURONS

In Chapter 9 we have discussed the concepts of membrane potential, depolarisation and repolarisation. The chemical and electrical aspects of these phenomena have been studied. These should be reviewed as they are equally applicable in neurons also. Some differences are given below.

1. The resting membrane potential in a neuron is −70mV.

2. Neurons have a lower threshold for excitation. The neuron 'fires' when depolarisation reaches −55mV.

3. When a neuron is stimulated an action potential is produced. This happens if the strength of the stimulus is adequate (i.e., it is above threshold value). The action potential obeys the all or none law. If the stimulus is adequate to produce a response, a maximal response is obtained, and further increase in strength of stimulation does not increase the response. The action potential is transmitted along the axon as a nerve impulse. As in muscle, the basis for a nerve impulse is the spread of a wave of depolarisation. In unmyelinated axons the impulse travels along the cell membrane, and such conduction is relatively slow. However, in myelinated axons conduction is much faster because depolarisation jumps from one node of Ranvier to the next. This is called saltatory conduction.

The Synapse

We have seen that synapses are sites of junction between neurons. Synapses may be of various types depending upon the parts of the neurons that come in contact. In the most common type of synapse, an axon terminal establishes contact with the dendrite of a receiving neuron to form an *axodendritic synapse.* The axon terminal may synapse with the cell body (*axosomatic synapse*) or, less commonly, with the axon of the receiving neuron (*axoaxonal synapse*).

A synapse transmits an impulse only in one direction. The two elements taking part in a synapse can, therefore, be spoken of as *presynaptic* and *postsynaptic*. In a typical synapse the terminal part of the axon is enlarged. It is called the *presynaptic bouton* (= button). Numerous vesicles are present in the presynaptic bouton. The dendrite terminal taking part in the synapse is called the *postsynaptic process*. The presynaptic bouton and the postsynaptic process are separated by a synaptic cleft (Fig. 10.8).

The transmission of impulses through synapses involves the release of chemical substances called *neurotransmitters* that are present within synaptic vesicles. When a nerve impulse reaches a terminal bouton neurotransmitter is released into the synaptic cleft. Under the influence of the neurotransmitter the postsynaptic surface becomes depolarized resulting in a nerve impulse in the postsynaptic neuron. The neurotransmitter released into the synaptic cleft acts only for a very short duration. It is either destroyed (by enzymes) or is withdrawn into the terminal bouton.

The best known neurotransmitters are acetylcholine, noradrenaline and adrenaline. Nerve fibres that release acetylcholine at their terminals are called cholinergic, and those that release noradrenaline are called adrenergic. Many other neurotransmitters are known.

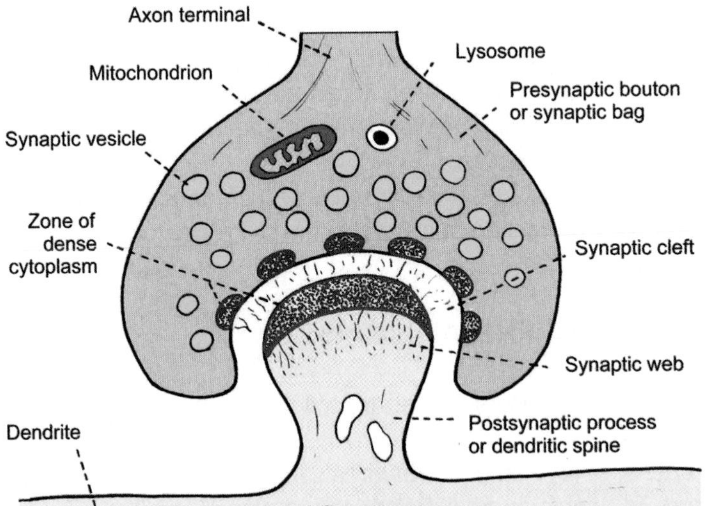

Synaptic transmission

1. When an action potential reaches an axon terminal (presynaptic process) permeability of presynaptic membrane increases allowing calcium ions to enter the axon terminal.

2. Entry of calcium ions triggers release of neurotransmitter (typically acetylcholine). Acetylcholine enters the synaptic cleft.

3. Acetylcholine binds with receptors on the postsynaptic membrane. Presence of acetylcholine-receptor complex increases permeability of postsynaptic neuron to sodium ions. As a result, there is influx of sodium ions. This causes mild depolarisation of postsynaptic membrane. This phenomenon is called ESPS. When ESPS is strong enough it triggers the development of an action potential in the

Fig. 10.8. Scheme showing the structure of a typical synapse as seen by EM.

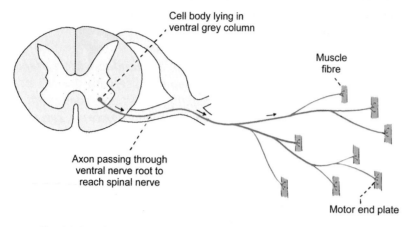

Fig. 10.9. Scheme to show the origin and course of a typical efferent nerve fibre.

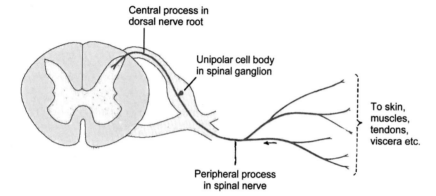

Fig. 10.10. Scheme to show the origin and course of a typical afferent nerve fibre.

postsynaptic neuron. This action potential travels down the axon as a nerve impulse.

Grey and White Matter

Sections through the spinal cord or through any part of the brain show certain regions that appear whitish, and others that have a darker greyish colour. These constitute the **white** and **grey matter** respectively. Microscopic examination shows that the cell bodies of neurons are located only in grey matter which also contains dendrites and axons starting from or ending on the cell bodies. Most of the fibres within the grey matter are unmyelinated. On the other hand the white matter consists predominantly of myelinated fibres. It is the reflection of light by myelin that gives this region its whitish appearance. Neuroglia and blood vessels are present in both grey and white matter.

The arrangement of the grey and white matter differs at different situations in the brain and spinal cord. In the spinal cord and brainstem the white matter is on the outside whereas the grey matter forms one or more masses embedded within the white matter. In the cerebrum and cerebellum there is an extensive, but thin, layer of grey matter on the surface. This layer is called the **cortex.** Deep to the cortex there is white matter, but within the latter several isolated masses of grey matter are present. Such isolated masses of grey matter present anywhere in the central nervous system are referred to as **nuclei.** As grey matter is made of cell bodies of neurons (and the processes arising from or terminating on them) nuclei can be defined as groups of cell bodies of neurons. Aggregations of the cell bodies of neurons may also be found outside the central nervous system. Such aggregations are referred to as **ganglia.** Some neurons are located in **nerve plexuses** present in close relationship to some viscera. These are, therefore, referred to as ganglionated plexuses.

The axons arising in one mass of grey matter very frequently terminate by synapsing with neurons in other masses of grey matter. The axons connecting two (or more) masses of grey matter are frequently numerous enough to form recognisable bundles. Such aggregations of fibres are called **tracts**. Larger collections of fibres are also referred to as **funiculi, fasciculi** or **lemnisci.** (A lemniscus is a ribbon-like band). Large bundles of fibres connecting the cerebral or cerebellar hemispheres to the brainstem are called **peduncles.**

Aggregations of processes of neurons outside the central nervous system constitute **peripheral nerves.**

PERIPHERAL NERVES

Peripheral nerves are collections of nerve fibres. These are of two types.

(a) Some nerve fibres carry impulses from the spinal cord or brain to peripheral structures like muscle or gland: they are called **efferent** or **motor** fibres. Efferent fibres are axons of neurons (the cell bodies of which are) located in the grey matter of the spinal cord or of the brainstem (Fig. 10.9).

(b) Other nerve fibres carry impulses from peripheral organs to the brain or spinal cord: these are called **afferent** fibres (Fig. 10.10). Many (but not all) afferent fibres are concerned in the transmission of sensations like touch or pain. They are, therefore, also called **sensory** fibres.

Afferent nerve fibres are processes of neurons that are located (as a rule) in sensory ganglia. In the case of spinal nerves these ganglia are located on the dorsal nerve roots. In the case of cranial nerves they are located on ganglia situated on the nerve concerned (usually near its attachment to the brain). The neurons in these ganglia are usually of the unipolar type. Each unipolar neuron gives off a peripheral process which passes into the peripheral nerve forming an afferent nerve fibre. It also gives off a central process that enters the brain or spinal cord.

From what has been said above it will be clear that the afferent nerve fibres in peripheral nerves are functionally dendrites. However, their histological structure is the same as that of axons.

Basic Structure of Peripheral Nerve Fibres

Each nerve fibre has a central core formed by the axon. This core is called the **axis cylinder**. The plasma membrane surrounding the axis cylinder is the **axolemma**. The axis cylinder is surrounded by a myelin sheath (Fig. 10.11). This sheath is in the form of short segments that are separated at short intervals called the **nodes of Ranvier** (Fig. 10.6). The part of the nerve fibre between two consecutive nodes is the **internode.** Each segment of the myelin sheath is formed by one Schwann cell. Outside the myelin sheath there is a thin layer of Schwann cell cytoplasm. This layer of cytoplasm is called the **neurilemma.**

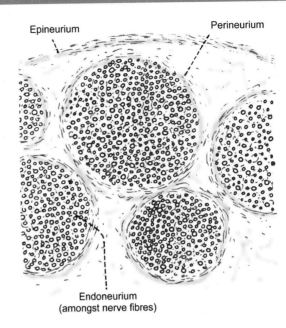

Fig. 10.12. Diagram to show the connective tissue supporting nerve fibres in a peripheral nerve.

Each nerve fibre is surrounded by a layer of connective tissue called the **endoneurium** (Fig.10.12). The endoneurium holds adjoining nerve fibres together and facilitates their aggregation to form bundles or **fasciculi**.

Each fasciculus is surrounded by a thicker layer of connective tissue called the **perineurium**.

A very thin nerve may consist of a single fasciculus, but usually a nerve is made up of several fasciculi. The fasciculi are held together by a fairly dense layer of connective tissue that surrounds the entire nerve and is called the **epineurium.**

DEGENERATION AND REGENERATION OF NEURONS

When the axon of a neuron is cut across a series of degenerative changes are seen in the axon distal to the injury, in the axon proximal to the injury, and in the cell body.

The changes in the part of the axon distal to the injury are referred to as **anterograde degeneration** or **Wallerian degeneration**. They take place in the entire length of this part of the axon. A few hours after injury the axon becomes swollen and irregular in shape, and in a few days it breaks up into small fragments (Fig. 10.13). The neurofibrils within it break down into granules. The myelin sheath breaks up into small segments. It also undergoes chemical changes that enable degenerating myelin to be stained selectively.

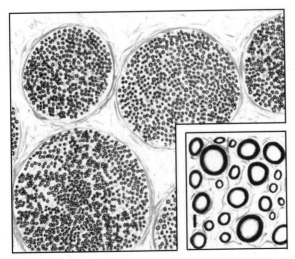

Fig. 10.11. Section through peripheral nerve stained by a method in which the myelin sheaths become black. The inset shows fibres at high magnification.

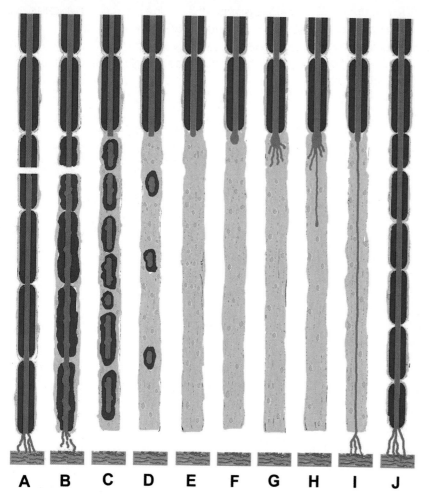

A B C D E F G H I J

Fig. 10.13. Stages in the degeneration of a nerve fibre after injury (A to E) and its subsequent regeneration (F to J). For explanation see text.

If the injury is sharp and clean the effects extend only up to one or two nodes of Ranvier proximal to the injury. If the injury is severe a longer segment of the axon may be affected. The changes in the affected part are exactly the same as described for the distal part of the axon. They are soon followed by active growth at the tip of the surviving part of the axon. This causes the terminal part of the axon to swell up (Fig. 10.13 F). It then gives off a number of fine branches. These branches grow into the connective tissue at the site of injury in an effort to reach the distal cut end of the nerve (Fig. 10.13 G.H). We have seen that the Schwann cells of the distal part of the nerve proliferate to form a series of tubes. When one of the regenerating axonal branches succeeds in reaching such a tube, it enters it and then grows rapidly within it. The tube serves as a guide to the growing fibre. The axon terminal growing through the Schwann cell tube ultimately reaches, and establishes contact with, an appropriate peripheral end organ. The new axon formed in this way is at first very thin and devoid of a myelin sheath (Fig. 10.13 I). However, there is progressive increase in its thickness and a myelin sheath is formed around it. (Fig. 10.13 J).

From the above account it will be clear that chances of regeneration of a cut nerve are considerably increased if the two cut ends are near each other, and if scar tissue does not intervene between them.

The region is invaded by numerous macrophages that remove degenerating axons, myelin and cellular debris. These macrophages probably secrete substances that cause proliferation of Schwann cells. The Schwann cells increase in size and produce a large series of membranes that help to form numerous tubes. We shall see later that these tubes play a vital role in regeneration of nerve fibres.

Degenerative changes in the neuron proximal to the injury are referred to as *retrograde degeneration*. These changes take place in the cell body and in the axon proximal to injury.

The cell body of the injured neuron undergoes a series of changes that constitute the phenomenon of *chromatolysis*. The cell body enlarges tending to become spherical. The nucleus moves from the centre to the periphery. The Nissl substance becomes much less prominent and appears to dissolve away: hence the term chromatolysis.

Changes in the proximal part of the axon are confined to a short segment near the site of injury (Fig. 10.13).

PERIPHERAL NERVE ENDINGS

We have seen that peripheral nerves contain afferent (or sensory) fibres, and efferent (or motor fibres). In relation to the peripheral endings of afferent nerve fibres there are *receptors* that respond to various kinds of stimuli. Most efferent nerve fibres supply muscle, and at the junction of a nerve fibre with muscle we see neuromuscular junctions. In this chapter we will study the structure of various kinds of sensory receptors, and of neuromuscular junctions

SENSORY RECEPTORS

Preliminary remarks about receptors and their classification

The peripheral terminations of afferent fibres are responsible for receiving stimuli and are, therefore, referred to as **receptors.** Receptors can be classified in various ways.

1. From a functional point of view receptors can be classified on the basis of the kind of information they provide. They may be of the following types.

(a) **Cutaneous receptors** are concerned with touch, pain, temperature and pressure. These are also called **exteroceptive receptors** or **exteroceptors** (Fig. 10.14).

(b) **Proprioceptive receptors** (or **proprioceptors**) provide information about the state of contraction of muscles, and of joint movement and position (Fig. 10.15). This information is necessary for precise control of movement and for maintenance of body posture. By and large these activities occur as a result of reflex action and the information from these receptors may or may not be consciously perceived.

(c) **Interoceptive receptors** (or **interoceptors**) are located in thoracic and abdominal viscera and in blood vessels. These include specialized structures like the carotid sinus and the carotid body.

(d) The above three categories also include receptors that are stimulated by damaging influences which are perceived as pain, discomfort or irritation. Such receptors are referred to as **nociceptors.**

(e) **Special sense receptors** of vision, hearing, smell and taste are present in the appropriate organs.

EXTEROCEPTIVE RECEPTORS
Free Nerve Endings

When the terminals of sensory nerves do not show any particular specialization of structure they are called free nerve endings. Such endings are widely distributed in the body. They are found in connective tissue. They are also seen in relation to the epithelial lining of the skin, cornea, alimentary canal, and respiratory system.

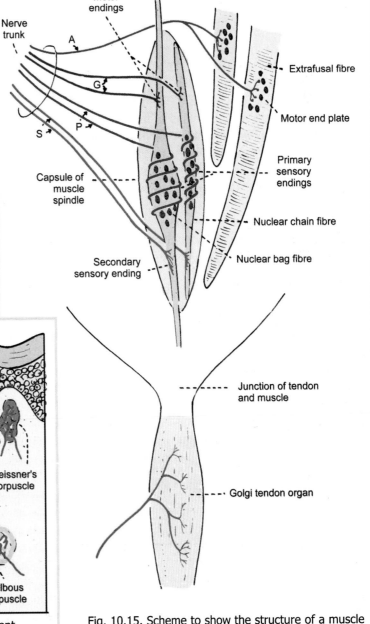

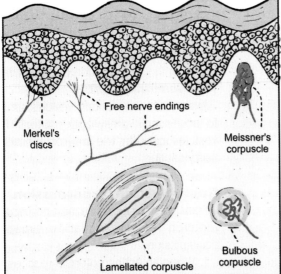

Fig. 10.14. Some sensory receptors present in relation to skin.

Fig. 10.15. Scheme to show the structure of a muscle spindle and of a Golgi tendon organ.

Tactile Corpuscles (of Meissner)

These are small oval or cylindrical structures seen in relation to dermal papillae in the hand and foot, and in some other situations. These corpuscles are believed to be responsible for touch.

Lamellated Corpuscles (of Pacini)

Pacinian corpuscles are circular or oval structures. These are much larger than tactile corpuscles. They may be up to 2 mm in length, and up to 0.5 mm across. They are found in the subcutaneous tissue of the palm and sole, in the digits, and in various other situations. Lamellated corpuscles are sensitive to vibration. They also respond to pressure.

PROPRIOCEPTIVE RECEPTORS

Golgi Tendon Organs

These organs are located at the junction of muscle and tendon. Each organ is about 500 μm long and about 100 μm in diameter. It consists of a capsule made up of concentric sheets of cytoplasm (Fig. 10.15). Inside the capsule there are small bundles of tendon fibres. The organ is innervated by one or more myelinated nerve fibres. These receptors are stimulated by pull upon the tendon during active contraction of the muscle, and to a lesser degree by passive stretching.

Muscle Spindles

These are spindle-shaped sensory end organs located within striated muscle (Fig. 10.15). The spindle is bounded by a fusiform connective tissue covering (forming an external capsule) within which there are a few muscle fibres of a special kind. These are called

intrafusal fibres in contrast to *extrafusal fibres* that constitute the main bulk of the muscle.

Each muscle spindle is innervated by sensory as well as motor nerves. Spindles provide information to the CNS about the extent and rate of changes in length of muscle.

NEUROMUSCULAR JUNCTIONS

We have seen that skeletal muscle fibres are supplied by ramifications of efferent neurons. We have also seen that axonal branches arising from one neuron may innervate a variable number of muscle fibres (that constitute a motor unit).

Each skeletal muscle fibre receives its own direct innervation. The site where the nerve ending comes into intimate contact with the muscle fibre is a *neuromuscular (or myoneural) junction*.

The nerve terminal comes in contact with a specialized area near the middle of the muscle fibre. This area is roughly oval or circular, and is referred to as the *sole plate*. The sole plate plus the axon terminal constitute the *motor end plate* (Fig. 10.16).

Structure of a typical Motor End Plate:

In the region of the motor end plate axon terminals are lodged in grooves in the sarcolemma covering the sole plate. Between the axolemma (over the axon) and the sarcolemma (over the muscle fibre) there is a narrow gap. It follows that there is no continuity between axoplasm and sarcoplasm.

Axon terminals are lodged in grooves in the sarcolemma covering the sole plate. In section (Fig. 10.17) this groove is seen as a semicircular depression.

This depression is the *primary cleft*. The sarcolemma in the floor of the primary cleft is thrown into numerous small folds resulting in the formation of *secondary (or subneural) clefts*.

Axon terminals contain vesicles similar to those seen in presynaptic boutons. The vesicles contain the neurotransmitter acetylcholine.

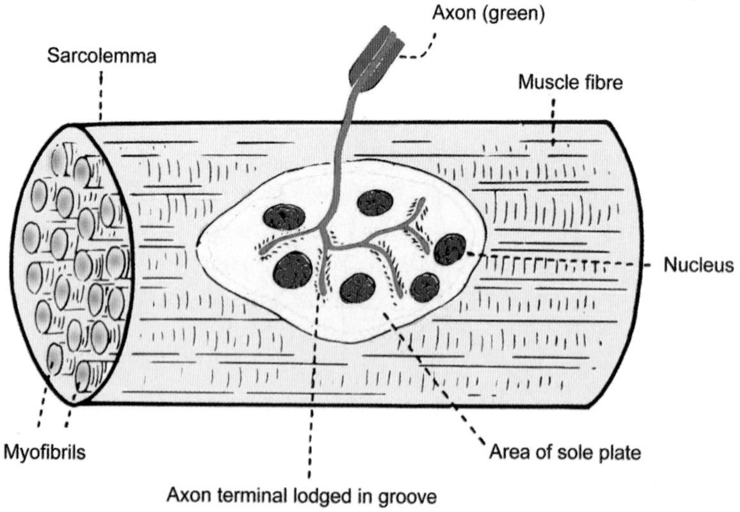

Neuromuscular transmission

Transmission across a neuromuscular junction is very similar to synaptic transmission.

1. When an action potential reaches an axon terminal (in a motor end plate) permeability of axon terminal (=

Fig. 10.16. Motor end plate seen in relation to a muscle fibre (surface view). Schwann cell cytoplasm covering the nerve terminal has not been shown for sake of clarity.

presynaptic membrane) increases, allowing calcium ions to enter the axon terminal.

2. Entry of calcium ions triggers the release of acetylcholine from vesicles in the terminal. This acetylcholine enters the cleft between axolemma and sarcolemma (= synaptic cleft).

3. Here acetylcholine binds with receptors present on the sarcolemma (= postsynaptic membrane) to form acetylcholine-receptor complex.

4. This complex increases permeability of sarcolemma to sodium ions, and these now enter the sarcoplasm at the neuromuscular junction.

5. Entry of sodium ions produces localised depolarisation in the sarcoplasm forming the end plate, resulting in creation of an action potential. This is the end plate potential.

6. The end plate potential triggers the development of action potential that spreads along the sarcolemma causing contraction of the entire muscle fibre.

7. Acetylcholine released into the synaptic cleft is destroyed rapidly (within 1 ms) by the enzyme acetylcholine esterase. This ensures that response to a stimulus reaching the neuromuscular junction is sharp and brief.

GANGLIA

Introductory Remarks

Aggregations of cell bodies of neurons, present outside the brain and spinal cord are known as ganglia. Ganglia are of two main types: sensory, and autonomic (Fig. 10.18).

Sensory ganglia are present on the dorsal nerve roots of spinal nerves, where they are called dorsal nerve root ganglia or spinal ganglia. They are also present on the 5th, 7th, 8th, 9th and 10th cranial nerves. We have seen that the neurons in these ganglia are of the unipolar type (except in the case of ganglia associated with the vestibulo-cochlear nerve in which they are bipolar). The peripheral process of each neuron forms an afferent (or sensory) fibre of a peripheral nerve. The central process enters the spinal cord or brain stem.

Autonomic ganglia are concerned with the nerve supply of smooth muscle or of glands. The pathway for this supply always consists of two neurons: preganglionic and postganglionic. The cell bodies of preganglionic neurons are always located within the spinal cord or brainstem. Their axons leave the spinal cord or brainstem and terminate by synapsing with postganglionic neurons, the cell bodies of which are located in autonomic ganglia. Autonomic ganglia are, therefore, aggregations of the cell bodies of postganglionic neurons. These neurons are multipolar. Their axons leave the ganglia as postganglionic fibres to reach and supply smooth muscle or gland. Autonomic ganglia are sub divisible into two major types: sympathetic and parasympathetic. Sympathetic ganglia are located on the right and left sympathetic trunks. Parasympathetic ganglia usually lie close to the viscera supplied through them.

NEUROGLIA

In addition to neurons, the nervous system contains several types of supporting cells. These are:

(i) **Neuroglial cells**, found in the parenchyma of the brain and spinal cord.

(ii) **Ependymal cells**, lining the ventricular system.

(iii) **Schwann cells**, forming sheaths for axons of peripheral nerves. They are also called **lemnocytes** or **peripheral glia**.

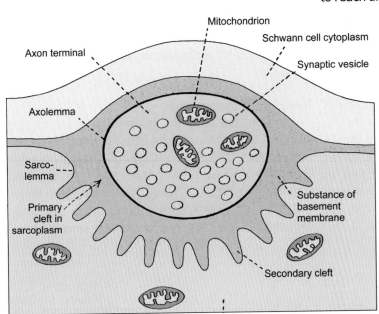

Fig. 10.17. Neuromuscular junction. This figure is a section across one of the axon terminals (and related structures) shown in Fig. 10.16. These details are seen only by EM.

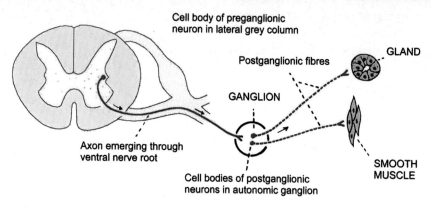

Fig. 10.18. Scheme to show the arrangement of visceral nerve fibres supplying glands and smooth muscle.

(iv) **Capsular cells** (also called **satellite cells** or **capsular gliocytes**) that surround neurons in peripheral ganglia.

(v) Various types of supporting cells found in relation to motor and sensory terminals of nerve fibres.

Functions of neuroglia

1. They provide mechanical support to neurons.

2. They serve as insulators.

3. Some neuroglial cells are concerned in providing myelin sheaths to nerve fibres.

4. Neuroglial cells help in regeneration of injured neurons. They also help in controlling the environment of neurons.

REFLEX ACTION

A reflex action is one that takes place automatically, without any conscious effort on our part. For example if you touch the sole of a sleeping person the leg is immediately drawn up. The nervous pathway for such an action is called a **reflex arc**. The pathway for a simple reflex arc is shown diagrammatically in Fig. 10.19. The stimulus is received by a receptor in skin. A nerve impulse is carried by an afferent nerve to a **reflex centre** (in spinal cord). From here an efferent neuron carries an impulse to a muscle (effector organ) causing its contraction. In most cases the actual pathways are more complex.

Reflexes can be classified in various ways.

1. In the reflex arc shown in Fig. 10.19 only one synapse (located in the reflex centre) is involved. Such a reflex is **monosynaptic**. When the pathway involves more than one synapse it is said to be **polysynaptic**.

2. **Location of reflex centre**: Depending on the location of the reflex centre a reflex may be spinal, bulbar (medulla), cerebellar, cortical etc.

3. Reflexes produced by stimulation of skin (or mucous membrane) are **superficial reflexes**. Those arising from deeper structures (e.g., tendons) are **deep reflexes**.

4. Reflexes are also named on the structures involved. Those elicited by stimulating skin are **cutaneous reflexes**, those from tendons are **tendon reflexes**. Similarly, we have **pupillary reflexes**, visceral reflexes etc.

5. Some reflexes are present at birth. These are **inborn reflexes**. Others develop as a result of experience. These are **acquired** (or **conditioned**) **reflexes**.

6. Some reflexes are protective e.g., withdrawal of the hand when a hot object is touched. In the movement of withdrawing joints of the extremity are flexed. Such reflexes are, therefore, also called **flexor reflexes**. When a person is standing a series of reflexes are active to prevent him from falling. As these keep the body straight (with hip and knee joints extended) these are called **extensor reflexes**, or **antigravity reflexes**.

Reciprocal innervation

In movements produced by reflexes, some muscles relax while others contract. In a flexor response, the flexors contract and extensors relax. It has been shown that afferent neurons of the reflex arc establish connections with motor neurons supplying both flexors and extensors, inhibiting one group while stimulating the other. This is the law of reciprocal innervation.

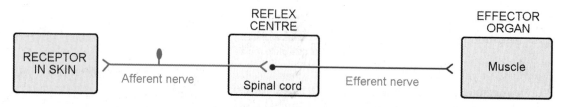

Fig. 10.19. Diagram showing the pathway for a simple reflex action.

11

Skin and Appendages

The skin consists of a superficial layer the **epidermis**, made up of stratified squamous epithelium; and a deeper layer, the **dermis**, made up of connective tissue (Fig. 11.1).

The Epidermis

The epidermis consists of stratified epithelium in which the following layers can be recognized (Fig. 11.2).

(**a**) The deepest or **basal layer** (**stratum basale**) is made up of a single layer of columnar cells.

The basal layer contains stem cells that undergo mitosis to give off cells called **keratinocytes**. Keratinocytes form the more superficial layers of the epidermis described below. The basal layer is, therefore, also called the **germinal layer**.

(**b**) Above the basal layer there are several layers of polygonal keratinocytes that constitute the **stratum spinosum** (or **Malpighian layer**).

(**c**) Overlying the stratum spinosum there are a few layers of flattened cells that are characterized by the presence of deeply staining granules in their cytoplasm. These cells constitute the **stratum granulosum**.

(**d**) Superficial to the stratum granulosum there is the **stratum lucidum** (lucid = clear). This layer is so called because it appears homogeneous, the cell boundaries being extremely indistinct.

(**e**) The most superficial layer of the epidermis is called the **stratum corneum**. This layer does not contain living cells. It is made up of flattened scale-like elements (squames) containing keratin filaments embedded in protein.

The thickness of the stratum corneum is greatest where the skin is exposed to maximal friction e.g., on the palms and soles. The superficial layers of the epidermis are being constantly shed off, and are replaced by proliferation of cells in deeper layers.

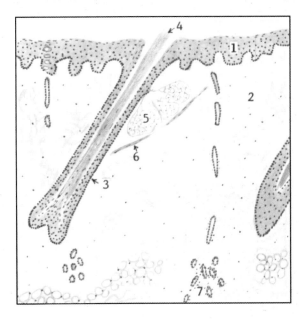

Fig. 11.1. Section through skin. 1-Epidermis. 2-Dermis. 3-Hair follicle. 4-Hair. 5-Sebaceous gland. 6- Arrector pili. 7-Sweat gland.

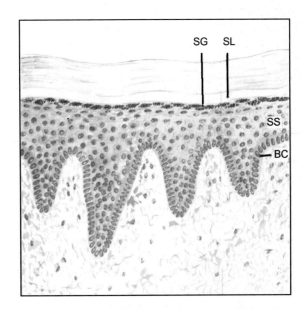

Fig. 11.2. Section through skin showing the layers of the epidermis. SC-Stratum corneum. SL-Stratum lucidum. SG-Stratum granulosum. SS-Stratum spinosum. BC-Basal cell layer.

The Dermis

The dermis is made up of connective tissue. Just below the epidermis the connective tissue is dense and constitutes the **papillary layer**. Deep to this there is a network of thick fibre bundles that constitute the **reticular layer** of the dermis.

The dermis rests on the superficial fascia through which it is attached to deeper structures.

We have seen that the dermis contains considerable amounts of elastic fibres. Atrophy of elastic fibres occurs with age and is responsible for loss of elasticity and wrinkling of the skin.

Pigmentation of the Skin

The cells of the basal layer of the epidermis, and the adjoining cells of the stratum spinosum contain a brown pigment called **melanin**. The pigment is much more prominent in dark skinned individuals. The cells actually responsible for synthesis of melanin are called **melanocytes**.

Blood supply

Blood vessels do not penetrate into the epidermis. The epidermis derives nutrition entirely by diffusion from capillaries in the dermal papillae. Veins from the dermal papillae drain (through plexuses present in the dermis) into a venous plexus lying on deep fascia.

A special feature of the blood supply of the skin is the presence of numerous arterio-venous anastomoses that regulate blood flow through the capillary bed and thus help in maintaining body temperature.

Nerve Supply

The skin is richly supplied with sensory nerves. Sensory nerves end in relation to various types of specialized terminals that present in the skin.

Apart from sensory nerves the skin receives autonomic nerves which supply smooth muscle in the walls of blood vessels and the arrectores pilorum muscles. They also provide a secretomotor supply to sweat glands.

FUNCTIONS OF THE SKIN

1. The skin provides mechanical protection to underlying tissues. In this connection we have noted that the skin is thickest over areas exposed to greatest friction.

The skin also acts as a physical barrier against entry of microorganisms and other substances. However, the skin is not a perfect barrier and some substances, both useful (e.g., ointments) or harmful (poisons), may enter the body through the skin.

2. The skin prevents loss of water from the body. The importance of this function is seen in persons who have lost extensive areas of skin through burns. One important cause of death in such cases is water loss.

3. The pigment present in the epidermis protects tissues against harmful effects of light (specially ultraviolet light). However, some degree of exposure to sunlight is essential for synthesis of vitamin-D. Ultraviolet light converts 7-dehydrocholesterol (present in skin) to vitamin-D.

4. The skin offers protection against damage of tissues by chemicals, by heat, and by osmotic influences.

5. The skin is a very important sensory organ, containing receptors for touch and related sensations.

6. The skin plays an important role in regulating body temperature as discussed later in this chapter.

APPENDAGES OF THE SKIN

The appendages of the skin are the hairs, nails, sebaceous glands and sweat glands.

In animals with a thick coat of hair (fur) the hair help to keep the animal warm. In man this function is performed by subcutaneous fat.

Hair

Each hair consists of a part (of variable length) that is seen on the surface of the body; and a part anchored in the thickness of the skin. The visible part is called the **shaft**, and the embedded part is called the **root**. The root has an expanded lower end called the **bulb**. The bulb is invaginated from below by part of the dermis that constitutes the **hair papilla**. The root of each

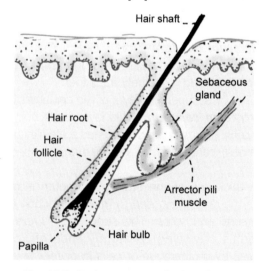

Fig. 11.3. Basic structure of a hair follicle.

hair is surrounded by a tubular sheath called the **hair follicle**. The follicle is made up of several layers of cells that are derived from the layers of the skin (Fig. 11.3).

Arrector Pili Muscles

These are bands of smooth muscle attached at one end to the dermis, just below the dermal papillae; and at the other end to the connective tissue sheath of a hair follicle. A sebaceous gland lies in the angle between the hair follicle and the arrector pili. Contraction of the muscle has two effects. Firstly, the hair follicle becomes almost vertical (from its original oblique position) relative to the skin surface). Simultaneously the skin surface overlying the attachment of the muscle becomes depressed while surrounding areas become raised. These reactions are seen during exposure to cold, or during emotional excitement, when the 'hair stand on end' and the skin takes on the appearance of 'goose flesh'. The second effect of contraction of the arrector pili muscle is that the sebaceous gland is pressed upon and its secretions are squeezed out into the hair follicle. The arrector pili muscles receive a sympathetic innervation.

Sebaceous Glands

Sebaceous glands are seen most typically in relation to hair follicles. Each gland consists of a number of alveoli that are connected to a broad duct that opens into a hair follicle (Fig. 11.1).

The secretion of sebaceous glands is called **sebum**. Its oily nature helps to keep the skin and hair soft. It helps to prevent dryness of the skin and also makes it resistant to moisture.

Nails

Nails are present on fingers and toes. The main part of a nail is called its **body**. The body has a free distal edge. The proximal part of the nail is implanted into a groove on the skin and is called the **root** (or **radix**). The tissue on which the nail rests is called the **nail bed**. The nail bed is highly vascular, and that is why the nails look pink in colour.

The nail represents a modified part of the zone of keratinization of the epidermis. The nail substance consists of several layers of dead, cornified, 'cells' filled with keratin.

When we view a nail in longitudinal section (Fig. 11.4) it is seen that the nail rests on the cells of the germinative zone (stratum spinosum and stratum basale). The germinative zone is particularly thick near the root of the nail where it forms the **germinal matrix**. The nail substance is formed mainly by proliferation of cells in the germinal matrix.

The germinative zone underlying the body of the nail (i.e., the nail bed) is much thinner than the germinal matrix. It does not contribute to the growth of the nail; and is, therefore, called the **sterile matrix**.

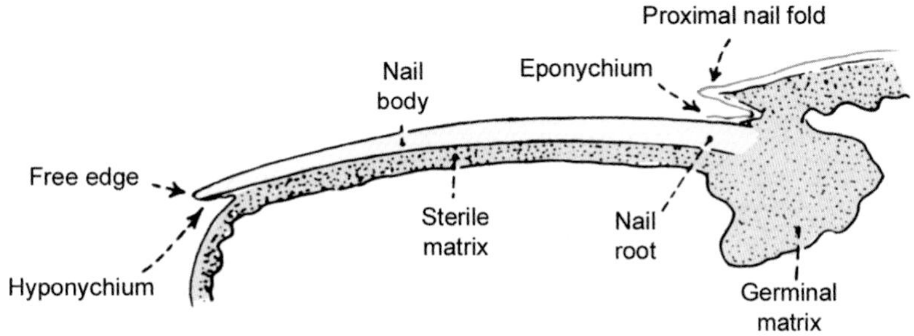

Sweat Glands

Sweat glands produce sweat or perspiration. They are present in the skin over most of the body. Their number and size varies in the skin over different parts of the body. They are most numerous in the palms and soles, the forehead and scalp, and the axillae.

The entire sweat gland consists of a single long tube (Fig. 11.5). The lower end of the tube is highly coiled on itself and forms the **body** (or **fundus**) or the gland. The body is made up of the secretory part of the gland.

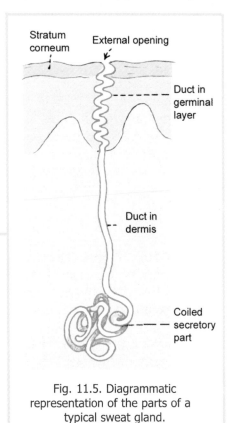

Fig. 11.5. Diagrammatic representation of the parts of a typical sweat gland.

Fig. 11.4. Parts of a nail and some related structures as seen in a longitudinal section.

It lies in the reticular layer of the dermis, or some-times in subcutaneous tissue. The part of the tube connecting the secretory element to the skin surface is the ***duct***. It runs upwards through the dermis to reach the epidermis.

As is well known the secretion of sweat glands has a high water content. Evaporation of this water plays an important role in cooling the body. Sweat glands are innervated by cholinergic nerves.

Regulation of body temperature

The average body temperature of a healthy person is roughly 37°C (= 98.4°F). Normal variation in temperature, between individuals, and at different times of the day is about 0.5°C. The temperature is maintained within these limits by balancing heat production and heat loss.

Heat is produced by the following ways:

1. Contraction of muscles. (That is why we shiver when exposed to cold).

2. Some metabolic processes produce heat. These take place mainly in the liver, in the intestines and in adipose tissue).

Heat is lost in the following ways:

1. Evaporation of sweat (from skin) is the most important method of cooling the body. That is why we perspire so much in hot weather.

2. Some heat is lost through expired air, and through urine and faeces.

Heat generated in the body is preserved in the following manner. These measures are necessary only if environmental temperature is lower than body temperature.

a). The clothes we wear prevent loss of heat from the surface of the body.

b). Vasoconstriction of blood vessels supplying the skin reduces blood flow, and hence reduces heat loss by radiation. Reduced blood flow also reduces perspiration and its evaporation.

Mechanisms controlling temperature

1. A collection of nerve cells in the brain (hypothalamus) constitutes a temperature regulatory centre. These cells respond to changes in temperature of blood. This centre sends out impulses that travel through autonomic nerves, influencing vasoconstriction and secretion of sweat.

2. In some diseases, substances called pyrogens are released. These act on the temperature regulating centre, and lead to rise in temperature, as in fever.

Hypothermia

Fall of temperature below 32°C is called hypothermia. Metabolic process show down and the mechanisms that normally increase temperature are unable to act. Extreme hypothermia causes death.

12

Blood

Blood is made up of a fluid base called the plasma, in which cellular elements are suspended.

The Plasma

Plasma consists of water in which **colloids** and **crystalloids** are dissolved. The colloids are proteins including prothrombin (associated with the clotting of blood), immunoglobulins (involved in immunological defence mechanisms), hormones, etc. The crystalloids are ions of sodium, chloride, potassium, calcium, magnesium, phosphate, bicarbonate etc. Several other substances like glucose and amino acids are also present.

About 55 per cent of the total volume of blood is plasma, the rest being constituted by the cellular elements described below.

CELLULAR ELEMENTS OF BLOOD

The cellular or formed elements of blood are of three main types. These are **red blood corpuscles** or **erythrocytes**, **white blood corpuscles** or **leucocytes**, and **blood platelets**. We refer to them as 'cellular' or 'formed' elements rather than as cells because of the fact that red blood corpuscles are not strictly cells (see below). However, in practice, the terms red blood cells and white blood cells are commonly used.

We have seen that about 55 per cent of the total volume of blood is accounted for by plasma. Most of the remaining 45 per cent is made up of red blood corpuscles, the leucocytes and platelets constituting less than 1 per cent of the volume. If we take one cubic millimetre (mm³ = microlitre or μl) of blood we find that it contains about five million erythrocytes. In comparison there are only about 7000 leucocytes in the same volume of blood.

ERYTHROCYTES (Red Blood Corpuscles)

When seen in surface view each erythrocyte is a circular disc having a diameter of about 7 μm (6.5-8.5 μm). When viewed from the side it is seen to be biconcave, the maximum thickness being about 2 μm (Fig. 12.1). Erythrocytes are cells that have lost their nuclei (and other organelles). They are bounded by a plasma membrane. They contain a red coloured protein called **haemoglobin**. It is because of the presence of haemoglobin that erythrocytes (and blood as a whole) are red in colour. Haemoglobin plays an important role in carrying oxygen from the lungs to all tissues of the body. In a healthy person there are about 15 g of haemoglobin in every 100 ml of blood.

When erythrocytes are seen in a film of blood spread out on a slide, they appear yellow (or pale red) in colour. Their rims (being thicker) appear darker than the central parts.

Erythrocytes are formed in bone marrow from where they enter the blood stream. Each erythrocyte has a life of about 100 to 120 days at the end of which it is

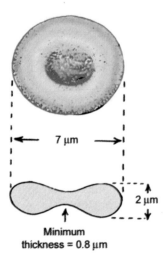

Fig. 12.1. Average dimensions of an erythrocyte. The erythrocyte is seen in surface view (A), and in profile (B)

removed from blood by cells of the mononuclear phagocyte system (specially in the spleen and bone marrow). The constituents of erythrocytes are broken down and reused to form new erythrocytes.

Like cell membranes of other cells, the plasma membranes of erythrocytes are composed of lipids and proteins. Several types of proteins are present, including **ABO antigens** responsible for a person's blood group.

LEUCOCYTES
(White Blood Corpuscles)

Differences between Erythrocytes and Leucocytes

Leucocytes are different from erythrocytes in several ways.

(**a**) They are true cells, each leucocyte having a nucleus, mitochondria, Golgi complex, and other organelles.

(**b**) They do not contain haemoglobin and, therefore, appear colourless in unstained preparations.

(**c**) Unlike erythrocytes, that do not have any mobility of their own, leucocytes can move actively.

(**d**) As a corollary of 'c' erythrocytes do not normally leave the vascular system, but leucocytes can move out of it to enter surrounding tissues. In fact, blood is merely a route by which leucocytes travel from bone marrow to other destinations.

(**e**) Most leucocytes have a relatively short life span.

Features of different types of leucocytes

Leucocytes are of various types. Some of them have granules in their cytoplasm and are, therefore, called **granulocytes**. Depending on the staining characters of their granules granulocytes are further divided into **neutrophil leucocytes** (or **neutrophils**), **eosinophil leucocytes** (or **eosinophils**), and **basophil leucocytes** (or **basophils**).

Apart from these granulocytes there are two types of agranular leucocytes. These are **lymphocytes** and **monocytes** (Fig. 12.4).

Apart from the presence or absence of granules, and their nature, the different types of leucocytes show various other differences. In describing the differences it is usual for text books to consider all features of one type of leucocyte together. However, in practice, it is more useful to take the features one by one and to compare each feature in the different types of leucocytes as given below.

Relative number

We have seen that there are about 7000 leucocytes (range 5000-10000) in every cubic millimetre (=mm³=μl) of blood. Of these about two thirds (60-70 per cent) are neutrophils, and about one fourth (20-30 per cent) are lymphocytes. The remaining types are present in very small numbers. The eosinophils are about 3 per cent, the basophils about 1 per cent, and the monocytes about 5 per cent. The relative and absolute numbers of the different types of leucocytes vary considerably in health; and to a more marked degree in disease. Estimations of their numbers provide valuable information for diagnosis of many diseases.

Relative size

In a blood film all types of granulocytes, and monocytes are about 10 μm in diameter. Most lymphocytes are distinctly smaller (6-8 μm) and are called small lymphocytes, but some (called large lymphocytes) measure 12-15 μm.

Nuclei

In lymphocytes the nucleus is spherical, but may show an indentation on one side. It stains densely in small lymphocytes, but tends to be partly euchromatic in large lymphocytes. In monocytes the nucleus is ovoid and may be indented: it is placed eccentrically. In basophils the nucleus is S-shaped. The nucleus of the eosinophil leucocyte is made up of two or three lobes that are joined by delicate strands. In neutrophil leucocytes the nucleus is very variable in shape and consists of several lobes (up to 6): that is why these cells are also called **polymorphonuclear leucocytes**, or simply **polymorphs**.

Cytoplasm

The cytoplasm of a lymphocyte is scanty and forms a thin rim around the nucleus. It is clear blue in stained preparations. In monocytes the cytoplasm is abundant. It stains blue, but in contrast to the 'transparent' appearance in lymphocytes the cytoplasm of monocytes is like frosted glass. Granules are not present in the cytoplasm of lymphocytes or of monocytes. The cytoplasm of granulocytes is marked by the presence of numerous granules. In neutrophils the granules are very fine and stain lightly with both acidic and basic dyes. The granules of neutrophils are really lysosomes: they are of various types depending upon the particular enzymes present in them. The granules of eosinophil leucocytes are large and stain brightly with acid dyes (like eosin). These are also lysosomes. In basophil leucocytes the cytoplasm contains large spherical granules that stain with basic dyes.

Motility and Phagocytosis

All leucocytes are capable of amoeboid movement. Neutrophils and monocytes are the most active. The eosinophil and basophil leucocytes move rather slowly. Lymphocytes in blood show the least power of movement. However, when they settle on solid surfaces they become freely motile and can pass through various tissues.

Because of their motility leucocytes easily pass through capillaries into surrounding tissues, and can migrate through the latter. Neutrophils collect in large numbers at sites of infection. Here they phagocytose bacteria and use the enzymes in their lysosomes to destroy the bacteria. Eosinophils are phagocytic, but their ability to destroy bacteria is less than that of neutrophils. The number of eosinophils is greatly increased in some allergic conditions. Monocytes are also actively phagocytic.

Life span

We have seen that erythrocytes have a life span of about 100-120 days. The life of a neutrophil leucocyte is only about 15 hours. Eosinophils live for a few days, while basophils can live for 9 to 18 months. The life span of lymphocytes is variable. Some live only a few days (**short-lived lymphocytes**) while others may live several years (**long-lived lymphocytes**).

FURTHER FACTS ABOUT LYMPHOCYTES

We have seen that lymphocytes are numerous and constitute about 20-30 per cent of all leucocytes in blood. Large numbers of lymphocytes are also present in bone marrow, and as aggregations in various lymphatic tissues.

Formation and Circulation of Lymphocytes

In the embryo lymphocytes are derived from mesenchymal cells present in the wall of the yolk sac, in the liver and in the spleen. These stem cells later migrate to bone marrow. Lymphocytes formed from these stem cells (in bone marrow) enter the blood. Depending on their subsequent behaviour they are classified into two types.

(**1**) Some of them travel in the blood stream to reach the thymus. Here they divide repeatedly and undergo certain changes.

They are now called **T-lymphocytes** ('T' from thymus). These T-lymphocytes, that have been 'processed' in the thymus re-enter the circulation to reach lymphoid tissue in lymph nodes, spleen, tonsils and intestines.

From these masses of lymphoid tissue many lymphocytes pass into lymph vessels, and through them they go back into the circulation. In this way lymphocytes keep passing out of blood into lymphoid tissue (and bone marrow), and back from these into the blood. About 85 per cent of lymphocytes seen in blood are T-lymphocytes (Fig. 12.2).

(**2**) Lymphocytes of a second group arising from stem cells in bone marrow enter the blood stream, but do not go to the thymus. They go directly to lymphoid tissues (other than the thymus). Such lymphocytes are called **B-lymphocytes**. Like T-lymphocytes, B-lymphocytes also circulate between lymphoid tissues and the blood stream (Fig. 12.3).

Lymphocytes play a very important role in the immune system which is considered in Chapter 18.

BLOOD PLATELETS

Blood platelets are round, oval, or irregular discs about 3 μm in diameter. They are also known as **thrombocytes**. Platelets are concerned with the clotting

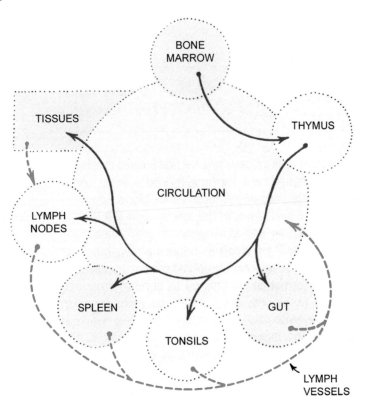

Fig. 12.2. Scheme to show the circulation of T-lymphoctes.

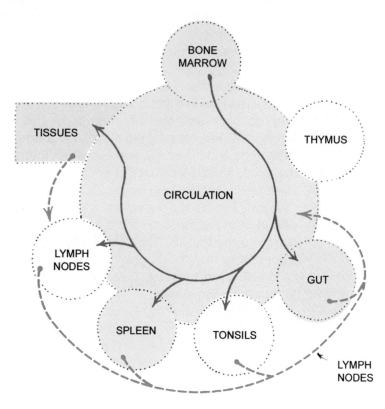

Fig. 12.3. Scheme to show the circulation of B-lymphocytes.

BLOOD VOLUME

The total amount of blood in a normal healthy male adult is about 5 litres.

Physiological factors that increase blood volume are as follows.

1. Greater body weight.
2. Male sex.
3. Higher environmental temperature.
4. Exercise.
5. Lying posture (in contrast to standing).
6. Emotional excitement.
7. Exposure to high altitude.
8. Pregnancy.

Factors that decrease blood volume are as follows.

1. Prolonged standing. Blood collects in the veins of the lower limb, and fluid passes out into tissues.
2. Loss of blood by bleeding, or by disease (haemolysis).
3. Loss of fluids for any reason including vomiting, diarrhoea, or excessive sweating.

of blood. As soon as blood is shed from a vessel, platelets stick to each other and to any available surfaces. Platelets break down into small granules and threads of fibrin appear around them.

FORMATION OF BLOOD (HAEMOPOIESIS)

In embryonic life blood cells are first formed in relation to mesenchymal cells surrounding the yolk sac. After the second month of intrauterine life blood formation starts in the liver; later in the spleen; and still later in the bone marrow. At first lymphocytes are formed along with other cells of blood in bone marrow, but later they are formed mainly in lymphoid tissues. In postnatal life blood formation is confined to bone marrow and lymphoid tissue. However, under conditions in which the bone marrow is unable to meet normal requirements, blood cell formation may start in the liver and spleen. This is referred to as **extramedullary haemopoiesis**.

Some steps in formation of blood cells are summarised in Fig. 12.4.

Regulation of blood volume

Blood volume is related to total fluid in the body. The latter is controlled by centres in the brain (in the hypothalamus). When there is decrease in body fluids the hypothalamus uses the following methods to bring it back to normal.

(a) There is increased thirst so that water intake increases.

(b) Urine output is decreased. The hypothalamus sends chemical signals to the hypophysis cerebri (or pituitary gland). These signals cause greater quantities of a hormone called ADH (antidiuretic hormone)to be secreted. This hormone reaches the kidneys. Under its influence reabsorption of water by renal tubules is greatly increased. As a result urine output decreases.

CLINICAL CORRELATIONS OF BLOOD

Clinical Examination of Blood

Examination of blood provides useful information about a patient. Some common tests done are as follows:

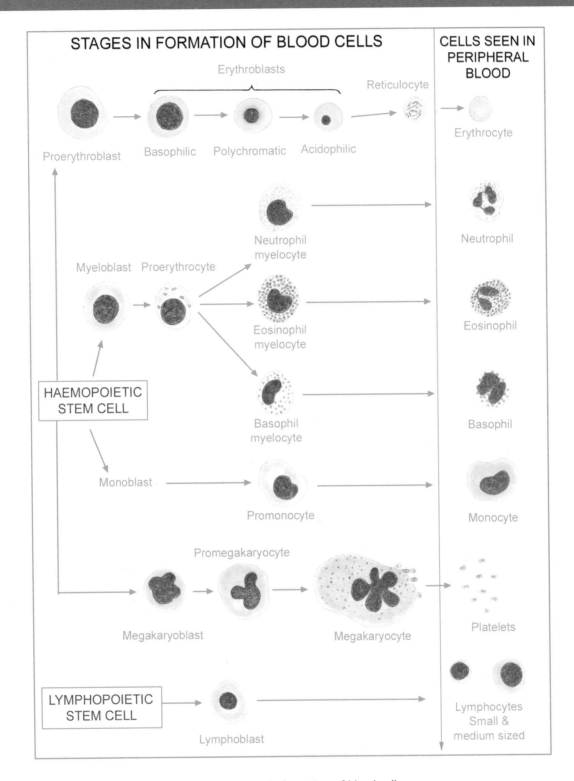

Fig. 12.4. Stages in formation of blood cells.

Investigations about Erythrocytes

1. *Total RBC count*. The number of erythrocytes is one cubic millimeter of blood is counted, The number is reduced in anaemia.

2. *Cell size*: Cells of normal size are normocytic. They may be too small (microcytic) or too large (macrocytic).

3. *Cell volume*: Mean cell volume is measured.

4. *Haemoglobin content*. Haemoglobin present in 100 ml of blood is estimated.

Investigations about Lymphocytes

1. *Total WBC count*. The count is increased in acute infections.

2. *Differential count*. The actual number of different types of lymphocytes is measured. In normal blood neutrophils are about 60 per cent, lymphocytes about 30 per cent. The remaining 1 per cent is made up by eosinophils, monocytes and basophils. These proportions can change in disease and may serve as pointers to diagnosis.

Blood Transfusion and Blood Groups

When blood of one person is introduced into the blood circulation of another individual this is called blood transfusion. However, some persons develop serious symptoms after transfusion, if the blood of the two individuals does not match for reason explained below.

Red blood cells bear proteins that function as antigens. If an antigen is introduced into a person, who does not already have it, the defense systems of the body produce **antibodies** that combine with antigen and try to destroy it. This is called an antigen-antibody reaction. In this process red blood cells are destroyed, leading to serious symptoms and even death.

Individuals can be classified on the basis of antigens present on their red blood cells. Such classification divides individuals on the basis of what we call **blood groups**.

There are many systems of blood groups, but the ones that are clinically important are the ABO system and the Rh system.

Bleeding and Clotting of Blood

It is common knowledge that any injury, small or big, can cause bleeding (also called haemorrhage). When this happens the body tries to stop the bleeding. As long as blood is within blood vessels it remains liquid. However once it comes out of vessels it undergoes a process of coagulation (clotting) which is an important factor in stopping bleeding, Blood platelets play an important role in the process.

The following changes are seen at the site of injury.

1. Platelets release chemicals that cause blood vessels to get constricted. This reduces blood flow.

2. Platelets collect in large number at site of injury. They stick to each other and to the wall of the damaged vessel, thus blocking it.

3. Clotting of blood takes place. Under the influence of platelets a mesh-work of fibres is formed and blood cells get trapped in it. This clot plugs the damaged vessel firmly. The process of clot formation is complex and many proteins and controlling factors are involved. Some of them are thrombin, fibrinogen and fibrin.

Vitamin K is essential for producing factors that control clotting of blood. Deficiency of Vitamin K, or reduced number of blood platelets (thrombocytopenia), can interfere with clotting.

Anaemia

Anaemia is a condition in which the quantity of haemoglobin in blood is less than normal. Depending on how low haemoglobin levels are, anaemia can be described as mild, moderate or severe.

As haemoglobin carries oxygen from lungs to tissues, a patient of anaemia complain of tiredness, and mild exertion can make the person breathless.

In anaemia the number of circulating red blood cells is less than normal. This can be a result of less production or of excessive loss. The concentration of haemoglobin in each RBC is also decreased.

Lukaemias

Lukaemia is a condition in which there is uncontrolled production of leucocytes by bone marrow. It is a malignant, life threatening, condition. Leucocyte precursors, normally confined to bone marrow, are seen in large numbers in peripheral blood.

PART THREE

BRIEF CONSIDERATION
OF
ORGAN SYSTEMS

13

Alimentary Canal, Liver and Pancreas, Nutrition and Digestion

A preliminary introduction to the parts of the alimentary canal has been given in Chapter 3. Those students who are new to the subject should read this introduction before proceeding further.

THE ORAL CAVITY

The lay person uses the word 'mouth' loosely both for the external opening and for the cavity it leads to. Strictly speaking, the term mouth should be applied only to the external opening which is also called the *oral fissure.* The cavity (containing the tongue and teeth) is the mouth cavity or *oral cavity*.

A basic idea of the boundaries of the oral cavity can be had from Fig. 13.1 which is a coronal section through it. Laterally the cavity is bounded by the cheeks; above by the palate (which separates it from the nasal cavity); and below it has a floor to which the tongue is attached. Projecting into the cavity from above and below, just medial to the each cheek, there are the alveolar processes of the upper and lower jaws which bear the teeth. When the mouth is closed bringing the upper and lower teeth into apposition, the oral cavity is seen to consist of a part between the teeth of the two sides (the *oral cavity proper*); and a part between the alveolar processes and the cheeks. The latter is called the *vestibule*.

The oral cavity proper communicates posteriorly with the oral part of the pharynx. The communication between the two is called the *oropharyngeal isthmus*. The roof of the cavity is formed by the palate (described below). The chief structure in the floor is the tongue.

Three pairs of salivary glands are present near the oral cavity and pour their secretions into it. These are the *parotid, submandibular* and *sublingual* glands.

LIPS AND CHEEKS

Some facts worth noting about the lips and cheeks are as follows.

The *lips* and *cheeks* are made up of an outer layer of skin, an inner layer of mucous membrane and an intervening layer of muscle, connective tissue and fat. Numerous glands are present in relationship to the lips and cheeks. They open into the vestibule of the mouth.

THE PALATE

The palate separates the oral cavity from the nasal cavity. It is divisible into an anterior, larger part the *hard palate*, and a posterior part the *soft palate*. The median part of the soft palate is prolonged downwards as a conical projection called the *uvula*.

THE TEETH

An individual has two sets of teeth. The teeth of the first set that appear in children and fall off with time are called *deciduous* (or milk) teeth. The teeth of the second set that gradually replace the deciduous teeth constitute the *permanent* teeth.

A set of deciduous teeth consists of the following. Beginning from the middle line (in front) there is a

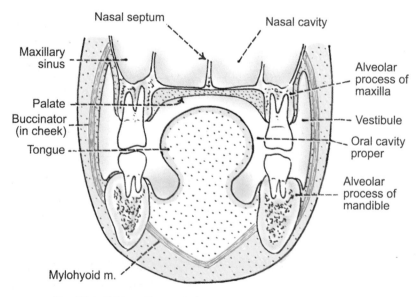

Fig. 13.1. Schematic coronal section through the oral cavity.

central incisor, a *lateral incisor* (i.e., two incisors); one *canine*; and two *molars*. There are, thus, five teeth in each half of each jaw i.e., twenty in all.

A set of permanent teeth consists of the following. Beginning from the middle line there is a *central incisor*, a *lateral incisor*, a *canine*, two *premolars* (first and second, that replace the deciduous molars), and three *molars* (first, second and third). Thus in each half of each jaw there are eight teeth, or thirty two in all.

THE TONGUE

The tongue lies in the oral cavity. The anterior part of the tongue (or *apex*) can be protruded out of the mouth. It has free upper and lower surfaces. The greater part of the tongue is attached below to the floor of the mouth. The attached part is called the *root* of the tongue. This part of the tongue has a free upper surface or *dorsum*. On either side, the tongue has *lateral edges* that are also free. The free surfaces of the tongue are lined by mucous membrane. The substance of the tongue is made up mainly of muscle.

The mucous membrane covering the dorsum of the tongue is rough because of the presence of numerous finger like projections or *papillae*.

The tongue bears *taste buds* which are end organs for taste. Sensations of taste from the anterior two-thirds of the tongue travel through the lingual nerve. Those for the posterior one third of the tongue pass through the glossopharyngeal nerve.

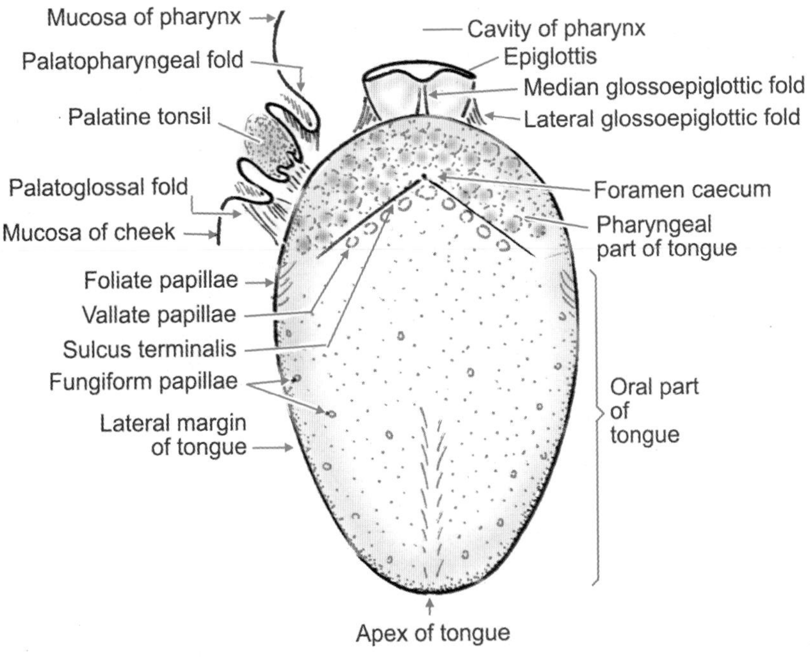

The movements of the tongue are produced by a number of muscles. These muscles are supplied by the hypoglossal nerve.

Swallowing

1. After food has been adequately chewed, and moistened by saliva, it is shaped (by pressure of tongue and cheeks) into a rounded mass or bolus.

2. The mouth closes and the tongue pushes the bolus into the pharynx.

3. Once food enters the pharynx, contraction of muscles in its wall pushes the bolus downward until it passes into the oesophagus. Food is prevented from going into the nasal cavity, into the larynx, or back into the mouth, by the actions of muscles that close these communications.

4. Once food enters the oesophagus, peristaltic contractions of muscle in its wall move food along its length until it reaches the stomach.

THE OESOPHAGUS

The oesophagus is a tubular structure which starts at the lower end of the oropharynx. It descends through the lower part of the neck, and enters the thorax through its inlet. After passing through the thorax the oesophagus enters the abdomen. After a very short course through the abdomen it ends by joining the cardiac end of the stomach.

THE STOMACH

The stomach is a sac-like structure that serves as a reservoir of swallowed food, and plays an important part in digesting it. It has a capacity of about one litre. It is the most dilated part of the alimentary canal. Its shape varies considerably depending upon whether it is full or empty; and is also influenced by posture. However, for purposes of description we can presume it to have the form shown in Fig. 13.3. The cranial end of the stomach is continuous with the oesophagus. As this end lies close to the heart it is named the *cardiac end*.

The caudal end of the stomach is continuous with the duodenum. This end is called the

Fig. 13.2. Tongue and some related structures seen from above.

Labels (left side, top to bottom): Mucosa of pharynx, Palatopharyngeal fold, Palatine tonsil, Palatoglossal fold, Mucosa of cheek, Foliate papillae, Vallate papillae, Sulcus terminalis, Fungiform papillae, Lateral margin of tongue

Labels (right side, top to bottom): Cavity of pharynx, Epiglottis, Median glossoepiglottic fold, Lateral glossoepiglottic fold, Foramen caecum, Pharyngeal part of tongue, Oral part of tongue

Apex of tongue

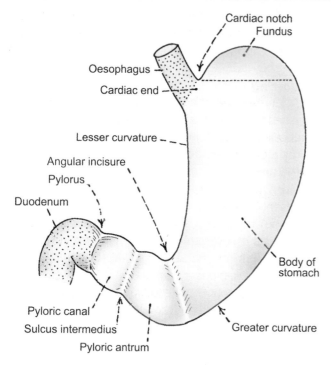

Fig. 13.3. Subdivisions of the stomach.

pyloric end, or simply the **pylorus**. The stomach has two surfaces, anterior and posterior. These surfaces meet at a concave upper border, and at a lower border that is convex. The concave upper border is called the **lesser curvature**, and the convex lower border is called the **greater curvature**.

The stomach is divided into a number of parts as follows (Fig. 13.3).

(a) At the junction of the left margin of the oesophagus with the greater curvature of the stomach there is a deep **cardiac notch**. Because of the upward convexity of the adjoining part of the greater curvature a part of the stomach lies above the level of the cardio-oesophageal junction. This part of the stomach is called the **fundus**.

(b) We have seen that the upper part of the lesser curvature faces to the right, while its lower part faces upwards. The junction of these parts of the curvature is often marked by a notch called the **angular incisure**. The part of the stomach to the left of the incisure is more or less rounded and is called the **body** (excluding the part already defined as the fundus).

(c) The part of the stomach to the right of the angular incisure is the **pyloric part**. It consists of a relatively dilated left part (continuous with the body) called the **pyloric antrum**; and a narrower right part called the **pyloric canal**.

Functions of the Stomach

The stomach is a reservoir for food. Its average capacity is between 1.0 to 1.5 litres.

Contractions of stomach muscle churn up the food and thoroughly mix it up with gastric juice secreted by the stomach, and thus liquefy it. The enzyme **pepsin** present in gastric juice is useful in digestion of proteins, which are broken down into polypeptides.

Gastric juice is highly acidic. The acid helps in digestion. It also kills microorganisms that enter the stomach.

The stomach plays an important role in digestion and absorption of iron. Hydrochloric acid dissolves iron salts. The stomach produces an intrinsic factor that is necessary for absorption of vitamin B_{12}.

After food is thoroughly liquefied, and has been acidified, it passes into the duodenum.

Gastric Juice contains water, mucous, hydrochloric acid, and pepsinogens (which are converted into the enzyme pepsin). Gastric juice also contains **intrinsic factor**, which is necessary for absorption of vitamin B_{12}. Some mineral salts are also present.

Water helps to liquefy food. Hydrochloric acid kills swallowed germs. It converts inactive pepsinogens into active pepsin, which digests proteins. Mucous protects the wall of the stomach from mechanical injury and from harmful effects of hydrochloric acid.

Secretion of Gastric Juice

1. The empty stomach contains a small quantity of gastric juice (fasting juice).
2. The mere thought of food produces secretion of some gastric juice (cephalic phase).
3. Presence of food in the stomach is the main stimulant for production of gastric juice (gastric phase).
4. A hormone, called **gastrin**, is secreted by cells in the pyloric antrum and in the duodenum. It stimulates production of gastric juice.

THE SMALL INTESTINE

The small intestine is a tube about five meters long. It is divided into three parts. These are (in cranio-caudal sequence) the **duodenum,** the **jejunum** and the **ileum.**

The Duodenum

The duodenum forms the first 25 cm (10 inches) of the small intestine. It is in the form of a roughly C-shaped loop which is retroperitoneal and, therefore, fixed to the posterior abdominal wall. It is continuous at its cranial end with the stomach. The junction between the two is called the **pyloroduodenal junction**. At its caudal end,

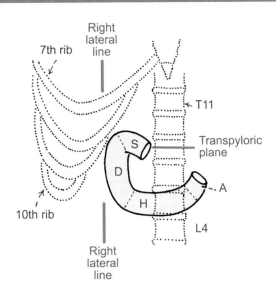

Fig. 13.4. Parts of the duodenum and their surface projection. S= superior part; D= descending part; H= horizontal part; A= ascending part.

the duodenum becomes continuous with the jejunum at the *duodenojejunal flexure*.

The duodenum is subdivided into four parts as follows (Fig. 13.4). The *first* or *superior part* begins at the pylorus and passes backwards, upwards and to the right. The *second or descending part* is about 8 cm long. It passes downwards. The *third* or *horizontal part* is about 10 cm long. It passes from right to left and crosses the midline at the level of the third lumbar vertebra. The *fourth* or *ascending part* runs upwards and to the left and ends by joining the jejunum at the *duodenojejunal flexure*. The junction of the superior and descending parts of the duodenum is called the *superior duodenal flexure*; while that between the descending and horizontal part is called the *inferior duodenal flexure*.

The bile duct bringing bile from the liver, and pancreatic ducts from the pancreas, open into the descending part of the duodenum.

The Jejunum and Ileum

The jejunum and ileum are in the form of a long coiled tube suspended from the posterior abdominal wall by a fold of peritoneum called the *mesentery*. The jejunum is proximal to the ileum. It is about two meters long, whereas the ileum is about three meters long.

The mucous membrane of the small intestine is marked by the presence of numerous, large, transverse, folds. These are few or absent in the ileum. The submucosa contains aggregations of lymphoid tissue

that can be seen with the naked eye and are called the *aggregated lymphatic follicles* or *Peyer's patches*.

THE LARGE INTESTINE

The large intestine is about one and a half meters long. The main subdivisions of the large intestine are shown in Fig. 13.5. These are the *caecum,* the *ascending colon,* the *transverse colon*, the *descending colon,* the *sigmoid* (or *pelvic*) *colon*, the *rectum* and the *anal canal*. The terminal part of the ileum becomes continuous with the large intestine at the *ileocaecal junction*. Near this junction the caecum is also joined by a short, narrow, blind tube called the *vermiform appendix*. The ascending colon meets the transverse colon at the *right colic flexure*. The junction of the transverse colon with the descending colon is called the *left colic flexure*.

The following differences enable a segment of the colon to be easily distinguished from a segment of small intestine.

(a) The colon is much wider than the small intestine. That is why it is called the 'large' intestine.

(b) The outer diameter of a segment of small intestine is more or less uniform. In contrast a segment of the colon shows a series of *sacculations* (also called *haustrations*).

(c) In the case of the small intestine the layer of longitudinal muscle is of uniform thickness all round its circumference. In the caecum and colon, however, the longitudinal muscle layer shows thickenings at three places on the circumference. These thickenings of muscle form three prominent bands that run along the

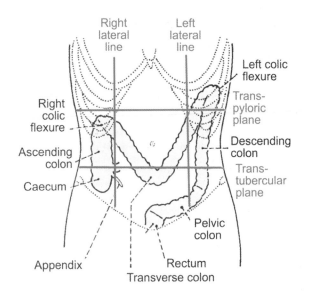

Fig. 13.5. Surface projection of the large intestine. Note that the position of the transverse colon, and of the pelvic (sigmoid) colon is highly variable.

length of the colon, approximately equidistant from each other. These bands are called the *taenia coli*. The taenia coli appear to be shorter than the rest of the wall of the colon. This may be one reason for presence of sacculations in the wall of the colon.

(d) Attached to the outer wall of the colon there are numerous irregular projections called the *appendices epiploicae*. Each of these consists of a small mass of fat enclosed by a covering of peritoneum.

BASIC PATTERN OF THE STRUCTURE OF THE ALIMENTARY CANAL

The structure of the alimentary canal, from the oesophagus up to the anal canal, shows several features that are common to all these parts. The alimentary canal has the form of a fibro-muscular tube. The wall of the tube is made up of the following layers (from inner to outer side) (Fig. 13.6).

A. The innermost layer is the *mucous membrane* which is made up of:

(i) A lining epithelium.

(ii) A layer of connective tissue, the *lamina propria*, that supports the epithelium.

(iii) A thin layer of smooth muscle called the *muscularis mucosae*.

B. The mucous membrane rests on a layer of loose areolar tissue called the *submucosa*.

C. The gut wall derives its main strength and form because of a thick layer of muscle (*muscularis externa*) that surrounds the submucosa.

D. At many places the muscularis externa is coveres by a *serous layer* (peritoneum).

Some general features of these layers are briefly considered below.

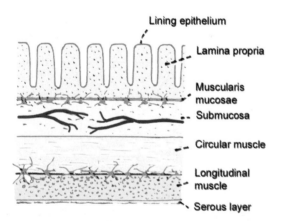

Fig. 13.6. Scheme to show the layers of the gut. Note the large blood vessels in the submucosa; the myenteric nerve plexus between the longitudinal and circular layers of muscle; and the subcutaneous nerve plexus near the muscularis mucosae.

It may be noted at the outset that the oesophagus and anal canal are merely transport passages. The part of the alimentary canal from the stomach to the rectum is the proper digestive tract, responsible for digestion and absorption of food. Reabsorption of secreted fluids is an important function of the large intestine.

The lining epithelium is columnar all over the gut; except in the oesophagus, and in the lower part of the anal canal, where it is stratified squamous. This stratified squamous epithelium has a protective function in these situations. The cells of the more typical columnar epithelium are either absorptive or secretory.

The epithelium of the gut presents an extensive absorptive surface. The factors contributing to the extent of the surface are as follows.

1. The *considerable length* of the alimentary canal, and specially that of the small intestine.

2. The presence of *numerous folds* involving the entire thickness of the mucous membrane. These folds can be seen by naked eye.

3. At numerous places the epithelium dips into the lamina propria forming *crypts* (see below).

4. In the small intestine the mucosa bears numerous finger-like processes that project into the lumen. These processes are called *villi*. Each villus has a surface lining of epithelium and a core formed by connective tissue.

5. The luminal surfaces of the epithelial cells bear numerous microvilli.

The epithelium of the gut also performs a very important secretory function. The secretory cells are arranged in the form of numerous glands as follows.

(a) Some glands are unicellular, the secretory cells being scattered among the cells of the lining epithelium.

(b) In many situations, the epithelium dips into the lamina propria forming simple tubular glands. (These are the crypts referred to above) .

(c) In other situations (e.g., in the duodenum) there are glands lying in the submucosa. They open into the lumen of the gut through ducts traversing the mucosa.

The muscle layer consists (typically) of an inner layer of circularly arranged muscle fibres, and an outer longitudinal layer.

The arrangement of muscle fibres shows some variation from region to region. In the stomach an additional oblique layer is present. In the colon the longitudinal fibres are gathered to form prominent bundles called the *taenia coli*.

Localised thickenings of circular muscle fibres form *sphincters* that can occlude the lumen of the gut. For example, the *pyloric sphincter* is present around the pyloric end of the stomach, and the ***internal anal sphincter*** surrounds the anal canal.

The gut is richly supplied with nerves.

Functioning of the small intestine

Muscle in the wall of the small intestine produces peristaltic movements that move intestinal contents onwards.

Intestinal juice, secreted by mucosal cells, helps in digestion of carbohydrates, proteins and fats. Digested food is absorbed into the circulation. Absorption is facilitated by the large surface area of the mucosa provided by the presence of villi.

Pancreatic juice produced by the pancreas, and bile produced by the liver are poured into the duodenum and play an important role in digestion. These juices are alkaline and neutralise the acid entering the intestine from the stomach.

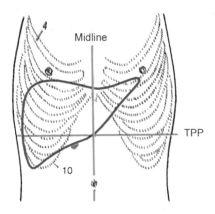

Fig. 13.7. Surface projection of the liver as seen from the front.

THE LIVER

The liver is one of the largest organs in the body weighing about 1.5 kg. It is included amongst the accessory organs of the alimentary system because it produces a secretion, the bile, which is poured into the duodenum (through the bile duct) and assists in the digestive process. All the blood circulating through the capillary bed of the abdominal part of the alimentary canal (excepting the lower part of the anal canal) reaches the liver through the portal vein and its tributaries. In this way all substances absorbed into the blood from the stomach and intestines are filtered through the liver, where some of them are stored; and some toxic substances may be destroyed. Numerous other functions essential to the well being of the individual are performed in the liver. It is, therefore, regarded as one of the vital organs.

The liver lies in the upper, right part of the abdominal cavity (Fig. 13.7). It lies immediately below the diaphragm. When seen from the front (Fig. 13.8) the liver is roughly triangular and appears to have upper, lower and right borders. Most of the liver is placed deep to the costal margin and only a small part of it comes into contact with the anterior abdominal wall.

Basically, the liver has two surfaces. Above it has a convex ***diaphragmatic surface***, and below it has an inferior or ***visceral surface***. The liver is divided into a larger right lobe and a much smaller left lobe.

The liver is covered almost all over by a layer of peritoneum. At many places this peritoneum is reflected on to the diaphragm in the form of so-called ligaments. These ligaments keep the liver in place.

The visceral surface of the liver shows a depression called the ***porta hepatis***. Blood vessels enter the liver here, and the hepatic ducts leave it.

The ***gall bladder*** It lies in a depression on the visceral surface of the liver.

Blood Vessels of the Liver

The liver receives oxygenated blood through the hepatic artery. This artery is a branch of the coeliac trunk. Entering the liver at the porta hepatis it divides into two main branches which are distributed to the right and left lobes.

The liver receives blood from the gastrointestinal tract through the portal vein. At the porta hepatis the portal

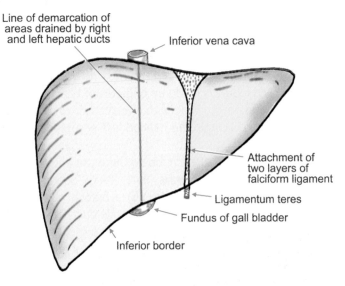

Fig. 13.8. Liver viewed from the front.

vein divides into right and left branches that accompany branches of the hepatic artery. Blood from the liver is drained by a number of hepatic veins that open directly into the inferior vena cava. They do not pass through the porta hepatis.

Histology of the liver

The liver substance is divisible into a large number of large lobes, each of which consists of numerous lobules. The exocrine secretion of the liver cells is called **bile**. Bile is poured out from liver cells into very delicate **bile canaliculi** that are present in intimate relationship to the cells. From the canaliculi bile drains into progressively larger ducts which end in the **bile duct**. This duct conveys bile into the duodenum where bile plays a role in digestion of fat.

All blood draining from the stomach and intestines (and containing absorbed food materials) reaches the liver through the portal vein and its branches. Within the liver this blood passes through sinusoids and comes into very intimate relationship with liver cells. The liver is thus able to 'screen' all substances entering the body through the gut. Some of them (e.g., amino acids) are used for synthesis of new proteins needed by the body. Others (e.g., glucose, lipids) are stored in liver cells for subsequent use; while harmful substances (e.g., drugs, alcohol) are detoxified. The portal vein also brings blood from the spleen to the liver. This blood contains high concentrations of products formed by breakdown of erythrocytes in the spleen. Some of these products (e.g., bilirubin) are excreted in bile, while some (e.g., iron) are stored for re-use in new erythrocytes.

In addition to deoxygenated blood reaching the liver through the portal vein, the organ also receives oxygenated blood through the **hepatic artery** and its branches.

The liver may be regarded as a modified exocrine gland that also has other functions. It is made up, predominantly, of liver cells or **hepatocytes**.

The liver is made up of a large number of **hepatic lobules**. Each lobule is made up of plates of liver cells that branch and anastomose with one another to form a network. Spaces within the network are occupied by sinusoids.

Along the periphery of each lobule there are angular intervals called **portal canals**. Each 'canal' contains (a) a branch of the portal vein; (b) a branch of the hepatic artery, and (c) an interlobular bile duct. These three structures collectively form a **portal triad**. Blood from the branch of the portal vein, and from the branch of the hepatic artery, enters the sinusoids at the periphery of the lobule and passes towards its centre.

Here the sinusoids open into a **central vein** which occupies the centre of the lobule. We have already seen that the central vein drains into hepatic veins (which leave the liver to end in the inferior vena cava).

Bile is secreted by liver cells into **bile canaliculi**. These canaliculi have no walls of their own. They are merely spaces present between plasma membranes of adjacent liver cells. At the periphery of a lobule the canaliculi become continuous with delicate **intralobular ductules**, which in turn become continuous with larger **interlobular ductules** of portal triads.

Functions of the Liver

The liver performs numerous functions. Some of these are as follows.

1. We have seen that the liver acts as an exocrine gland for the secretion of bile. However, the architecture of the liver has greater resemblance to that of an endocrine gland, the cells being in intimate relationship to blood in sinusoids. This is to be correlated with the fact that liver cells take up numerous substances from the blood, and also pour many substances back into it.

2. The liver plays a prominent role in metabolism of carbohydrates, proteins and fats. Metabolic functions include synthesis of plasma proteins fibrinogen and prothrombin, and the regulation of blood glucose and lipids.

3. The liver acts as a store for various substances including glucose (as glycogen), lipids, vitamins and iron. When necessary the liver can convert lipids and amino acids into glucose (**gluconeogenesis**).

4. The liver plays a protective role by detoxifying substances (including drugs and alcohol). Removal of bile pigments from blood (and their excretion through bile) is part of this process. Amino acids are deaminated to produce urea, which enters the blood stream to be excreted through the kidneys.

5. During fetal life the liver is a centre for haemopoiesis.

Functions of Bile

1. Bile is alkaline. It helps to neutralise acidic food entering the duodenum from the stomach.

2. Bile contains bile salts (sodium taurocholate and sodium glycocholate). They emulsify fat and thus help in its digestion.

3. When erythrocytes finish their useful life they are destroyed (mainly in the spleen). One of the by products of their destruction is a pigment called bilirubin. Bilirubin is excreted by the liver through bile, and reaches the intestine. In the large intestine bilirubin is converted

into stercobilin, which is responsible for the brownish colour of faeces. Some bilirubin is converted into urobilinogen, which is absorbed into blood and is excreted though urine.

EXTRAHEPATIC BILIARY APPARATUS

The passages through which bile, produced in the liver, passes before entering the duodenum are seen in Fig. 13.9. The *right* and *left hepatic ducts* emerge at the porta hepatis and join to form the *common hepatic duct*. At its lower end the common hepatic duct is joined by the *cystic duct* (from the *gall bladder*) to form the *bile duct*. The bile duct opens into the duodenum.

THE GALL BLADDER

The gall bladder is a small sac attached to the visceral surface of the liver. The lowest part of the gall bladder, which is called the *fundus*, projects beyond the inferior border of the liver (Fig. 13.8). The central part of the gall bladder is called the *body*. The narrow part succeeding the body is called the *neck*. The neck is connected to the *cystic duct* through which the gall bladder drains into the bile duct.

The gall bladder stores and concentrates bile. This bile is discharged into the duodenum when required. The wall of the gall bladder is made up of a mucous membrane, a fibromuscular coat, and a serous layer that covers part of the organ.

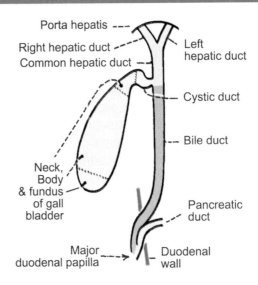

Fig. 13.9. Scheme to show the parts of the extrahepatic biliary apparatus.

THE BILE DUCT

The bile duct extends from just below the porta hepatis to the middle of the descending part of the duodenum. It is about 7 cm long. Just outside the duodenal wall the bile duct is joined by the pancreatic duct. The bile and pancreatic ducts open into the duodenum. The opening lies on a prominence called the *major duodenal papilla*.

THE PANCREAS

The pancreas is a large gland present in close relationship to the duodenum and stomach. It lies obliquely on the posterior abdominal wall. Its right end is enlarged and is called the *head*. Next to the head there is a short, somewhat constricted part called the *neck*. The neck is continuous with the main part of the gland which is called the *body*. The left extremity of the pancreas is thin and is called the *tail.*

Ducts of the Pancreas

Secretions of the pancreas are poured into the duodenum through two ducts (Fig. 13.10). These are the *main pancreatic duct* and the *accessory pancreatic duct.*

Histology of the Pancreas

The pancreas is a gland that is partly exocrine, and partly endocrine, the main bulk of the gland being constituted by its exocrine part. The exocrine pancreas

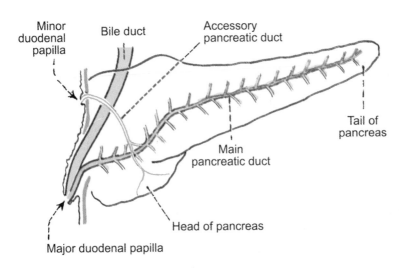

Fig. 13.10. Schematic diagram of the ducts of the pancreas.

secretes enzymes that play a very important role in the digestion of carbohydrates, proteins and fats. The endocrine part of the pancreas produces two very important hormones, *insulin* and *glucagon*. These two hormones are also carried through the portal vein to the liver where they have a profound influence on the metabolism of carbohydrates, proteins and fats.

The endocrine part of the pancreas is in the form of numerous rounded collections of cells that are embedded within the exocrine part. These collections of cells are called the *pancreatic islets*, or the *islets of Langerhans*. Three main types of cells can be distinguished in these islets.

(**a**) The *alpha cells* (or *A-cells*) secrete the hormone *glucagon*.

(**b**) The *beta cells* (or *B-cells*) secrete the hormone *insulin*.

(**c**) The *delta cells* (or *D-cells*) probably produce the hormones *gastrin* and *somatostatin*.

Pancreatic Juice

It consists of water, some mineral salts, and enzymes which are as follows:

1. Amylase helps in digestion of carbohydrates.

2. Lipase helps in digestion of fats. This process is helped by emulsification of fats by bile salts.

3. Trypsinogen, chymotrypsinogen and procarboxypeptidase are inactive precursors of protein digesting enzymes. They become active only after reaching the intestine. Here they are acted upon by enterokinase (produced by mucosal cells of small intestine) and are converted to trypsin and chymotrypsin. These enzymes are responsible for digestion of proteins. The production of pancreatic juice is stimulated by the hormones secretin and CCK produced by cells in the intestine.

NUTRITION

The energy required by the body for performing various functions is obtained from food. Food is also required for growth, for repair of tissues after injury or disease, and for replacement of tissues that have a limited life. The food taken by a person constitutes his diet.

Substances in food that can be utilised by the body are called nutrients, and the use of nutrients is called nutrition. Any food contains one or more of the following.

(a) Carbohydrates
(b) Proteins
(c) Fats
(d) Vitamins
(e) Mineral salts
(f) Water

The body requires all these in appropriate proportion. The greater part of the diet of most persons is made up of carbohydrates (in the form of *chappatis*, bread or rice). Protein requirements are met through milk, eggs, or the flesh of animals. In vegetarians, lentils (*dal*) and beans are important sources of protein. Fats are obtained through milk and milk products (butter or *ghee*), or from vegetable oils (mustard oil, groundnut oil, sunflower oil, etc.,).

Fresh vegetables and fruits are important constituents of diet. Apart from carbohydrates, they provide vitamins and mineral salts which are essential for the body.

An adequate intake of water is essential, more so in a hot country like India.

A diet containing all necessary constituents in appropriate amount is called a balanced diet. A person not receiving such a diet shows signs of deficiency of one or more substances.

Carbohydrates

Food grains such as wheat and rice are made up predominantly of starch, which is a complex form of carbohydrate. Another form of carbohydrate, which is well known to us, is sugar.

Carbohydrates are so called because they contain carbon, oxygen and hydrogen.

The simplest form in which carbohydrates exist is that of glucose. Carbohydrates in food are ultimately broken down (by the process of digestion) to glucose. Glucose is absorbed into blood and reaches all part of the body. The chemical structure of glucose is shown in Fig. 13.11. The carbon atoms are arranged in the form of a ring. Atoms of hydrogen and oxygen are attached to the carbon atoms.

Sugars, like glucose, which exist as single molecules, are called monosaccharides. Another example of a monosaccharide is fructose (fruit sugar). Sugars made up of two molecules are called disaccharides. The sugar we use in homes is a disaccharide called sucrose. It is made up of one molecule of glucose plus one of fructose.

Carbohydrates, derived from food, constitute the must important source of energy required for various needs. When available in excess, glucose is converted to glycogen, which is stored in the body. Excess carbohydrate is also converted into fat.

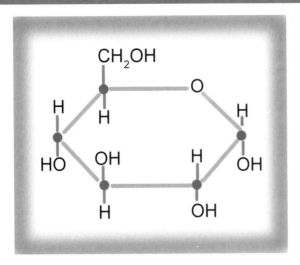

Fig. 13.11. Structure of glucose.

Proteins

Animal flesh is made up mainly of proteins. Egg white (albumin) is also a common form of protein. Proteins are also present in many plant foods specially beans and lentils.

Proteins in food are broken down by digestion, into amino acids. Each amino acid contains carbon, hydrogen, oxygen, and nitrogen. Some of them contain sulphur. The simplest amino acid is glycine. Its structure is shown in Fig. 13.12.

Amino acids join together to form proteins. Proteins exist in various forms. Some proteins form the structural basis of cells and tissues, while others serve as enzymes, hormones, antibodies and many other biologically active substances.

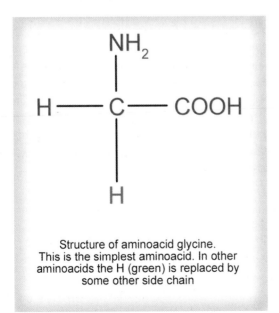

Structure of aminoacid glycine.
This is the simplest aminoacid. In other aminoacids the H (green) is replaced by some other side chain

Fig. 13.12. Basic structure of an aminoacid.

Proteins are essential for growth and repair of tissues. When available in excess, proteins can be used to provide energy, or for storage as fat, but normally carbohydrates are used for this purpose.

Fats or Lipids

Lipids are important constituents of cells and tissues. We obtain fats through milk and milk products (butter, cheese, ghee, cream) and also through vegetable oils (groundnut oil, mustard oil, sunflower oil and many others). Considerable fat is also present in many non-vegetarian foods.

Like carbohydrates, fats also contain carbon, hydrogen and oxygen. Some lipids contain phosphorus (phospholipids).

The basic structure of a molecule of fat is shown in Fig. 13.13. It consists of a core of glycerol to which three

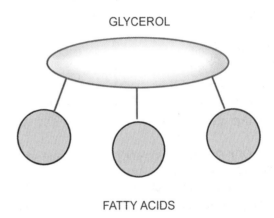

Fig. 13.13. Basic structure of a molecule of fat.

fatty acids are attached. During digestion, fats are broken down into fatty acids and glycerol. Fats present in food are absorbed in the form of these end products.

Like carbohydrates, lipids are a source of energy for the body. When available in excess, fat is stored in the body. Fats are essential constituents of many tissues e.g., of cell membranes and of myelin sheaths of nerves.

Vitamins

Vitamins are substances (present in some foods) that are essential for health. They are needed in small amounts. Vitamins are of two types (1) water soluble, (2) fat soluble. The fat-soluble vitamins are vitamins A, D, E and K. Water-soluble vitamins, are B (made up of several components), and C. The fat-soluble vitamins are present in fatty foods like milk, cheese and eggs. They are also present in some vegetables and fruits. Water-soluble vitamins are present in vegetables, liver, meat, etc. Some vitamins are stable but many are destroyed by heat or by exposure to light.

Vitamin A is necessary for vision, specially in poor light. When this vitamin is deficient the patient suffers from *night blindness*. The vitamin is also important for growth (specially in bone and in epithelia) and for resistance to infection.

Vitamin B complex consists of the following components.

Vitamin B1, (thiamine) is necessary for utilization of carbohydrate. It is also necessary for functioning of the nervous system. Deficiency of this vitamin causes a disease called *beri beri*. The person becomes very weak, and does not grow normally. The person may develop oedema and degeneration of nerves.

Vitamin B2 (riboflavine) is necessary to keep the eyes and vision normal. In deficiency there is blurred vision and cataract may form. Cracks appear in skin at the angles of the mouth (*angular stomatitis*).

Folic acid is synthesised by bacteria in the colon. Deficiency can occur if these bacteria are destroyed by antibiotics. Folic acid is essential for synthesis of DNA and cell multiplication (specially in bone marrow). Deficiency leads to megaloblastic anaemia.

Niacin (or nicotinic acid) is important in fat metabolism. Deficiency causes a disease called pellagra. There are disturbances in skin, mouth and nervous system.

Vitamin B6 (or pyridoxine) plays a role in amino acid metabolism.

Vitamin B12 (or cyanacobalamin) is required in DNA synthesis. Deficiency leads to megaloblastic anaemia and to degenerative changes in the nervous system.

Other components of vitamin B-complex are pantothenic acid and biotin.

Vitamin C

This is needed in protein metabolism and in production of collagen. It is an antioxidant. It is therefore, useful in wound repair and in resistance to infections. In vitamin C deficiency (*scurvy*) the gums get swollen and bleed easily.

Vitamin D

This vitamin is essential for metabolism of calcium and phosphorus, and for maintaining strength of bones. Deficiency in children causes rickets. Deficiency in adults causes osteomalacia. The bones become soft and deformities develop, e.g., in the pelvis.

Vitamin E

This vitamin is an antioxidant. It protects the body from infections by improving immunity.

Vitamin K

This vitamin is required for production of various factors that are important for normal clotting of blood. This vitamin is synthesised by bacteria in the colon.

Mineral Salts

In addition to vitamins, the body requires adequate intake of several inorganic chemical salts.

Calcium and phosphorus are essential for normal bone growth. Calcium is obtained mainly from milk.

Sodium and potassium play an essential role in contraction of muscle, transmission of nerve impulse, and for maintaining electrolyte balance of the body.

Iron is essential for normal formation of blood. Deficiency leads to anaemia.

Iodine is essential for production of hormones by the thyroid gland.

Fibre

After food has been digested and nutrients in it absorbed, some residue is left. This residue is referred to as fibre. Fibre increases the bulk of food eaten and this bulk increases the feeling of satisfaction that comes after eating. Fibre also adds to the bulk of faeces and helps to soften them, thus preventing constipation. Vegetables are rich in fibre.

Water

Water is essential for life. About 70% of body weight is made up of water. All tissues, including blood and lymph contain water. Cell function is impossible without water. Adequate intake of water is essential to replace water lost through perspiration, urine, faeces and expired air. Excessive water loss through vomiting or diarrhoea, through loss of blood or through oozing of fluid in extensive burns, leads to dehydration. Severe dehydration is a life-threatening condition that has to be treated or prevented by intravenous administration of fluids.

DIGESTION

Digestion of carbohydrates

1. Amylase present in saliva, converts some starches into dissacharides.

2. Pancreatic amylase present in the small intestine converts starch into disaccharides.

3. Enzymes present in epithelial cells lining the small intestines contain enzymes that convert disaccharides (sucrose, maltose, lactose) into glucose.

4. Glucose is absorbed into blood circulating through villi.

Digestion of proteins

1. Digestion of proteins begins in the stomach. Pepsinogen secreted by chief cells of the stomach is converted to pepsin by the action of hydrochloric acid. Pepsin converts proteins to polypeptides.

2. Chymotrypsinogen and trypsinogen are produced in the pancreas and reach the small intestines through pancreatic juice. Enterokinase present in the small intestine converts these into active protein digesting enzymes chymotrypsin and trypsin. These enzymes break down polypeptides into smaller units (dipeptides, tripeptides).

3. Peptidase present in epithelial cells lining the small intestine, convert dipeptides and tripeptides into amino acids.

4. Amino acids are absorbed into blood circulating through intestinal villi.

Digestion of fats

1. Bile poured into the duodenum contains bile salts, which emulsify fat and prepare it for digestion.

2. Pancreatic lipase present in pancreatic juice, and lipase produced by intestinal mucosa break down fats into fatty acids and glycerol.

3. Fatty acids and glycerol cannot be absorbed directly into blood. They pass into lymph vessels (lacteals) present in villi, and then into larger lymph vessels. Ultimately they reach the blood circulation

METABOLISM

In simple terms, metabolism tells us what happens to nutrients that are absorbed. It consists of numerous chemical reactions. These reactions release energy, which is utilised for various purposes. Metabolism also includes a study of chemical reactions through which various molecules required for repair and growth of tissues are produced.

ATP

Adenosine triphosphate (usually abbreviated to ATP) is one of the most important molecules in the body. ATP serves as a source of energy. When energy is available it is stored in the form of ATP. When energy is required ATP is converted into energy (Figs. 9.19, 9.20).

Catabolism and Anabolism

Metabolism consists of two basic processes. In catabolism large molecules are broken down into smaller ones. Energy is released and is stored as ATP.

In anabolism small molecules are joined together to form large molecules. Energy is needed for this, and is taken from stored ATP.

A proper balance of catabolism and anabolism is necessary for good health.

The energy that a food can generate is usually expressed in calories, or kilocalories (kcal).

Basal Metabolic Rate

The breaking down of large molecules for release of energy requires the presence of oxygen (Compare with the need of oxygen, present in air, for burning fuel). In the process oxygen combines with carbon (e.g., in carbohydrate) to form carbon dioxide. The speed at which oxygen is utilised, and carbon dioxide produced, tells us how fast metabolism is taking place. This is referred to as metabolic rate.

The metabolic rate is lowest when a person is at rest (so that no energy is being used by muscles); when the body is warm (so that energy is not needed for producing heat); and when the person has not had anything to eat for several hours (so that energy is not being used for digestion or absorption of food). This level of metabolism is called the basal metabolic rate (BMR). BMR is higher in the young (as compared to the old), higher in men than in women. Some diseases (e.g., hyperactivity of the thyroid gland) raise BMR.

Carbohydrate Metabolism

We have seen that carbohydrates ingested in food, are ultimately broken down into glucose. Glucose is the most important source of energy. When glucose is not available amino acids, fatty acids and glycerol can also be converted into glucose. This is called gluconeogenesis.

Glucose absorbed into blood (in the intestine) reaches the liver. When available in excess glucose is converted to glycogen, and is stored in that form. When required glycogen is reconverted into glucose. Apart from the liver, glycogen is also stored in skeletal muscle. If availability of glucose is more than what can be stored as glycogen, it is converted into fat, which gets deposited at various sites in the body.

How glucose is used to release energy

See Chapter 9 (Figs. 9.19 to 9.21)

Protein Metabolism

We have seen that in the process of digestion, proteins are broken down into amino acids. Conversely, when a protein is required in the body (e.g., for growth or repair of tissue), it is synthesised by joining together amino acids.

There are about twenty amino acids in the body. We obtain them through proteins present in diet. Some of these can also be synthesised in the body. However, there are some that cannot be synthesised and their presence in diet is essential. That is why they are called essential amino acids.

Each protein is made up of polypeptides. Each polypeptide is made up of amino acids joined to form chains. One protein differs from another because of the amino acids present, and the sequence in which they are arranged.

We have seen that amino acids are used to synthesise proteins required for cell growth and replacement. Many hormones, antibodies and enzymes are also proteins.

The body maintains a small reserve of amino acids for use as required. This is called the amino acid pool. Amino acids released by protein breakdown are added to the pool and those required for synthesis are removed. However, the amino acid pool can hold only a small quantity of amino acids. When in excess amino acids are disposed off as follows.

1. When other sources are not available, amino acids can be converted to glucose for obtaining energy. Other amino acids form products used in glucose metabolism (acetyl coenzyme A, oxaloacetic acid).

2. Amino acid can be broken down by the process of deamination. As a result, urea is formed and is excreted through urine.

3. Some proteins are lost in faeces.

Fat Metabolism

We have seen that fat present in food is broken down into fatty acids and glycerol. These are absorbed into lacteals (in villi). They pass into larger lymph vessels to ultimately reach the thoracic duct. This duct opens into large veins in the neck. In this way fatty acids and glycerol reach the bloodstream. Their fate is as follows.

1. Some fatty acids and glycerol are used by cells to provide energy (see below).

2. Some are used in synthesis of some secretions.

3. In the liver fatty acids combine with glycerol to form triglycerides (a form in which fat can be stored). When required triglycerides can be broken down into glycerol and fatty acids and these can be used to provide energy.

How fatty acids are used to provide energy

While discussing the production of energy from glucose we have seen that one intermediate product of glucose utilization is acetyl coenzyme A which is then used in reactions involving the citric acid cycle. Fatty acids can be converted into acetyl coenzyme A, which can be used to provide ATP (just as in glucose metabolism).

Sometimes (as in a fasting individual) acetyl coenzyme A produced from fatty acids may be more than can be utilised. The enzyme is then converted into ketone bodies (in the liver). Ketone bodies can be excreted through lungs and kidneys. High concentrations of ketone bodies are toxic.

14

Respiratory System

INTRODUCTION

The respiratory system is meant, primarily, for the oxygenation of blood. The chief organs of the system are the right and left **lungs**. Oxygen contained in air reaches the lungs by passing through a series of respiratory passages, which also serve for removal of carbon dioxide released from the blood.

The respiratory passages are shown in Figs. 14.1 and 14.2. Air from the outside enters the body through the right and left **anterior nares** (or **external nares**) which open into the right and left **nasal cavities.** Apart from their respiratory function, the nasal cavities have olfactory areas that act as end organs for smell. At their posterior ends the nasal cavities have openings called the **posterior nares** (or **internal nares**) through which they open into the **pharynx.** The pharynx is a single cavity not divided into right and left halves. It is divisible, from above downwards, into an

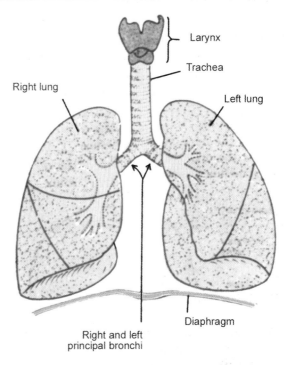

Fig. 14.2. Diagram to show the main parts of the respiratory system.

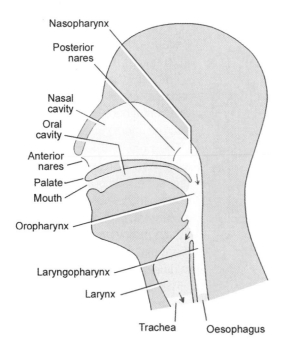

Fig. 14.1. Simplified diagram showing intercommunications between the nasal cavities, the mouth, the pharynx, the larynx and the oesophagus.

upper part the **nasopharynx** (into which the nasal cavities open); a middle part the **oropharynx** (which is continuous with the posterior end of the oral cavity); and a lower part the **laryngopharynx**. Air from the nose enters the nasopharynx and passes down through the oropharynx and laryngopharynx. Air can also pass through the mouth directly into the oropharynx and from there to the laryngopharynx. Air from the laryngopharynx enters a box-like structure called the **larynx.** The larynx is placed on the front of the upper part of the neck. Apart from being a respiratory passage it is the organ where voice is produced: it is, therefore, sometimes called the voice-box.

Inferiorly the larynx is continuous with a tube called the **trachea.** The trachea passes through the lower part of the neck into the upper part of the thorax. At the level of the lower border of the manubrium sterni the trachea bifurcates into the right and left **principal bronchi**, which carry air to the right and left lungs.

Within the lung each principal bronchus divides, like the branches of a tree, into smaller and smaller *bronchi* that ultimately end in microscopic tubes that are called *bronchioles.* The bronchioles open into microscopic sac-like structures called *alveoli.* The walls of the alveoli contain a rich network of blood capillaries. Blood in these capillaries is separated from the air in the alveoli by a very thin membrane through which oxygen can pass into the blood and carbon dioxide can pass into the alveolar air.

Nasal cavity

The nasal cavity is divided by a median septum into right and left halves. Each half of the nasal cavity opens to the exterior through the external (or anterior) nares; and posteriorly it opens into the nasopharynx. A schematic coronal section through the nasal cavity is shown in Fig. 14.3. It is seen that each half of the cavity is triangular. It has a vertical medial wall formed by the *nasal septum*; a sloping lateral wall; a relatively broad floor formed by the *palate* (which separates the nasal cavity from the oral cavity); and a narrow roof which lies at the junction of the medial and lateral walls.

These walls have a skeletal basis that is made up predominantly of bone, but is cartilaginous at some places. The skeletal basis is covered by mucous membrane. Typically, the mucosa is moist and highly vascular. It serves to warm inspired air and also helps to remove dust (which sticks to the moist wall). For these reasons the mucosa is referred to as *respiratory.* The mucosa lining the uppermost part of the septum and the adjoining part of the lateral wall differs from that present elsewhere in the nasal cavity. It is characterised by the presence of receptor cells that are sensitive to smell: the mucosa in this region is, therefore, called the *olfactory mucosa.* Olfactory nerves arise from this mucosa. A small area of the nasal cavity (near the anterior nares) is lined not by mucous membrane, but by skin. This skin bears hair which serve to trap dust present in inspired air.

The nasal septum is fairly often deflected to one side so that one half of the nasal cavity may be larger than the other.

The lateral wall of the nasal cavity is shown in Fig. 14.4. There are three antero-posterior elevations on the lateral wall. These are the superior, middle and inferior nasal *conchae.* Each concha has an upper border attached to the rest of the lateral wall and a free lower margin. The spaces deep to the superior, middle and inferior conchae are called the superior, middle and inferior *meatuses* respectively (2, 3, 4 in Fig. 14.3). There is a triangular space above the superior concha (1 in Fig. 14.3). This is the *sphenoethmoidal recess*.

The part of the nasal cavity just above the anterior nares is called the *vestibule.* The vestibule is lined by skin.

Some additional features are labeled in Fig. 14.4.

The Paranasal Sinuses

These are spaces present in the substance of bones related to the nasal cavities. Each sinus opens into the nasal cavity, and is lined by mucous membrane continuous with that of the latter. Because of this communication each sinus is normally filled with air.

The right and left *frontal sinuses* are present in the part of the frontal bone. Each sinus opens into the middle meatus.

The right and left *sphenoidal sinuses* are present in the body of the sphenoid bone. Each sinus opens into the corresponding *sphenoethmoidal recess*.

Each *maxillary sinus* lies within the maxilla. The sinus opens into middle meatus of the nasal cavity.

The *ethmoidal air sinuses* are located within the ethmoid bone. They can be divided into anterior, middle and posterior groups.

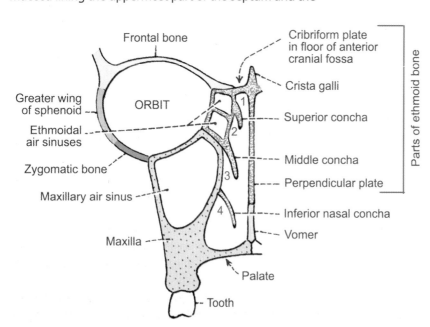

Frontal bone

Cribriform plate in floor of anterior cranial fossa

Crista galli

Superior concha

Greater wing of sphenoid

ORBIT

Ethmoidal air sinuses

Middle concha

Zygomatic bone

Perpendicular plate

Maxillary air sinus

Inferior nasal concha

Vomer

Maxilla

Palate

Tooth

Parts of ethmoid bone

Fig. 14.3. Schematic coronal section through the nasal cavity to show some bones forming its walls. The orbit is also shown.

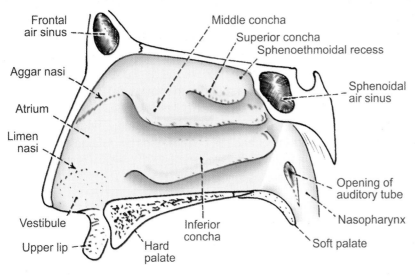

Fig. 14.4. Lateral wall of the nasal cavity.

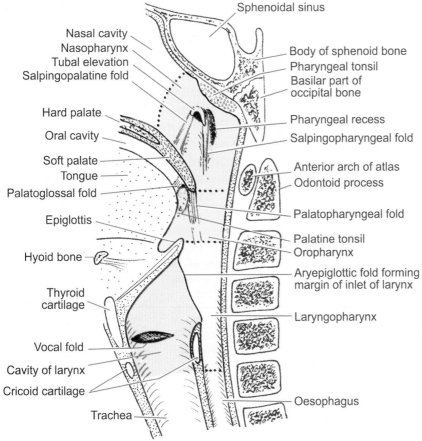

Fig. 14.5. Schematic median section through the pharynx (and neighbouring structures) to show its lateral wall. The limits of the subdivisions of the pharynx are indicated in dotted lines.

The Pharynx

The pharynx is a median passage that is common to the alimentary and respiratory systems (Fig. 14.5). It is divisible (from above downwards) into a nasal part (or nasopharynx) into which the nasal cavities open; an oral part (or oropharynx) which is continuous with the posterior end of the oral cavity; and a laryngeal part (or laryngopharynx) which is continuous in front with the larynx, and below with oesophagus.

The communication between the nasopharynx and the oropharynx is called the *pharyngeal isthmus*. This isthmus can be closed (e.g., during swallowing) by elevation of the soft palate.

The communication between the oral cavity and the pharynx is called the *oropharyngeal isthmus* (Fig. 14.6). It is bounded above by the soft palate, below by the posterior part of the tongue, and on either side by the palatoglossal arches. The oropharyngeal isthmus can be closed by contraction of muscles. This closure plays an important part in deglutition.

In Fig. 14.6 observe the palatine tonsil lying close to the isthmus.

The laryngopharynx lies just behind the larynx. The opening from pharynx into larynx is called the *inlet of the larynx*.

Note the following additional features.

(a) On each lateral wall of the nasopharynx there is an opening which leads into the auditory tube. This tube connects the nasopharynx to the middle ear.

(b) The mucosa of the median part of the roof of the nasopharynx shows a bulging produced by a mass of lymphoid tissue. This lymphoid tissue constitutes the *pharyngeal tonsil*. (When enlarged, the pharyngeal tonsil is referred to as *adenoids*). Some lymphoid tissue is also present

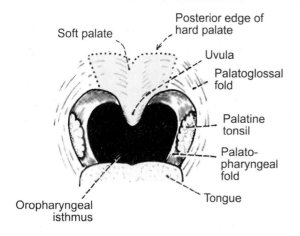

Fig. 14.6. Soft palate as seen through the mouth. The dotted line indicates its upper and lateral limits.

behind the opening of the auditory tube. This collection of lymphoid tissue is called the **tubal tonsil**.

(c) The palatine tonsil lies in the lateral wall of the oropharynx.

The Larynx

The larynx is a space that communicates above with the laryngeal part of the pharynx, and below with the trachea. Apart from being a respiratory passage the larynx is the organ where voice is produced. Near the middle of the larynx there are a pair of **vocal folds** (one right and one left) that project into the laryngeal cavity (Fig.14.7). Between these folds there is an interval called the **rima glottidis.** The rima is fairly wide in ordinary breathing. When we wish to speak the two vocal folds come close together narrowing the rima glottidis. Expired air passing through the narrow gap causes the vocal folds to vibrate resulting in the production of sound. Variation in the loudness of sound is produced by the force with which air is expelled through the rima glottidis.

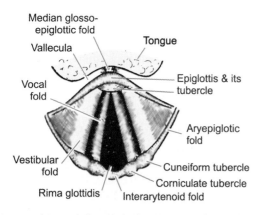

Fig. 14.7. Some features of the larynx as seen through a laryngoscope (i.e., from above). The gap between the two vestibular folds is the rima vestibuli.

The Trachea

The trachea is a wide tube lying on the front of the neck more or less in the middle line. The upper end of the trachea is continuous with the lower end of the larynx. At the root of the neck the trachea passes into the thorax (superior mediastinum).

The lumen of the trachea is kept patent because of the presence of a series of cartilaginous rings in its wall. At its lower end the trachea ends by dividing into the right and left principal bronchi. Each principal bronchus enters the corresponding lung (Fig. 14.1).

THE LUNGS

The right and left lungs lie in the corresponding halves of the thorax. They are separated from each other by structures in the mediastinum (including the heart, the great vessels entering or leaving the heart, the trachea, and the oesophagus). A general idea of the shape of the lungs can be had from Fig. 14.1 in which both lungs are shown as seen from the front. A basic idea of the surfaces and borders of the lungs can be obtained from Fig. 14.9.

Each lung has a relatively narrow upper end, or **apex**; a much broader inferior surface or **base**; a rounded **lateral** or **costal surface**; and a **medial surface**. The costal surface meets the medial surface, in front at the **anterior border** and behind at the **posterior border**. The costal and medial surfaces end, below, in an **inferior border** by which they are separated from the base. The surface of the lung is free all round and is covered by pleura (visceral layer) except at an area of the medial surface called the **hilum**. The principal bronchus and the pulmonary artery enter the lung, and the pulmonary veins leave it, at the hilum.

Fissures and Lobes of The Lungs

Both the right and left lungs have a prominent **oblique fissure**. The right lung has an additional **horizontal fissure**. These fissures divide the left lung into **superior** and **inferior lobes**. The right lung has an additional **middle lobe**.

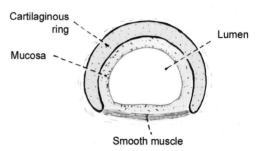

Fig. 14.8. Low power view of a section through the trachea.

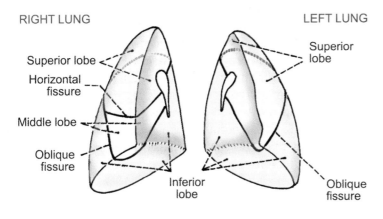

RIGHT LUNG
LEFT LUNG

Superior lobe

Horizontal fissure

Middle lobe

Oblique fissure

Superior lobe

Inferior lobe

Oblique fissure

Fig. 14.9. Simplified drawings of right and left lungs as seen from the anteromedial aspect to show fissures and lobes.

On entering the lung the principal bronchus divides into secondary, or **lobar bronchi** (one for each lobe). Each lobar bronchus divides into tertiary, or **segmental bronchi** (one for each segment of the lobe). The segmental bronchi divide into smaller and smaller bronchi, which ultimately end in **bronchioles**. The lung substance is divided into numerous lobules each of which receives a **lobular bronchiole**. The lobular bronchiole gives off a number of **terminal bronchioles** (Fig. 14.10). As indicated by their name the terminal bronchioles represent the most distal parts of the conducting passage. Each terminal bronchiole ends by dividing into **respiratory bronchioles**. Each respiratory bronchiole ends by dividing into a few **alveolar ducts**. Each alveolar duct ends in a passage, the **atrium**, which leads into a number of rounded **alveolar sacs**. Each alveolar sac is studded with a number of air sacs or **alveoli**. The alveoli are blind sacs having very thin walls through which oxygen passes from air into blood, and carbon dioxide passes from blood into air.

The amount of muscle in the bronchial wall increases as the bronchi become smaller. The presence of muscle in the walls of bronchi is of considerable clinical significance. Spasm of this muscle constricts the bronchi and can cause difficulty in breathing. This is specially likely to occur in allergic conditions and leads to a disease called **asthma**.

Blood vessels of the Lungs

The blood supply of the lungs is peculiar in that two sets of arteries carry blood to them.

(**1**) The pulmonary arteries convey deoxygenated blood from the right ventricle. This blood circulates through a capillary plexus intimately related to the walls of the alveoli, and receives oxygen from the alveolar air. This blood which is now oxygenated is returned to the heart (left atrium) through the pulmonary veins.

(**2**) The lungs also receive oxygenated blood like any other tissue in the body. This is conveyed through the bronchial arteries. This blood supplies the walls of the bronchi and the connective tissue of the lung.

THE PLEURA

The right and left pleurae (singular = pleura) are thin serous membranes which are closely related to the corresponding lungs and to the corresponding half of the thoracic wall. The arrangement of the pleura is best understood by thinking of it as a closed sac that is invaginated (from the medial side) by the corresponding lung. As a result of this invagination the pleura of each side comes to have an inner or **visceral layer** that is closely adherent to the surface of the lung; and an outer, or **parietal layer** that lines the wall of the thoracic cavity.

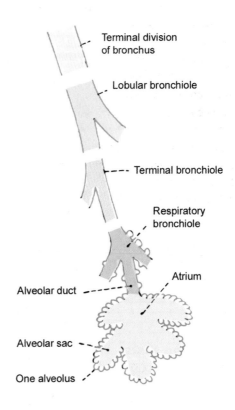

Terminal division of bronchus

Lobular bronchiole

Terminal bronchiole

Respiratory bronchiole

Atrium

Alveolar duct

Alveolar sac

One alveolus

Fig. 14.10. Scheme to show some terms used to describe the terminal ramifications of the bronchial tree.

SOME PHYSIOLOGICAL CONSIDERATIONS

RESPIRATORY CYCLE

Each respiratory cycle consists of:

(a) *inspiration* in which air is taken into the lungs;

(b) *expiration* in which air is breathed out; and

(c) a short pause before the next inspiration.

Mechanism of respiration
Mechanism of respiration

The pumping of air in and out of the lungs is a result of respiratory movements performed by respiratory muscles. The most important of these is the *diaphragm*. The diaphragm is so called because it forms a partition between the thorax and the abdomen. Another important set of respiratory muscles are the *intercostal muscles* that occupy the intercostal spaces (intervals between adjacent ribs).

When the thoracic cavity expands, a negative pressure is created within the pleural cavity. This negative pressure exerts a pull on elastic tissue within the lungs causing the lungs to expand. Expansion of the lungs draws air into them. The reverse happens in expiration.

The main force for expansion of the thoracic cavity (in inspiration) is provided by the diaphragm. When this muscle contracts its central part (which is tendinous) is pulled downwards. This increases the vertical diameter of the thorax. When the diaphragm relaxes, pressure of abdominal contents pushes it upwards.

The second force for expansion of the thorax is provided by intercostal muscles that move the ribs. These movements, along with movements of the sternum, increase the lateral and anteroposterior dimensions of the thorax.

For proper breathing it is necessary that the airway should be normal. In patients of asthma contraction of muscle in the walls of bronchi leads to broncho-constriction. The person has to make greater effort to breathe.

Lung Function tests

In investigating a patient with a respiratory problem some tests are done. You should be familiar with the following terms.

1. The air taken into the lungs in one inspiration is called *tidal volume*. It is about 500 ml.

2. In normal breathing the thoracic cavity does not expand to its full extent. Full expansion takes place when we inspire as forcefully as we can. The quantity of air then inspired is called *inspiratory capacity*.

3. The difference between inspiratory capacity and tidal volume is *inspiratory reserve volume*.

4. During normal expiration all air in the lungs is not expelled. The air remaining is called *functional residual capacity*.

5. After a normal expiration, more air can be expelled by force. However, some air remains in the lungs even after forceful expiration. The air that remains is *residual volume*.

6. The maximum volume of air that can be inspired, and expired, in one respiratory cycle is called *vital capacity*.

External and Internal Respiration

The exchange of gases between air in alveoli of the lungs, and blood is called *external respiration*.

Exchange of gases between blood (in tissues), and body cells is called *internal respiration*. When blood circulates through a tissue oxygen passes from blood to tissue fluid, and from tissue fluid to cells. Carbon dioxide passes from cells to tissue fluid, and from there to blood. This process is the reverse of what happens in the lungs.

Transport of blood gases

Oxygen absorbed in the lungs combines with haemoglobin to form oxyhaemoglobin and travels through blood in this form. In the tissues oxygen is released from oxyhaemoglobin. Carbon dioxide is produced in tissue. Some of it combines with haemoglobin to form carbamino-haemoglobin. However most of the CO_2 combines with hydrogen to form bicarbonate ions and these travel in plasma.

Control of respiration

Respiration is controlled by the nervous system. In the medulla and pons there is a respiratory centre that influences respiration. The respiratory centre receives input from chemoreceptors (carotid body, aortic body). When CO_2 content of blood increases chemoreceptors send impulses to the respiratory centre. The respiratory centre sends impulses that increase the rate and depth of respiration, so that CO_2 levels return to normal. The respiratory centre ensures that necessary changes in respiration are made to meet the extra requirements (or altered requirements) in exercise, fever, speech, singing, or coughing. Respiration becomes faster in respiratory infections (e.g., pneumonia), and in circulatory disturbances, produced by heart failure.

Respiratory quotient

This is an expression to show how much carbon dioxide is produced when one molecule of oxygen is used for metabolism. In a person at rest, one molecule of oxygen used for metabolism of carbohydrate produces one molecule of CO_2. Hence respiratory quotient is 1.0. (For fats the quotient is 0.7 and for proteins it is 0.8).

The respiratory quotient increases during exercise. From 1.0 it becomes 1.5 to 2.0 After termination of exercise it falls to 0.5.

Effect of exercise on respiration

More oxygen is required during exercise. The factors that increase oxygen supply are as follows.

1. *Increased pulmonary ventilation*: This is a result of increase in rate and depth of respiration. This is produced by stimulation of the respiratory centre, stimulation of chemoreceptors, by hypoxia, by increase of body temperature and by acidosis.

2. *Increased blood flow* through pulmonary capillaries increases the diffusion capacity for oxygen.

3. *Increased consumption of oxygen*: The oxygen consumed by tissues, specially by muscle, greatly increases during exercise. This is possible because of increased availability of oxygen through blood.

Hypoxia

Hypoxia is a condition in which the oxygen available to tissues is less than normal. Hypoxia can be caused by the following factors.

1. Decreased oxygen content of blood because of decreased availability of oxygen in air (e.g., at high altitude, or in some respiratory and cardiac diseases). This is called *hypoxic hypoxia*.

2. Inability of blood to carry enough oxygen (as in anaemia). This is called *anaemic hypoxia*.

3. Decreased flow of blood as in heart failure or shock. This is *stagnant hypoxia*.

4. Inability of tissue to utilize oxygen (as in poisoning). This is *histotoxic hypoxia*.

Severe hypoxia can result in death. It is treated with immediate oxygen therapy.

The body reacts to hypoxia by:
1. Increased production of blood cells.
2. Increased heart rate and blood pressure.
3. Increased rate of respiration.

Effect of high altitude

As atmospheric pressure is less, there is reduced pressure of oxygen, and this leads to hypoxia. This is the cause of mountain sickness. Breathlessness develops with mild exertion. Headache, depression and irritation are common. There is loss of appetite, nausea and vomiting.

Adaptation to high altitude takes place in a few weeks. The mechanisms for this are as follows:
1. Increase in number of erythrocytes.
2. Increased haemoglobin content of blood.
3. Increased heart rate and cardiac output.
4. Increased pulmonary ventilation because of increase in rate and force of respiration.
5. Increased flow of blood through the lungs.
6. Increased diffusing capacity of alveoli.

Artificial respiration

This is required when breathing stops (but heart keeps beating) in cases of drowning, accidents, poisoning or electric shock. The methods used are as follows.
1. Mouth to mouth breathing.
2. Application of intermittent pressure on the back of the chest.
3. Use of machines.

ACID BASE BALANCE

Acids and Alkalis

Some naturally occurring substances have a sour taste, e.g., lemon juice and vinegar. Such substances are said to be acidic and contain acids. In contrast, some other substance are bitter in taste e.g., sodium bicarbonate used in cooking. Sodium bicarbonate is an alkali. Water is neither acidic nor alkaline.

We know that water contains two atoms of hydrogen and one of oxygen. However, these exist as two ions H^+ and OH^-. H^+ ions are responsible for making a solution acidic. The more the number of free H^+ in the solution, the stronger the acid. The OH^- ion is called a hydroxyl ion. It is responsible for alkalinity. Water is neither acid or alkaline as it contains equal number of H^+ and OH^- ions.

The acidity of a solution is related to the number of free H^+ ions in it. This is spoken of as *hydrogen ion concentration*. For sake of convenience hydrogen ion concentration is expressed in a scale from zero to fourteen. This is called the pH scale. Water has a pH of 7 and is neutral. The strongest acid has a pH of zero and the strongest alkali has a pH of 14.

Fluids presents within the body vary considerably in pH and most of them are mildly acidic or alkaline. For example pH of blood is about 7.4. Gastric juice, present in the stomach, is highly acidic, (about pH 2), the acidity being necessary for digestion of food. Urine is normally acidic but can sometimes be alkaline. It is very important that pH of blood and other blood fluids be maintained within narrow limits.

Acidosis and alkalosis

If the pH of body fluids become more acidic than normal the condition is called *acidosis*. If the fluid is more alkaline than normal the condition is called *alkalosis*.

Some of the factors responsible for these conditions are as follows.

1. CO_2 is produced by metabolism of carbohydrates and lipids. It is removed from the body by the lungs. Hypoventilation reduces excretion and tends to cause acidosis. Hyperventilation tends to produce alkalosis.

2. The pH of body fluids is kept within normal limits by *buffers*. When H^+ ions are in excess, these get attached to some buffers and this prevents the fluid from becoming too acidic. In a similar manner OH^- (hydroxyl) ions get fixed to some buffers preventing the solution from becoming too alkaline.

Some substances that act as buffers are phosphates, bicarbonates and certain proteins. The extent to which buffers can control pH is limited by the availability of buffers. Under certain circumstances all available buffer is used up, and further formation of acid leads to acidosis.

3. Various acids are produced by metabolism of amino acids, and by anaerobic metabolism of glucose. They are excreted through urine. Urine is acidic because renal tubules excrete H^+ ions and reabsorb HCO_3^- ions. Impaired renal excretion of H^+ ions leads to acidosis. Drugs that increase production of urine (diuretics) can produce alkalosis because of excessive loss of H^+ ions. Alkalosis can also be caused by vomiting.

15

Cardiovascular System

The cardiovascular system consists of the heart and of blood vessels. The blood vessels that take blood from the heart to various tissues are called *arteries*. The smallest arteries are called *arterioles*. Arterioles open into a network of *capillaries* that pervade the tissues. Exchanges of various substances between the blood and the tissues take place through the walls of capillaries. In some situations, instead of capillaries there are slightly different vessels called *sinusoids*. Blood from capillaries (or from sinusoids) is collected by small *venules* that join to form *veins*. The veins return blood to the heart (Fig. 15.1).

THE HEART

The heart is a muscular pump designed to ensure the circulation of blood through the tissues of the body. Both structurally and functionally it consists of two halves, right and left. The 'right heart' circulates blood only through the lungs for the purpose of oxygenation (i.e., through the pulmonary circulation). The 'left heart' circulates blood to tissues of the entire body (i.e., through the systemic circulation). Each half of the heart consists of an inflow chamber called the *atrium*, and of an outflow chamber called the *ventricle* (Fig. 15.2). The right and left atria are separated by an *interatrial septum.* The right and left ventricles are separated by an *interventricular septum*. The right atrium opens into the right ventricle through the *right atrioventricular orifice*: this orifice is guarded by the *tricuspid valve.* The left atrium opens into the left ventricle through the *left atrioventricular orifice*: this orifice is guarded by the *mitral valve.* These valves allow flow of blood from atrium to ventricle, but not in the reverse direction.

Each chamber of the heart is connected to one or more large blood vessels (Fig. 15.2). The right atrium receives deoxygenated blood from tissues of the entire

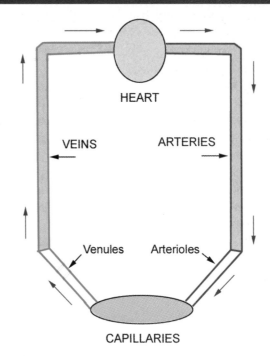

Fig. 15.1. Blood vessels of the body.

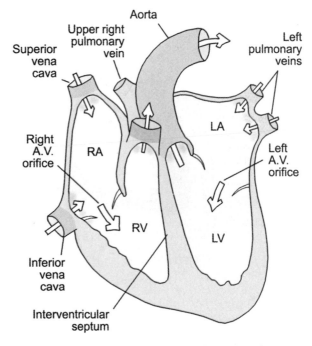

Fig. 15.2. Schematic diagram of the heart, to show its chambers and their communications.

body through the *superior and inferior venae cavae.* This blood passes into the right ventricle. It leaves the right ventricle through a large outflow vessel called the *pulmonary trunk.* This trunk divides into right and left *pulmonary arteries* that carry blood to the lungs. Blood oxygenated in the lungs is brought back to the heart by four *pulmonary veins* (two right and two left) that end in the left atrium. This blood passes into the left ventricle. The left ventricle pumps this blood into a large outflow vessel called the *aorta*: the aorta and its branches distribute blood to tissues of the entire body. It is returned to the heart (right atrium) through the venae cavae, thus completing the circuit.

Blood from many parts of the body has to return to the heart against the force of gravity. The negative intrathoracic pressure created during inspiration has a sucking effect on blood and is an important factor in facilitating venous return to the heart.

The heart is enclosed in the pericardium (Figs. 15.3). The pericardium consists of an outer fibrous layer, and two layers (visceral and parietal) of serous pericardium. The visceral serous pericardium lines the external surface of the heart, while the parietal serous pericardium lines the inside of the fibrous pericardium.

The two layers are separated by a thin film of fluid which prevents friction during contractions of the heart.

Some relationships of the heart can be seen in Fig. 15.3. Anteriorly the heart is related to the body of the sternum and to costal cartilages. This aspect of the heart is, therefore, called the *sternocostal surface*. Inferiorly, the heart is related to the diaphragm (*diaphragmatic surface*). The posterior aspect, or *base*, of the heart is related to structures in the posterior mediastinum (aorta, oesophagus). Towards the right and left sides the heart is related to the corresponding pleura and lung.

In Fig. 15.4, note that the sternocostal surface of the heart is formed by the right atrium, the right ventricle, and the left ventricle. Note also that the apex of the heart is formed by the left ventricle. In Fig. 15.5, observe that the diaphragmatic surface is formed only by the right and left ventricles. The base of the heart is formed by the right and left atria (mainly the left).

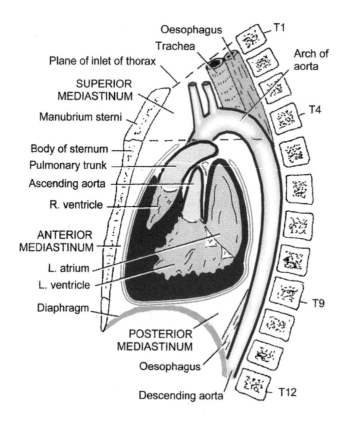

Fig. 15.3. Schematic sagittal section across the thorax to show the heart and some related structures.

Structure of walls of the heart

There are three layers in the wall of the heart.

(**a**) The innermost layer is called the *endocardium*. It corresponds to the tunica intima of blood vessels.

The cavities of the heart (and of all blood vessels) are lined by flattened *endothelial cells* or *endotheliocytes*.

(**b**) The main thickness of the wall of the heart is formed by cardiac muscle. This is the *myocardium*. The structure of cardiac muscle has already been described.

(**c**) The external surface of the myocardium is covered by *epicardium* (or *visceral layer of serous pericardium*). The epicardium consists of a layer of connective tissue which is covered, on the free surface, by a layer of flattened mesothelial cells.

The *valves of the heart* are folds of endocardium that enclose a plate-like layer of dense fibrous tissue.

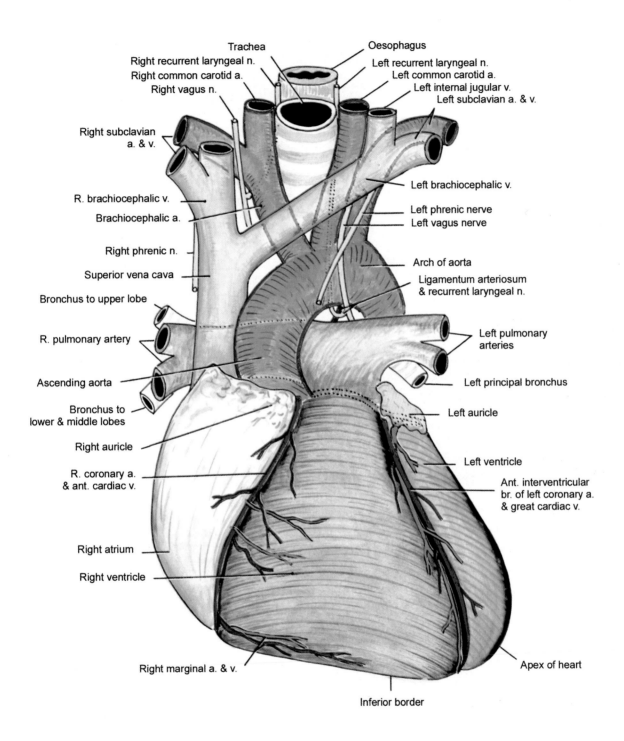

Trachea
Right recurrent laryngeal n.
Right common carotid a.
Right vagus n.
Oesophagus
Left recurrent laryngeal n.
Left common carotid a.
Left internal jugular v.
Left subclavian a. & v.
Right subclavian a. & v.
R. brachiocephalic v.
Brachiocephalic a.
Right phrenic n.
Superior vena cava
Bronchus to upper lobe
R. pulmonary artery
Ascending aorta
Bronchus to lower & middle lobes
Right auricle
R. coronary a. & ant. cardiac v.
Right atrium
Right ventricle
Left brachiocephalic v.
Left phrenic nerve
Left vagus nerve
Arch of aorta
Ligamentum arteriosum & recurrent laryngeal n.
Left pulmonary arteries
Left principal bronchus
Left auricle
Left ventricle
Ant. interventricular br. of left coronary a. & great cardiac v.
Right marginal a. & v.
Apex of heart
Inferior border

Fig. 15.4. Heart and some related structures viewed from the front.

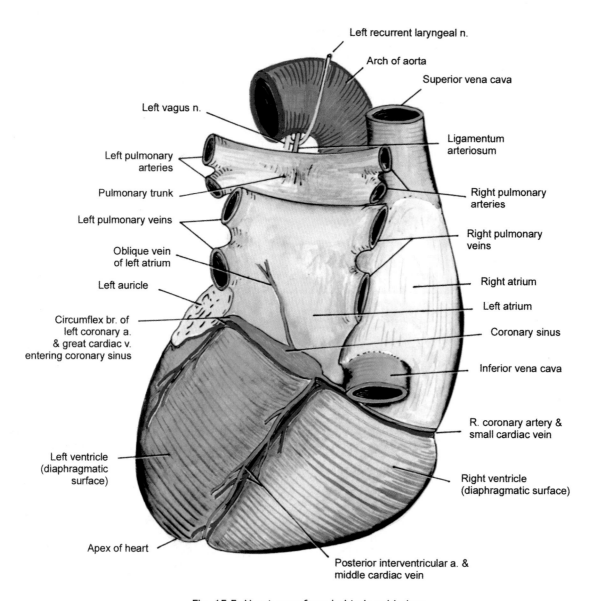

Fig. 15.5. Heart seen from behind and below.

ARTERIES

Basic Structure of Arteries

The histological structure of an artery varies considerably with its diameter. However, all arteries have some features in common which are as follows (Figs. 15.6, 15.7).

The wall of an artery is made up of three layers.

(**1**) The innermost layer is called the **tunica intima** (tunica = coat). It is lined by endothelium. It is separated from the tunica media by the **internal elastic lamina** (a membrane formed by elastic fibres).

(**2**) Outside the tunica intima there is the **tunica media** or middle layer. The media may consist predominantly of elastic tissue or of smooth muscle. Some connective tissue is usually present. On the outside the media is limited by a membrane formed by elastic fibres: this is the **external elastic lamina**.

(**3**) The outermost layer is called the **tunica adventitia**. This coat consists of connective tissue in which collagen fibres are prominent. This layer prevents undue stretching or distension of the artery.

Elastic and Muscular Arteries

On the basis of the kind of tissue that predominates in the tunica media, arteries are often divided into elastic arteries and muscular arteries. Elastic arteries include the aorta and the large arteries supplying the head and neck (carotids) and limbs (subclavian, axillary, iliac). The remaining arteries are muscular.

Although all arteries carry blood to peripheral tissues, elastic and muscular arteries play differing additional roles. When the left ventricle of the heart contracts, and blood enters the large elastic arteries with considerable force, these arteries distend significantly. They are able to do so because of much elastic tissue in their walls. During diastole (i.e., relaxation of the left ventricle) the walls of the arteries come back to their original size because of the elastic recoil of their walls. This recoil acts as an additional force that pushes the blood into smaller arteries. It is because of this fact that blood flows continuously through arteries (but with fluctuation of pressure during systole and diastole). In contrast a muscular artery has the ability to alter the size of its lumen by contraction or relaxation of smooth muscle in its wall. Muscular arteries can, therefore, regulate the amount of blood flowing into the regions supplied by them.

ARTERIOLES

When traced distally, muscular arteries progressively decrease in diameter. They then become continuous with arterioles. Arterioles have a few layers of muscle in their wall (Fig. 15.7). They are important in controlling flow of blood into the capillary bed.

Arterioles having a diameter between 50 to 100 μm are called **muscular arterioles**. Those having a

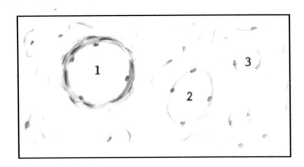

Fig. 15.7. Section showing an arteriole (1), a venule (2), and a capillary (3)

diameter less than 50 μm are called **terminal arterioles**.

VEINS

The basic structure of veins is similar to that of arteries. The tunica intima, media and adventitia can be distinguished specially in large veins. The structure of veins differs from that of arteries in the following respects (Fig. 15.7).

1. The wall of a vein is distinctly thinner than that of an artery having the same sized lumen.

2. The tunica media contains a much larger quantity of collagen than in arteries. The amount of elastic tissue or of muscle is much less.

3. Because of the differences mentioned above, the wall of a vein is easily compressed. After death veins are usually collapsed. In contrast arteries retain their patency.

4. In arteries the tunica media is usually thicker than the adventitia. In contrast the adventitia of veins is thicker than the media (specially in large veins).

5. A clear distinction between the tunica intima, media and adventitia cannot be made out in small veins as all these layers consist predominantly of fibrous tissue.

Valves of Veins

Most veins contain valves that allow the flow of blood towards the heart, but prevent its regurgitation in the opposite direction. Typically each valve is made up of two semilunar cusps (Fig. 15.10). Each cusp is a fold of endothelium within which there is some connective tissue that is rich in elastic fibres. Valves are absent in very small veins; in veins within the cranial cavity, or within the vertebral canal; in the venae cavae; and in some other veins.

Flow of blood through veins is assisted by contractions of muscle in their walls. It is also assisted by contraction of surrounding muscles specially when the latter are enclosed in deep fascia.

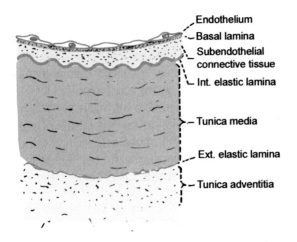

Endothelium
Basal lamina
Subendothelial connective tissue
Int. elastic lamina

Tunica media

Ext. elastic lamina

Tunica adventitia

Fig. 15.6. Scheme to show the layers in the wall of a typical artery.

VENULES

The smallest veins, into which capillaries drain, are called venules. They are 20 to 30 μm in diameter. Their walls consist of endothelium, basal lamina, and a thin adventitia consisting of longitudinally running collagen fibres. Flattened or branching cells called **pericytes** may be present outside the basal laminae of small venules (called **post-capillary venules**), while some muscle may be present in larger vessels (**muscular venules**).

Functionally, venules have to be distinguished from true veins. The walls of venules (specially those of postcapillary venules) have considerable permeability and exchanges between blood and surrounding tissues can take place through them. In particular venules are the sites at which lymphocytes and other cells may pass out of (or into) the blood stream.

CAPILLARIES

We have seen that terminal arterioles are continued into a capillary plexus which pervades the tissue supplied. The arrangement of the capillary plexus and its density varies from tissue to tissue, the density being greatest in tissues having high metabolic activity. Exchanges (of oxygen, carbon dioxide, fluids and various molecules) between blood and tissue take place through the walls of the capillary plexus (and through postcapillary venules).

The average diameter of a capillary is 8 μm. The wall of a capillary is formed essentially by endothelial cells which are lined on the outside by a basal lamina (glycoprotein). Overlying the basal lamina there may be isolated branching perivascular cells (pericytes), and a delicate network of reticular fibres and cells.

SINUSOIDS

In some tissues the 'exchange' network is made up of vessels that are somewhat different from capillaries, and are called sinusoids. The main differences between capillaries and sinusoids are as follows.

(1) The wall of a sinusoid consists only of endothelium supported by a thin layer of connective tissue. The wall may be incomplete at places, so that blood may come into direct contact with tissue cells.

(2) Sinusoids have a broader lumen (about 20 μm) than capillaries. The lumen may be irregular. Because of this fact blood flow through them is relatively sluggish.

(3) Sinusoids are found typically in organs that are made up of cords or plates of cells. These include the liver, the adrenal cortex, the hypophysis cerebri, and the parathyroid glands. Sinusoids are also present in the spleen, in the bone marrow, and in the carotid body.

Blood Vessels, Lymphatics and Nerves supplying Blood Vessels

The walls of small blood vessels receive adequate nutrition by diffusion from blood in their lumina. However, the walls of large and medium sized vessels are supplied by small arteries called **vasa vasorum** (literally 'vessels of vessels': singular = **vas vasis**). These vessels supply the adventitia and the outer part of the media. These layers of the vessel wall also contain many lymphatic vessels.

Blood vessels have a fairly rich supply by autonomic nerves (sympathetic). The nerves are unmyelinated. Most of the nerves are vasomotor and supply smooth muscle. Their stimulation causes vasoconstriction in some arteries, and vasodilatation in others. Some myelinated sensory nerves are also present in the adventitia.

SOME PHYSIOLOGICAL AND CLINICAL CONSIDERATIONS

MECHANISMS CONTROLLING BLOOD FLOW THROUGH THE CAPILLARY BED

The requirements of blood flow through a tissue may vary considerably at different times. For example, a muscle needs much more blood when engaged in active contraction, than when relaxed. Blood flow through intestinal villi needs to be greatest when there is food to be absorbed. The mechanisms that adjust blood flow through capillaries are considered below.

Blood supply to relatively large areas of tissue is controlled by contraction or relaxation of smooth muscle in the walls of muscular arteries and arterioles. Control of supply to smaller areas is effected through arteriovenous anastomoses, and some other similar mechanisms.

Arteriovenous Anastomoses

In many parts of the body small arteries and veins are connected by direct channels that constitute arteriovenous

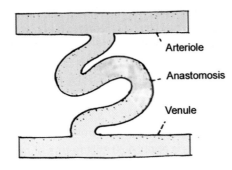

Fig. 15.8. Diagram to show an arteriovenous anastomosis (glomus).

anastomoses (Fig.15.8). These channels may be straight or coiled. Their walls have a thick muscular coat which is richly supplied with sympathetic nerves. When the anastomoses are patent, blood is short circuited from the artery to the vein so that very little blood passes through the capillary bed. However, when the muscle in the wall of the anastomosing channel contracts its lumen is occluded so that all blood now passes through the capillaries. Arteriovenous anastomoses are found in the skin specially in that of the nose, lips and external ear; and in the mucous membrane of the alimentary canal and nose. They are also seen in the tongue, in the thyroid, in sympathetic ganglia, and in the erectile tissues of sex organs.

Arteriovenous anastomoses in the skin help in regulating body temperature, by increasing blood flow through capillaries in warm weather; and decreasing it in cold weather to prevent heat loss.

Factors influencing blood flow through vessels

Blood flow can be influenced by contraction or relaxation of muscle in the walls of arteries (specially of medium size. Contraction of muscle makes the lumen narrower (vasoconstriction) reducing flow. Relaxation makes the lumen wider (vasodilatation). Most of the time blood vessels are slightly constricted. Increased sympathetic stimulation constricts them while decreased stimulation dilates them. Vasoconstriction increases resistance (called *peripheral resistance*) to blood flow. Therefore, the heart works harder to overcome this resistance leading to increased blood pressure. Apart from sympathetic stimulation, blood flow through tissues can be influenced by chemicals like lactic acid (produced by muscle contraction), by tissue damage, or by reduced oxygen supply.

Control of Heart Rate

1. Basically, heart rate is controlled by impulses arising in the SA node which is, therefore, called the pace maker.

2. Stimulation of sympathetic nerves increases heart rate, while parasympathetic (or vagal) stimulation decreases it.

3. Heart rate is influenced by some hormones. The most important of these are adrenaline and noradrenaline.

4. Physical exertion and emotional stress also influence heart rate.

5. Heart rate is increased in fever.

An abnormal increase in heart rate (as in fever) is called tachycardia. Abnormal slowness is called bradycardia.

Cardiac Cycle

The power for flow of blood is provided by the heart, which acts as a pump. This pump-like action is produced by alternate contraction and relaxation of heart muscle. Contraction is called systole. Relaxation is called diastole. The direction of flow of blood is determined by valves. The chambers of the heart contact and relax in a definite sequence.

1. First there is contraction of atria (right and left). This is atrial systole. This pushes blood into the ventricles.

2. Next, there is contraction of ventricles (right and left). This is ventricular systole. This pushes blood into the aorta and the pulmonary trunk.

3. Finally, both atria and ventricles relax. This is diastole. In this stage, blood from veins enters the atria and fills them.

The amount of blood ejected from the heart in one heart beat is called the stroke volume. By multiplying stroke volume with heart rate we can calculate the cardiac output i.e., the amount of blood thrown into the circulation in one minute. It is normally about 5 litres per minute.

Pulse

When the left ventricle contracts a considerable volume of blood is forced into the initial part of the aorta. The wall of the aorta is elastic and it, therefore, undergoes dilatation. As blood flows into a more distal part of the aorta, the initial part returns to normal size, and the next part gets dilated. In this way, a wave of distention travels down the vessel, once for each heart beat. The same wave of dilatation passes into all arteries. This periodic dilatation of arteries is called the pulse. It can be felt by placing ones fingers over any artery that is superficial, specially where it lies over a bone.

The commonest artery used for feeling the pulse is the radial artery, just above the wrist. Other useful sites are the superficial temporal artery (just in front of the ear), and the dorsalis pedis artery (in the foot).

By examining the pulse we can count the heart rate. The degree of dilatation of the vessel with each heart beat is referred to as pulse volume. An experienced person can get some idea of blood pressure from pulse volume. Irregularity in the pulse can also be known.

Heart Sounds

Using a stethoscope we can hear two heart sounds during each heart beat. The first sound is heard at the beginning of ventricular systole and is caused by closure of atrioventricular valves. The second sound is caused by closure of aortic and pulmonary valves.

Electrocardiogram (ECG)

Contractions of heart muscle generate minute electrical currents. These can be recorded using electrodes applied to the surface of the body. Such a record is called an electrocardiogram (Fig. 15.9). The up and down deflections of the recording are referred to as waves.

1. An upward deflection occurs when the SA node produces as impulse. This is the P-wave.

2. Three waves appear close together. The Q-wave is a downward deflection. The R-wave is defected upwards. The S-wave is again downward. The three are referred to as the QRS complex. It is produced by activity of ventricular muscle.

3. After a short interval there is another upward deflection called the T-wave. It is caused by relaxation of ventricles.

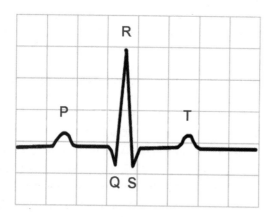

Fig. 15.9. Basic pattern of ECG tracing.

Blood Pressure

When the left ventricle contracts blood is forced into the aorta, and its branches , under pressure. This pressure provides the driving force that makes blood flow through arteries. The pressure is highest just after ventricular systole. This is called systolic blood pressure. The pressure gradual falls and is lowest during diastole. This is called diastolic blood pressure. Normal systolic blood pressure is about 120 millimeters of mercury (120 mmHg). Normal diastolic pressure is about 80 mmHg.

Blood pressure can be measured using an instrument called a sphygmomanometer (or simply blood pressure instrument).

Normal Variations in Blood Pressure

In a healthy person blood pressure increases or decreases from time to time within narrow limits. Blood pressure increases during muscular activity as more blood is required by muscles. Even mental activity can increase blood pressure. Blood pressure rises when a person is excited or angry. It is lowest when a person is resting in bed.

We have seen that activity of the heart can be expressed in terms of cardiac output (amount of blood thrown into the aorta in one minute). We have also seen that cardiac output = (stroke volume × heart rate). To pump blood through tissues the heart has to work against resistance to flow offered by blood vessels. This peripheral resistance is increased when smooth muscle in the walls of small arteries contracts. Conversely it falls when the vessels dilate. When peripheral resistance increases the heart has to work harder (to push the same amount of blood through tissues). Hence blood pressure rises.

Mechanisms Controlling Blood Pressure

1. Some nerve cells present in the brain (in the medulla and pons) constitute a cardiovascular centre or vasomotor centre.

2. The vasomotor centre is connected to the heart and to blood vessels through sympathetic and parasympathetic nerves.

3. Some large arteries (aorta, carotid) contain areas that are sensitive to changes in blood pressure. These areas are called baroreceptors. Nerves arising in these baroreceptors carry this information to the vasomotor centre.

4. Some small organs present close to of blood vessels (carotid body and aortic body) are sensitive to concentration of oxygen or CO_2 in blood. These are called chemoreceptors. Nerves carry information from these chemoreceptors to the vasomotor centre.

5. The vasomotor centre responds to impulses from baroreceptors and chemoreceptors by sending impulses through sympathetic or parasympathetic nerves. The effect is to increase or decrease heart rate; and to cause vasoconstriction or vasodilatation. These in turn lead to variations in blood pressure.

DISORDERS OF BLOOD PRESSURE

Hypertension

In some persons blood pressure remains persistently higher than normal. This condition is referred to simply as high blood pressure, or more correctly, as hypertension. A person whose blood pressure remain persistently above 140/90 mmHg is said to be hypertensive.

In hypertension the heart has to work harder than normal. Over a period of time, the left ventricle enlarges. If hypertension is untreated the heart is eventually unable to pump adequate quantity of blood. Such a condition if referred to as heart failure.

Persons with hypertension are more prone to heart attacks (myocardial infarction); and to stroke (in which an artery in the brain get blocked, leading to paralysis or death).

Hypotension

Persistently low blood pressure is called hypotension. When severe it can lead to shock (see below).

Blood pressure can fall when a person suddenly stands up from a lying position. This is *orthostatic hypotension*, or *postural hypotension*. It is more pronounced in the elderly, and in persons taking medication for hypertension.

Shock

In some of the above sections we have seen that adequate cardiac output is essential for maintaining blood pressure, and this is in turn responsible for maintaining adequate supply of oxygen and of nutrients to cells. If the circulation is unable to maintain this supply the patient goes into a condition of *shock*. The person becomes restless and may become unconscious. Severe shock often leads to death.

Some of the conditions that can lead to shock are as follows:

1. Reduction in volume of blood can lead to *hypovolaemia shock*. Reduction in volume can result from severe bleeding; loss of water from the body because of vomiting or diarrhoea; and loss of blood and plasma because of extension burns.

2. Shock can result from direct damage to the heart. This occurs if blood supply to a part of heart muscle is blocked. This muscle dies (myocardial infarction). This is what is called a heart attack.

3. Shock can occur in severe infections (bacteraemic shock or septacaemic shock); in severe allergic reactions (anaphylactic shock); or by severe disturbances in the nervous system (neurogenic shock).

If shock is mild compensatory increase in blood pressure takes place by stimulation of baroreceptors, by stimulation of adrenaline release by adrenal glands; and by increase in heart rate. The body tries to conserve water by reducing urine formation. These measures can help in recovery. However, if shock is severe, and enough fluid does not reach the brain, brain cells undergo permanent damage. Lack of oxygen and the accumulation of harmful substances (e.g. lactic acid) in blood, disrupts cellular activity and death often follows.

Effect of exercise on Cardiovascular system

1. Exercise leads to some degree of hypoxia (because of heavy demand for oxygen). This stimulates the juxtaglomerular apparatus (in the kidney)to produce erythropoietin. Erythropoietin stimulates mechanisms that result in *release of erythrocytes from bone marrow* into blood.

2. Muscular activity produces considerable heat. Sweating increases and fluid is lost from the body. This leads to *reduced blood volume*.

3. *Heart rate is increased* by increased sympathetic tone and reduced vagal tone. In severe exercise heart rate can reach up to 250 beats per minute. Increased sympathetic tone is a result of proprioceptive impulses from muscles, increased carbon dioxide tension, raised body temperature, and increased secretion of catecholamines.

4. *Cardiac output* is increased.

5. *Venous return* to the heart is increased.

6. *Blood flow* through muscles increase many times.

7. In isotonic exercise, systolic *blood pressure is raised* but diastolic pressure remains normal. In isometric exercise both systolic and diastolic pressures are increased.

Some Diseases of blood Vessels

1. The walls of the arteries of a young person are elastic. They are soft to feel and the vessels can expand or constrict easily. With increasing age the walls gradually become harder, and elasticity is reduced. The intima (which is normally smooth) becomes rough. This occurs because of infiltration of the intima with fat

(including cholesterol) and collagen. These changes are referred to as *atheroma*.

The thickenings formed are *atheromatous plaques*. Atheroma leads to narrowing of the arterial lumen, and consequently to reduced blood flow.

2. Normally, blood does not clot within a blood vessel as platelets do not adhere to the smooth vessel wall. When the wall becomes rough clots of blood can form. These can obstruct a vessel. This is called *thrombosis*. Thrombosis in a coronary artery supplying heart muscle is called *coronary thrombosis*. It leads to *myocardial infarction* (which manifests as a heart attack).

Thrombosis in an artery supplying the brain leads to *stroke*.

3. An artery in which the wall is weakened by atheroma can rupture, leading to haemorrhage (bleeding). Such an event in the brain (*cerebral haemorrhage*) is another cause of stroke, which is frequently fatal.

4. Dilatation of a part of a blood vessel is called an *aneurysm*.

5. Localised narrowing of a vessel (e.g., aorta) is called *coarctation*.

6. Thrombosis can occur in veins (*venous thrombosis*). It can result in swelling (e.g., in a leg) and pain, and in obstruction of circulation through the part.

7. In some people (specially those who have to stand for long periods) the superficial veins of the legs become enlarged and tortuous. They are called *varicose veins*.

Some Disorders of the Heart

1. *Congenital malformations.*

Some children are born with abnormalities of the heart, or of large blood vessels arising from it. The interatrial or interventricular septa may have defects in them so that blood of the two atria or of the two ventricles gets mixed. The valves may not be formed properly.

2. When the heart is unable to pump enough blood into the circulation the condition is called heart failure. The failure can be left-sided or right-sided.

3. We have seen that heart valves can be congenitally abnormal. They can also be damaged by infection (*endocarditis*). If the opening guarded by the valve becomes too narrow this is called *stenosis*. Mitral stenosis is one of the commonest valvular diseases of the heart. In an effort to push blood through a narrowed atrioventricular opening, the left atrium first enlarges, and ultimately fails. When this happens, return of blood from the lungs to the heart is interfered with.

4. Changes in walls of coronary arteries, with age, lead to their narrowing. Enough blood does not reach cardiac muscle. This condition is called *coronary insufficiency*.

At first the cardiac muscle may receive enough blood during normal activity, but not during exertion e.g., climbing stairs. When such activity in attempted the patient has pain in the chest and left shoulder. This is called *angina pectoris*.

The state of the coronary arteries can be studied by a procedure called *coronary angiography*, and site of narrowing or blockage can be localised. In suitable cases a segment of the blocked artery can be replaced to restore the circulation and prolong life. This procedure is called *coronary bye-pass surgery*.

ARTERIES AND VEINS OF THE BODY

Details about the various arteries and veins of the body will be considered in Chapters 26, 31 and 36.

16

Urinary System

Introduction To The Urinary System

The organs of the body that are concerned with the formation of urine and its elimination from the body are referred to as urinary organs. They consist (Fig. 16.1) of the right and left **kidneys**, in which urine is formed; the right and left **ureters**; the **urinary bladder**, in which urine is stored temporarily and is also concentrated; and the **urethra** which carries urine from the urinary bladder to the exterior.

Many harmful waste products (that result from metabolism) are removed from blood through urine. These include urea and creatinine which are end products of protein metabolism.

Many drugs, or their breakdown products, are also excreted in urine. In diseased conditions urine can contain glucose (as in diabetes mellitus), or proteins (in kidney disease), the excretion of which is normally prevented. Considerable amount of water is excreted through urine. The quantity is strictly controlled being greatest when there is heavy intake of water, and least when intake is low or when there is substantial water loss in some other way (for example by perspiration in hot weather). This enables the water content of plasma and tissues to remain fairly constant.

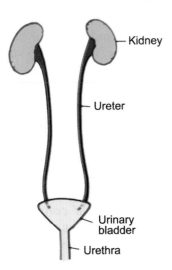

Urine production, and the control of its composition, is done exclusively by the kidneys. The urinary bladder is responsible for storage of urine until it is voided. The ureter and urethra are simple passages for transport of urine.

Fig. 16.1. The urinary organs.

THE KIDNEYS

Each kidney has a characteristic bean-like shape (Fig. 16.2). It has a convex lateral margin; and a concavity on the medial side which is called the **hilum**. Terminal branches of the renal artery enter the kidney at the hilum, and the veins emerge from it. The hilum also gives attachment to the upper expanded end of the ureter (miscalled the **renal pelvis**).

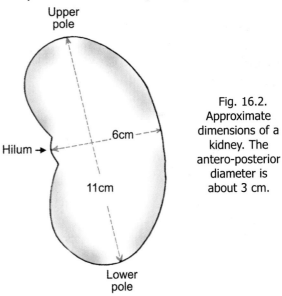

Fig. 16.2. Approximate dimensions of a kidney. The antero-posterior diameter is about 3 cm.

Gross Internal Structure

When we examine a transverse section across a kidney it is seen that the hilum leads into a space called the **renal sinus** (Fig. 16.4). The renal sinus is occupied by the upper expanded part of the ureter which is called the **renal pelvis**; by renal vessels, and by some fat. Within the renal sinus the pelvis divides into two (or three) parts called **major calices** (singular = calyx) (Fig. 16.3). Each major calyx divides into a number of minor calices (Fig. 16.5). The end of each minor calyx is shaped like a cup. A projection of kidney tissue called a **papilla** fits into the cup.

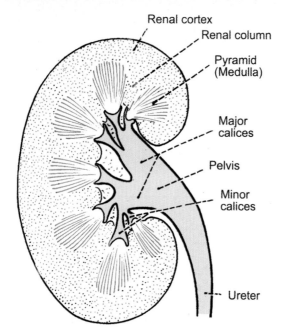

Fig. 16.3. Some features to be seen in a coronal section through the kidney.

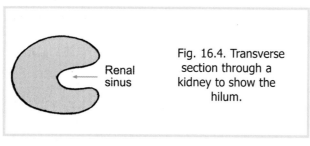

Fig. 16.4. Transverse section through a kidney to show the hilum.

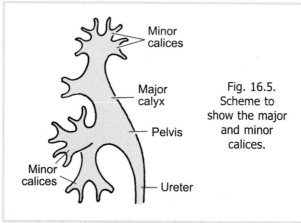

Fig. 16.5. Scheme to show the major and minor calices.

Some features of the internal structure of the kidney can be seen when we examine a coronal section through the organ (Fig.16.3). Kidney tissue consists of an outer part called the **cortex**, and an inner part called the **medulla**.

The medulla is made up of triangular areas of renal tissue that are called the **renal pyramids**. Each pyramid has a base directed towards the cortex; and an apex (or papilla) which is directed towards the renal pelvis, and fits into a minor calyx. Pyramids show striations that pass radially towards the apex.

The renal cortex consists of the following:

(**a**) Tissue lying between the bases of the pyramids and the surface of the kidney, forming the **cortical arches** or **cortical lobules**. This part of the cortex shows light and dark striations. The light lines are called **medullary rays**.

(**b**) Tissue lying between adjacent pyramids is also a part of the cortex. This part constitutes the **renal columns**.

(**c**) In this way each pyramid is surrounded by a 'shell' of cortex. The pyramid and the cortex around it constitutes a lobe of the kidney. This lobulation is obvious in the fetal kidney.

Kidney tissue is intimately covered by a thin layer of fibrous tissue which is called the **capsule**. The capsule of a healthy kidney can be easily stripped off, but it becomes adherent in some diseases.

The Uriniferous Tubules

From a functional point of view the kidney may be regarded as a collection of numerous **uriniferous tubules** that are specialised for the excretion of urine. Each uriniferous tubule consists of an excretory part called the **nephron**, and of a **collecting tubule**. The collecting tubules draining different nephrons join to form larger tubules called **papillary ducts**, each of which opens into a minor calyx at the apex of a renal papilla. Each kidney contains one to two million nephrons.

Parts of the Nephron

The nephron consists of a **renal corpuscle** (or **Malpighian corpuscle**), and a long complicated **renal tubule** (Fig. 16.6). The renal corpuscle is a rounded structure consisting of (a) a rounded tuft of blood capillaries called the **glomerulus**; and (b) a cup-like, double layered covering for the glomerulus called the **glomerular capsule** (or **Bowman's capsule**). The glomerular capsule represents the cup-shaped blind beginning of the renal tubule. Between the two layers of the capsule there is a **urinary space** which is continuous with the lumen of the renal tubule.

The renal tubule is divisible into several parts that are shown in Fig. 16.6. Starting from the glomerular capsule there are: (**a**) the **proximal convoluted tubule**; (**b**) the **loop of Henle** consisting of a **descending limb**, a **loop**, and an **ascending limb**; and (**c**) the **distal convoluted tubule**, which ends by joining a collecting tubule.

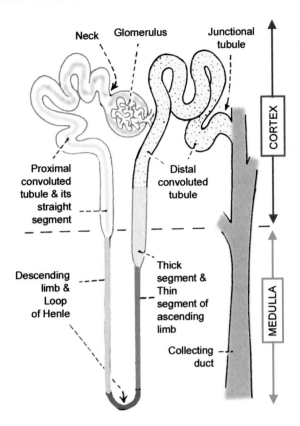

Fig. 16.6. Parts of a nephron. A collecting duct is also shown.

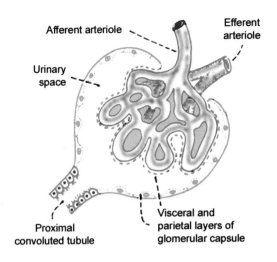

Fig. 16.7. Scheme to show the basic structure of a renal corpuscle.

Renal corpuscles, and (the greater parts of) the proximal and distal convoluted tubules are located in the cortex of the kidney. The loops of Henle and the collecting ducts lie in the medullary rays and in the substance of the pyramids.

The Renal Corpuscle

We have seen that the glomerulus is a rounded tuft of anastomosing capillaries (Figs. 16.7, 16.9). Blood enters the tuft through an afferent arteriole and leaves it through an efferent arteriole (Fig. 16.7). (Note that the efferent vessel is an arteriole, and not a venule. It again breaks up into capillaries as described below). The afferent and efferent arterioles lie close together at a point that is referred to as the *vascular pole* of the renal corpuscle.

We have seen that the glomerular capsule is a double layered cup, the two layers of which are separated by the urinary space. The urinary space becomes continuous with the lumen of the renal tubule at the *urinary pole* of the renal corpuscle.

The Renal Tubule

We have seen that the renal tubule is made up (in proximo-distal sequence) of the proximal convoluted tubule, the loop of Henle, and the distal convoluted

tubule. The distal convoluted tubule ends by opening into a collecting tubule. The following additional details may be noted.

(**a**) The junction of the proximal convoluted tubule with the glomerular capsule is narrow and is referred to as the *neck*.

(**b**) The proximal convoluted tubule is made up of an initial part having many convolutions (lying in the cortex), and of a terminal straight part that descends into the medulla to become continuous with the descending limb of the loop of Henle.

(**c**) The descending limb, the loop itself, and part of the ascending limb of the loop of Henle are narrow and thin walled. They constitute the *thin segment* of the loop. The upper part of the ascending limb has a larger diameter and thicker wall and is called the *thick segment*.

(**d**) The distal convoluted tubule has a straight part continuous with the ascending limb of the loop of Henle, and a convoluted part lying in the cortex. At the junction between the two parts, the distal tubule lies very close to the renal corpuscle of the nephron to which it belongs. The terminal part of the distal convoluted tubule is again straight. This part is called the *junctional tubule* or *connecting tubule*, and ends by joining a collecting duct.

Renal circulation

A knowledge of some features of the arrangement of blood vessels within the kidney is essential to the understanding of renal function.

At the hilum of the kidney each renal artery divides into a number of *lobar arteries* (one for each pyramid) (Fig. 16.7). Each lobar artery divides into two (or more)

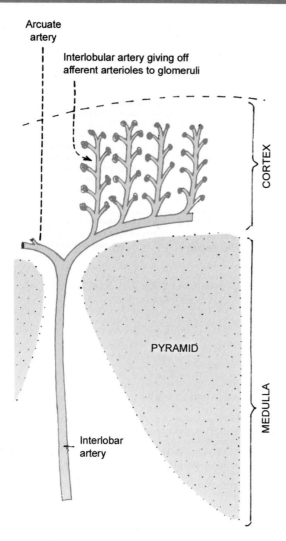

Fig. 16.8. Scheme to show the arrangement of arteries within the kidney.

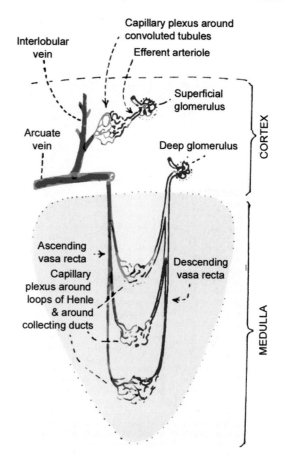

Fig. 16.9. Scheme to show behaviour of efferent arterioles of glomeruli in the superficial and deeper parts of the renal cortex.

interlobar arteries that enter the tissue of the renal columns and run towards the surface of the kidney. Reaching the level of the bases of the pyramids, the interlobar arteries divide into **arcuate arteries**. The arcuate arteries run at right angles to the parent interlobar arteries.

They lie parallel to the renal surface at the junction of the pyramid and the cortex. They give off a series of **interlobular arteries**. Each interlobular artery gives off a series of arterioles that enter glomeruli as **afferent arterioles**.

Blood from these arterioles circulates through gomerular capillaries which join to form **efferent arterioles** that emerge from glomeruli.

Efferent arterioles arising from the majority of glomeruli (superficial) divide into capillaries that surround the proximal and distal convoluted tubules. These capillaries drain into **interlobular veins**, and through them into **arcuate veins** and **interlobar veins**. Efferent arterioles arising from glomeruli nearer

the medulla (**juxtamedullary glomeruli**) divide into several straight vessels that descend into the medulla. These are the **descending vasa recta** (Figs. 16.9, 16.7). These form a capillary plexus that surrounds the descending and ascending limbs of the loop of Henle. It is drained by **ascending vasa recta** that run upwards parallel to the descending vasa recta to reach the cortex. Here they drain into interlobular or arcuate veins.

Juxtaglomerular apparatus

The juxtaglomerular apparatus is a mechanism that controls the degree of resorption of ions by the renal tubule. Its cells monitor the ionic constitution of the fluid passing across them (within the tubule). The cells of the macula densa appear to influence the release of renin by the juxtaglomerular cells. Renin influences aldosterone production (through angiotensin II) and hence controls tubular resorption. In this way it helps to regulate plasma volume and blood pressure.

The juxtaglomerular cells also probably act as baroreceptors reacting to a fall in blood pressure by release of renin. Secretion of renin is also stimulated by low sodium blood levels and by sympathetic stimulation.

Renal Capsule

Kidney tissue is intimately covered by a thin layer of fibrous tissue which is called the capsule. In the healthy kidney the capsule can be easily stripped off; but it become adherent in some diseases.

KIDNEY FUNCTION

The function of the kidney is to produce urine. Many substances not required by the body, or harmful to it, are removed from blood through urine. The process of urine formation is complex. A simplified account is given below.

1. Blood circulating through glomeruli is separated from the cavity of the glomerular capsule by a very thin membrane. Water and many types of molecules pass through this membrane by the simple process of filtration. This fluid has a composition similar to that of plasma except that it does not contain plasma proteins. The fluid is called the glomerular filtrate. The volume of filtrate formed every minute (by both kidneys) is the glomerular filteration rate. This is about 125 ml per minute. Note that this works out to about 180 litres per day. An average person passes only about 1.0 to 1.5 litres of urine per day. It follows that most of the water in the glomerular filtrate has to be reabsorbed.

2. A more or less constant glomerular filtration rate is maintained. It is not influenced by variations in blood present (unless systolic blood pressure falls below 80 mmHg, as in shock), or by nervous influences.

3. As the glomerular filtrate pass through the convoluted tubules, water and many other substances are reabsorbed into the circulation.

(a) When blood glucose levels are normal, all glucose in glomerular filtrate is completely reabsorbed. If blood glucose levels are higher than normal, all the glucose cannot be reabsorbed. It then appears in urine (as in diabetes).

(b) Amino acids, sodium, potassium, phosphate and chloride are also reabsorbed.

Reabsorption of water is influenced by the antidiuretic hormones (ADH) produced by the posterior lobe of the hypophysis cerebri.

Parathyroid hormone, and calcitonin (produced by the thyroid gland) control reabsorption of calcium. Aldosterone (produced by the adrenal cortex) controls reabsorption of sodium.

Some substances that do not pass into the glomerular filtrate, are secreted in to urine by collecting tubules. These include many drugs. Maintenance of the pH of blood is helped secretion of hydrogen ions by tubules (Correlate this with the fact that urine is normally acidic).

Composition of urine

Ninety-six per cent of urine is water. The remaining four per cent is made up of salts dissolved in water. The main salt is urea (formed by protein beak down). Other substances present are sodium, potassium, uric acid, creatinine, ammonia, chlorides, phosphates, sulphates, and oxalates.

Maintenance of water balance

The body has to maintain a balance between water intake and water loss. Water intake is for all practical purposes equal to the water contained in what we eat and drink. (A small quantity called metabolic water is released during chemical reactions within the body).

Some water is excreted through expired air and some in faeces. In hot weather considerable water is lost through perspiration (sweating). However, the most important water loss is through the kidneys.

Nature tries to maintain a more or less constant concentration of water within the body. Some cells in the brain (hypothalamus) are sensitive to osmotic pressure of blood (which is in turn a reflection of its water content). These cells are osmoreceptors. When water content of plasma is less than normal, these cells send impulses to the positive lobe of the hypophysis cerebri (pituitary). These impulses lead to increased secretion of antidiuretic hormone (ADH). This hormone acts or renal tubules, increasing reabsorption of water.

In some diseases urine output is increased (polyurea). This happens in diabetes, but water loss is compensated for by increased thirst and drinking of water.

Maintenance of sodium and potassium concentrates ions

Sodium and potassium ions are essential for the body and their concentration has to be maintained at proper level. Intake of sodium takes place through food. Excess sodium is excreted in urine, and through sweat (when environmental temperature is high). Excretion of sodium is controlled though the hormone aldosterone which is secreted by the adrenal cortex.

Role of kidney in control of blood pressure

Some cells of the kidneys, located near the afferent arteries of glomeruli, produce a substance called renin.

Renin enters the blood stream. Here it interacts with angiotensinogen to form angiotensin-1. Other enzymes convert angiotensin-1 to angiotensin-2. The action of angiotension is to increase blood pressure.

When blood pressure is low the production of renin and of angiotensin is stimulated and this increases blood pressure. Low blood volume stimulates secretion of aldosterone, which increases reabsorption of sodium and of water, to restore blood volume.

Role of kidney in maintaining pH has already been mentioned.

THE URETERS

The ureter (right or left) is a long tube that connects the lower end of the renal pelvis with the urinary bladder. It is about 25 cm (10 inches) long. The upper half of this length lies on the posterior abdominal wall and the lower half in the true pelvis.

THE URINARY BLADDER

In the adult, the urinary bladder lies in the pelvis. However, when distended with urine, part of it extends above the level of the pubic symphysis and comes in contact with the anterior abdominal wall.

Urine is formed continuously in the kidneys and is conveyed to the urinary bladder through the ureters. The urinary bladder acts as a reservoir. When it is distended beyond a certain limit the desire for passing urine is felt. This limit is usually reached when the

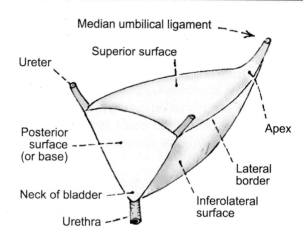

Fig. 16.10. Scheme to show the surfaces of the urinary bladder.

bladder contains about 300 ml of urine. The maximum capacity of the urinary bladder is about 500 ml.

The shape and surfaces of the empty urinary bladder are shown in Fig. 16.10.

The right and left ureters join the urinary bladder at its posterolateral angles. The lowest part of the bladder is called the neck. The urethra emerges from the bladder here. The wall of the urinary bladder consists of an outer serous layer, a thick coat of smooth muscle, and a mucous membrane.

The mucous membrane is lined by transitional epithelium.

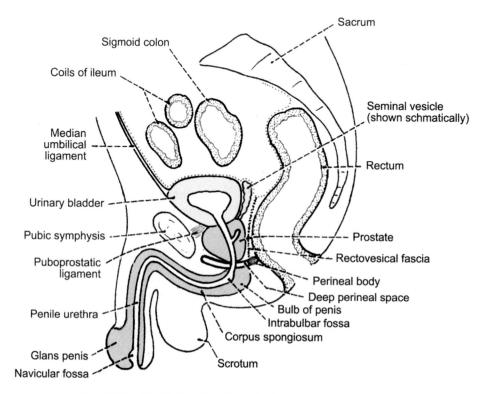

Fig. 16.11. Sagittal section through the male pelvis.

The muscle layer is thick. The smooth muscle in it forms a meshwork. Internally and externally the fibres tend to be longitudinal. In between them there is a thicker layer of circular (or oblique) fibres. Contraction of this muscle coat is responsible for emptying of the bladder. That is why it is called the **detrusor muscle**. Just above the junction of the bladder with the urethra the circular fibres are thickened to form the **sphincter vesicae**.

THE URETHRA

The urethra is a tube that connects the lower end (or neck) of the urinary bladder to the exterior: urine stored in the bladder is passed out through it. The urethra is much longer in the male (about 20 cm) as compared to the female (4 cm). In both sexes its average diameter is about 6 mm.

The parts of the male urethra are shown in Fig. 16.11. The female urethra is much shorter than the male urethra. It opens to the exterior at the perineum.

At the junction with the urinary bladder the urethra is surrounded by a ring of smooth muscle called the **sphincter vesicae**. While passing through the perineum the urethra is surrounded by striated muscle of the **sphincter urethrae** (or external urethral sphincter).

Micturition

Emptying of the urinary bladder leads to passing of the urine, or micturition. For this purpose detrusor muscle in the bladder wall contracts, and sphincters (internal and external) relax. Urine produced by kidneys travels down the ureters and gets stored in the urinary bladder. As the volume of urine increases the walls of the bladder are gradually stretched. When this stretching reaches a certain limit nerve endings present in the walls are stimulated.

In infants, emptying of the bladder takes place automatically in response to stimuli from the bladder wall. It is not under voluntary control. Nerve impulses from the bladder reach the lower part of the spinal cord. Here nerve cells are stimulated and impulses pass down from them to the bladder muscle, causing it to contract. This is an example of a spinal reflex.

As the child grown up, and the nervous system matures, nervous inputs reaching the spinal cord (from the bladder wall) are relayed to the brain. They make the person conscious of the desire to urinate. If the time and place are not convenient, urination can be postponed for sometime. When the time is convenient, suitable signals pass from the brain to the spinal cord, and from there to the bladder, leading to micturition.

17

Reproductive System

The Reproductive System

Both in the male and in the female the reproductive system consists of genital organs that are concerned with the function of reproduction. These organs may be divided into the ***primary sex organs,*** or ***gonads,*** which are responsible for the production of gametes; and the ***accessory sex organs,*** which play a supporting role. The genital organs are also divided into the ***internal genital organs*** (or ***internal genitalia***) which include the gonads and those supporting organs that cannot be seen from the outside of the body; and the ***external genital organs*** (or ***external genitalia***) which are visible on the outside. In human beings (as in many other animal groups) fertilization takes place within the female body. This requires that male gametes be introduced into the female body through the process of ***copulation*** or ***coitus*** (commonly referred to as sexual intercourse). The male and female organs that are concerned with copulation are referred to as ***copulatory organs.*** The region of the body where the external genitalia (and anus) are located is referred to as the ***perineum***.

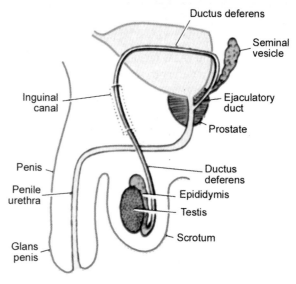

Fig. 17.1. Diagram to show the male reproductive organs.

The testis, epididymis and the initial part of the ductus deferens of both sides lie in a sac-like structure covered by skin: this sac is called the ***scrotum.*** From here the ductus deferens passes upwards and enters the abdomen by passing through an oblique passage in the anterior abdominal wall: this passage is called the ***inguinal canal.*** Here the ductus deferens is surrounded by several structures that collectively form the ***spermatic cord.***

As spermatozoa pass through the genital ducts, named above, they undergo maturation. They get mixed up with secretions produced by the seminal vesicle and the prostate to form the ***seminal fluid*** or ***semen.*** The process of ejection of semen from the body is called ***ejaculation.*** In this process semen is poured into the urethra and passes through it to the exterior. The male urethra is, therefore, both a urinary and a genital passage.

The ***penis*** is the male external genital organ. It is the organ of copulation. Because it is capable of becoming rigid it can be introduced into the vagina of the female, and semen can be injected into the vaginal cavity.

MALE REPRODUCTIVE ORGANS

The male gonads are the right and left ***testes*** (singular = testis) (Fig. 17.1). They produce the male gametes, which are called ***spermatozoa*** (singular = ***spermatozoon***). From each testis the spermatozoa pass through a complicated system of genital ducts. The most obvious of these are the ***epididymis*** and the ***ductus deferens***. Near its termination, the ductus deferens is joined by the duct of the ***seminal vesicle*** (a sac-like structure), to form the ***ejaculatory duct.*** The right and left ejaculatory ducts open into the urethra.

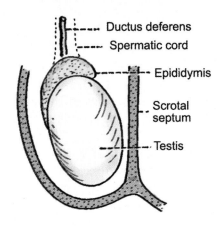

Fig. 17.2. Right testis seen from the front.

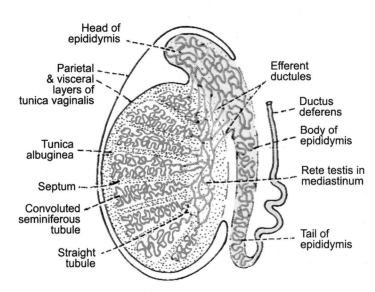

Fig. 17.3. Schematic coronal section through testis.

The Scrotum

The scrotum is a sac that has a wall made up of by skin. Closely united to the skin there is a layer of smooth muscle, which constitutes the **dartos muscle**. The scrotum consists of two halves, right and left that are separated from each other by a septum. Each half of the scrotum is lined by a number of membranes. These are the coverings of the testis (Fig. 17.5). Each half of the scrotum contains the corresponding testis, epididymis, and the initial part of the ductus deferens.

THE TESTIS AND EPIDIDYMIS

Each testis (right or left) is an oval shaped structure about 4 cm in its longest (vertical) diameter. It is about 2.5 cm broad and about 3 cm in anteroposterior diameter. The two testes lie in the scrotum (Fig. 17.2).

The epididymis is a mass formed by tortuous tubules (Fig. 17.3). Its upper end lies near the upper pole of the testis: it is enlarged and is called the **head**. The middle part of the epididymis is of medium size and called the **body**. Its lower part is thin and is called the **tail**.

On each side the testis and epididymis lie in a closed sac which is called the **tunica vaginalis** (Fig. 17.3).

Deep to the visceral layer of the tunica vaginalis, the outermost layer of the testis is formed by a dense fibrous membrane called the **tunica albuginea**. In the posterior part of the testis the connective tissue forming the tunica albuginea is thicker than elsewhere and projects into the substance of the testis: this projection is called the **mediastinum testis**. Numerous septa pass from the mediastinum testis to the tunica albuginea, and divide the substance of the testis into a large number of lobules. Each lobule contains one or more highly convoluted **seminiferous tubules**. These tubules are lined by an epithelium the

cells of which are concerned with the production of spermatozoa. From Fig. 17.3 it will be seen that each lobule is roughly conical, the apex of the cone being directed towards the mediastinum testis. Near the apex of the lobule the seminiferous tubules lose their convolutions and join one another to form about twenty to thirty larger **straight tubules**. These enter the fibrous tissue of the mediastinum testis and unite to form a network called the **rete testis**. The rete testis gives off twelve to twenty **efferent ductules**. These ductules pass from the upper part of the testis into the head of the epididymis. Within the head these tubules become highly convoluted. The **head of the epididymis** is in fact nothing but a mass of these convoluted tubules. At the lower end of the head of the epididymis these tubules end in a single tube called the **duct of the epididymis**. The body and tail of the epididymis are formed by convolutions of this duct. At the lower end of the tail the duct of the epididymis becomes continuous with the ductus deferens.

Seminiferous tubules

Each tubule a lined by several layers of cells that represent stages in the formation of spermatozoa. They are therefore called **germ cells**. The process of formation of spermatozoa is called **spermatogenesis**. Seminiferous tubules also contain cells that perform a supporting function. These are the Sertoli cells.

THE DUCTUS DEFERENS

A good idea of the course of the ductus deferens can be had by examining Fig. 17.1. It is seen that beginning in the scrotum (as a continuation of the epididymis) the ductus deferens passes through the inguinal canal

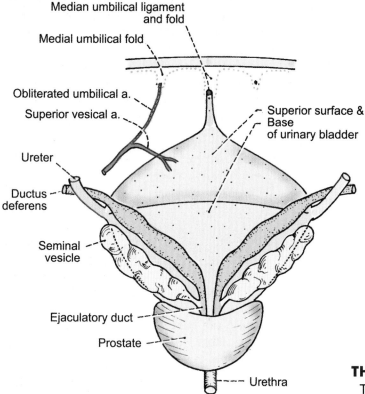

Fig. 17.4. Male urinary bladder and some related structures seen from behind.

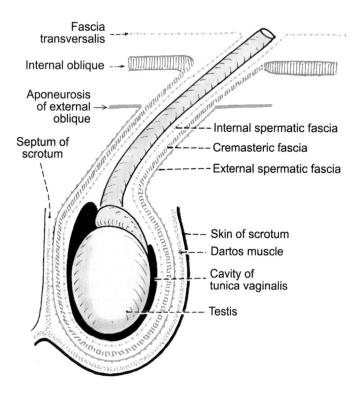

Fig. 17.5. Scheme to show the coverings of the spermatic cord and testis.

to enter the abdomen. It reaches the posterior aspect of urinary bladder. Here the ductus deferens terminates by joining the duct of the seminal vesicle to form the ejaculatory duct (Fig. 17.4). The part of the ductus deferens that lies in the inguinal canal forms part of the spermatic cord.

THE SPERMATIC CORD

The spermatic cord extends from the upper pole of the testis, through the inguinal canal, to the deep inguinal ring. Apart from the ductus deferens it contains blood vessels, lymphatics and nerves.

Seminal vesicle

The seminal vesicle is a sac-like mass that is really a convoluted tube. The seminal vesicles produce a thick secretion, which forms the bulk of semen.

THE PENIS

The penis consists of a *root* that is fixed to the perineum, and of a free part, which is called the *corpus* (or body) (Fig. 17.6). The free part is lined all round by skin. The apical part of the penis is enlarged and conical: this part is called the *glans penis.*

The skin covering the penis is loosely attached except over the glans. Here it is firmly attached to underlying tissues. The glans is also covered by a fold of skin, which extends from the neck of the penis towards the tip. This fold is called the *prepuce*. The prepuce normally covers the greater part of the glans, but can be retracted to expose the latter. The space between the surface of the glans and the prepuce is called the *preputial sac*.

A transverse section through the free part of the penis is shown in Fig. 17.6. The substance of the penis is made up of three masses of spongy tissue, two dorsal and one ventral. The dorsal masses are the right and left *corpora cavernosa* (singular = corpus cavernosum). They lie side by side and are separated only by a median fibrous septum. The *corpus spongiosum* is placed in the midline ventral to the corpora cavernosa. It is traversed by the penile part of the urethra.

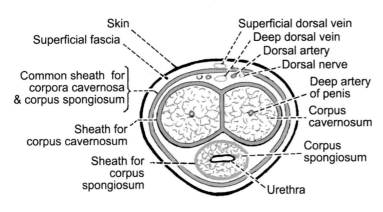

Fig. 17.6. Schematic cross section through the free part of the penis.

THE PROSTATE

The prostate is a glandular organ. It lies just below the urinary bladder and is traversed by the prostatic part of the urethra (Fig. 17.4). The prostate is divided into a number of lobes. The substance of the prostate consists of glandular tissue. The secretions are poured into prostatic part of the urethra.

FEMALE REPRODUCTIVE ORGANS

The female reproductive organs are shown in Fig. 17.7. The female gonads are the right and left *ovaries*. The female internal genital organs are the *uterus*, the *uterine tubes* and the *vagina*. The vagina is the female organ of copulation. It opens to the exterior through a depression in the perineum called the *vestibule*. The female external genital organs are present around the vestibule. They are the *labia majora,* the *labia minora* and the *clitoris*; and some deeper structures that are associated with them. The *mammary glands* are accessory organs of reproduction.

In a mature female one ovum is produced every month (in the right or left ovary). It travels into the uterine tube towards the uterus. Spermatozoa introduced into the vagina can travel from the vagina into the uterus to reach the uterine tube. If a spermatozoon encounters an ovum fertilization can take place. (Fertilization normally takes place in the uterine tube).

The fertilized ovum then travels to the uterus where it gets lodged and starts developing into a fetus (unborn child in the process of development).

The uterus provides the fetus with nutrition and with a suitable environment for its growth. The period during which a fetus is growing in the uterus is called *pregnancy*. During pregnancy a fetus receives nutrition and oxygen from the mothers' blood. Transfer of these from mother to fetus takes place through an organ called the *placenta*.

The uterus enlarges greatly during pregnancy. At the end of pregnancy the fetus is expelled out of the uterus. It passes through the vagina to the exterior as a new born infant. The process of childbirth is called *parturition*. The mammary glands provide the newborn baby with nourishment in the form of milk.

Female External Genitalia

The region of the female external genitalia is referred to as the *vulva* or the *pudendum.* When viewed from the surface we see a midline *pudendal cleft.* The vagina and the urethra open to the exterior through this cleft.

The cleft is bounded on either side by an elevation called the *labium majus.* When the labia majora are

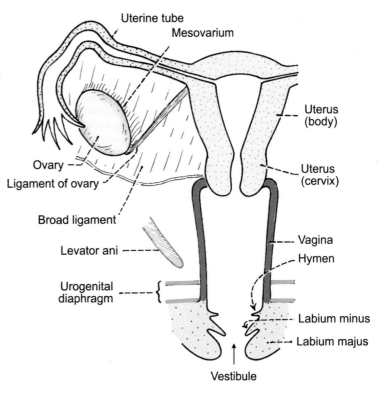

Fig. 17.7. Scheme to show the female reproductive organs.

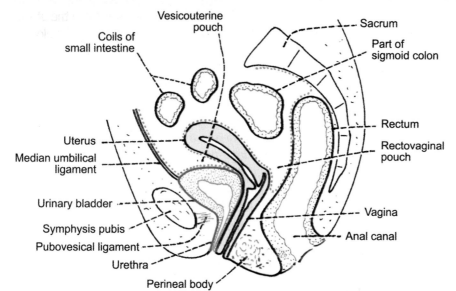

Fig. 17.8. Sagittal section through female pelvis.

THE OVARIES

The right and left ovaries are the female gonads. Female gametes, called *ova* (singular = ovum), are produced in them. The ovary also produces female sex hormones (oestrogens).

The free surface of the ovary is covered by a single layer of cuboidal cells (*germinal epithelium*). The substance of the ovary is divisible into a thick cortex and a much smaller medulla (Fig. 17.9).

separated we see two smaller and thinner folds of skin deep to them. These are the *labia minora* placed on either side of the vaginal orifice. The space between the right and left labia minora is called the *vestibule.*

The external orifice of the female urethra is located a short distance in front of the vaginal opening.

Immediately deep to the germinal epithelium the *cortex* is covered by a condensation of connective tissue called the *tunica albuginea*. Deep to the tunica albuginea the cortex has a stroma. Scattered in this stroma there are *ovarian follicles* at various stages of development. Each follicle contains a developing ovum.

The *medulla* consists of connective tissue in which numerous blood vessels (mostly veins) are seen.

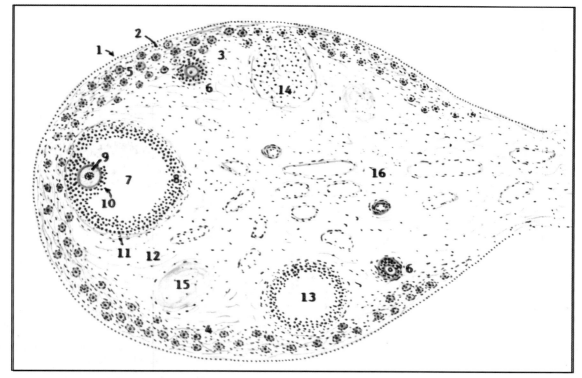

Fig. 17.9. Ovary, panoramic view. 1-Cuboidal epithelium over surface. 2-Tunica albuginea. 3, 4-Cortex. 5-Primordial follicle. 6-Secondary follicle. 7-Follicular cavity. 8-Granulosa cells. 9-Ovum. 10-Cumulus oophoricus. 11-Capsule of follicle. 12-Stroma. 14-Corpus luteum.

Oogenesis

The stem cells from which ova are derived are called **oogonia**. These are large round cells present in the cortex of the ovary. Oogonia are derived (in fetal life) from **primordial germ cells**.

An oogonium enlarges to form a **primary oocyte** (Fig. 17.10). The primary oocyte contains the diploid number of chromosomes i.e., 46. It undergoes the first meiotic division to form two daughter cells each of which has 23 chromosomes. However, the cytoplasm of the primary oocyte is not equally divided. Most of it goes to one daughter cell which is large and is called the **secondary oocyte**. The second daughter cell has hardly any cytoplasm, and forms the **first polar body**. The secondary oocyte now undergoes the second meiotic division, the daughter cells being again unequal in size. The larger daughter cell produced as a result of this division is the **mature ovum**.

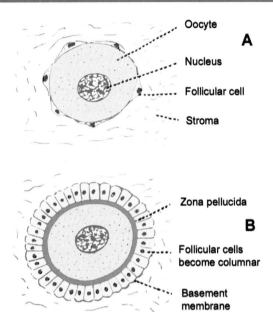

Fig. 17.11. Diagrammatic presentation of: A. Primordial follicle. B. Primary follicle.

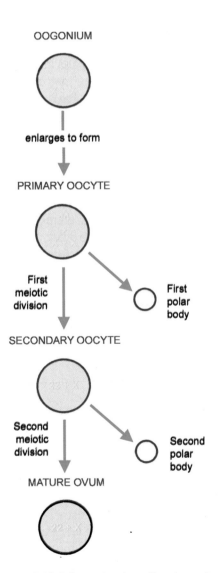

Fig. 17.10 Scheme to show the stages in oogenesis.

The smaller daughter cell (which has hardly any cytoplasm) is the **second polar body**. From the above it will be seen that one primary oocyte ultimately gives rise to only one ovum.

Formation of Ovarian Follicles

Ovarian follicles (or **Graafian follicles**) are derived from stromal cells that surround developing ova as follows.

1. Some cells of the stroma become flattened and surround an oocyte (Fig. 17.11A). These stromal cells are now called **follicular cells**.

The ovum and the flat surrounding cells form a **primordial follicle**.

2. The flattened follicular cells become columnar (Fig. 17.11B). Follicles at this stage of development are called **primary follicles**.

3. A homogeneous membrane, the **zona pellucida**, appears between the follicular cells and the oocyte (Fig.17.11B).

4. The follicular cells proliferate to form several layers of cells which constitute the **membrana granulosa**. The cells are now called **granulosa cells**. This is a **secondary follicle**.

5. So far the granulosa cells are in the form of a compact mass. However, the cells to one side of the ovum soon partially separate from one another so that a **follicular cavity** (or **antrum folliculi**) appears between them. The follicular cavity is filled by a fluid, the **liquor folliculi** (Fig. 17.12).

6. The follicular cavity rapidly increases in size. As a result, the wall of the follicle (formed by the granulosa cells) becomes relatively thin (Fig. 17.12). The oocyte now lies eccentrically in the follicle surrounded by some granulosa cells that are given the name of **cumulus oophoricus**. The granulosa cells that attach the oocyte to the wall of the follicle constitute the **discus proligerus**.

7. As the follicle expands the stromal cells surrounding the membrana granulosa become condensed to form a covering called the **theca interna** (theca = cover). The cells of the theca interna later secrete a hormone called **oestrogen**, and they are then called the cells of the **thecal gland**.

8. Outside the theca interna some fibrous tissue becomes condensed to form another covering for the follicle. This is the **theca externa**.

9. The ovarian follicle is at first very small. It gradually increases in size. Ultimately it ruptures and the ovum is shed from the ovary. The shedding of the ovum is called **ovulation**.

10. After ovulation, the remaining part of the follicle undergoes changes that convert it into an important structure called the **corpus luteum**.

Corpus Luteum

The corpus luteum secretes a hormone, **progesterone**.

(**a**) If the ovum is not fertilized, the corpus luteum persists for about 14 days. During this period it secretes progesterone. It remains relatively small and is called the **corpus luteum of menstruation**.

(**b**) If the ovum is fertilized and pregnancy results, the corpus luteum persists and becomes large. It is called the **corpus luteum of pregnancy**. The progesterone secreted by it is essential for the maintenance of pregnancy in the first few months. After the fourth month, the corpus luteum is no longer needed, as the placenta begins to secrete progesterone.

The series of changes that begin with the formation of an ovarian follicle, and end with the degeneration of the corpus luteum constitute what is called an **ovarian cycle**.

The changes taking place during the ovarian cycle are greatly influenced by certain hormones produced by the hypophysis cerebri. The hormones produced by the ovarian follicle and the corpus luteum in turn influence other parts of the female reproductive system, notably the uterus, resulting in a cycle of changes referred to as the **uterine cycle** or **menstrual cycle**.

THE UTERINE TUBES

Each uterine tube (right or left) lies in the free margin of the corresponding broad ligament. It has medial and lateral ends (Fig. 17.7). The **medial end** is attached to the corresponding side of the uterus. Here its lumen communicates with the cavity of the uterus. The **lateral end** of the tube lies near the ovary. At this end it has an opening through which its lumen is in communication with the peritoneal cavity: this opening is called **abdominal ostium** (Fig. 17.7).

Ova discharged from the ovary enter the uterine tube through the infundibulum and pass into the ampulla. They

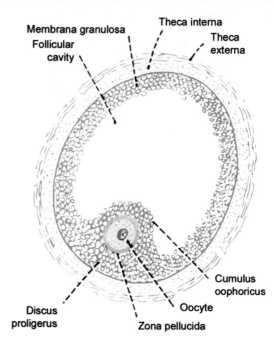

Fig. 17.12. Mature ovarian follicle.

slowly travel towards the uterus. If sexual intercourse takes place at the appropriate time, spermatozoa enter the uterine tube through the vagina and uterus, and meet the ovum in the ampulla of the tube. Fertilisation normally takes place here. The fertilised ovum travels through the uterine tube towards the uterus to enter its cavity. Here, it gets implanted in the uterine wall. If fertilisation does not occur the unfertilised ovum degenerates.

Each uterine tube has a medial or uterine end, attached to (and opening into) the uterus, and a lateral end that opens into the peritoneal cavity near the ovary. The tube has (from medial to lateral side) a **uterine part** that passes through the thick uterine wall; a relatively narrow, thick walled part called the **isthmus**; and a thin walled dilated part called the **ampulla**. The lateral end of the tube is funnel-shaped and is called the **infundibulum**. It is prolonged into a number of finger like processes or **fimbria**.

THE UTERUS

A general idea of the form of the uterus is presented in Fig. 17.7. It is seen that the organ is piriform. It is broader above and narrows down below. The uterus is about 7.5 cm (3 inches) in length. Its maximum width (near its upper end) is about 5 cm (2 inches). Its thickness (anteroposterior) is about 2.5 cm (1 inch). The exterior of the uterus shows a constriction at the junction of its upper two thirds with the lower one third. The part above the constriction is called the **body**: it is broad above and narrow below. The part below the constriction is called the **cervix**: this part is more or less cylindrical.

Sections across the uterus show that it has a thick wall, and a relatively narrow lumen. The wall is made up of a thick layer of muscle (called the **myometrium**) and of an inner lining of mucosa (called the **endometrium**). In a sagittal section (Fig. 17.7) the lumen is seen to be only a narrow slit, the anterior and posterior walls being close to each other. In the coronal plane the lumen of the body of the uterus is triangular (Fig. 17.7). The lumen of each uterine tube join the lateral angle of this triangle. The part of the body of the uterus that lies above the level of the openings of the uterine tubes is called the **fundus**. The cavity of the cervix (or **canal of the cervix**) is roughly cylindrical. However, its upper and lower ends are somewhat narrower than the central part. The upper narrow end of the canal is called the **internal os** and the narrow lower end is called the **external os**.

The Myometrium

The muscle layer of the uterus is also called the **myometrium**. The muscle cells of the uterus are capable of undergoing great elongation in association with the great enlargement of the organ in pregnancy. New muscle fibres are also formed. Contractions of the myometrium are responsible for expulsion of the fetus at the time of child birth.

The Endometrium

The mucous membrane of the uterus is called the **endometrium**. The endometrium consists of a lining epithelium that rests on a stroma. Numerous uterine glands are present in the stroma.

Menstrual cycle

The endometrium undergoes marked cyclical changes that constitute the **menstrual cycle**. The most prominent feature of this cycle is the monthly flow of blood from the uterus. This is called **menstruation**.

Hormones influencing Ovulation and Menstruation

We have seen that the changes taking place in the uterine endometrium during the menstrual cycle occur under the influence of:

(**a**) Oestrogens produced by the ovarian follicle.
(**b**) Progesterone produced by the corpus luteum.

The development of the ovarian follicle, and of the corpus luteum, is in turn dependent on hormones produced by the anterior lobe of the hypophysis cerebri. These are:

(**a**) The **follicle stimulating hormone** (FSH) which stimulates the formation of follicles and the secretion of oestrogens by them; and

(**b**) The **luteinising hormone** (LH) which helps to convert the ovarian follicle into the corpus luteum, and stimulates the secretion of progesterone. Secretion of FSH and LH is controlled by a **gonadotropin releasing hormone** (GnRH) produced by the hypothalamus.

THE VAGINA

The vagina is a tubular structure with a muscular wall. Its lower end opens to the exterior through the vestibule (Fig. 17.7). At its upper end it is attached to the cervix of the uterus. The cervix projects into the upper part of the vagina through the uppermost part of its anterior wall (Fig. 17.8); and that the space between the cervix and the adjoining part of the vaginal wall is divided (for descriptive purposes) into the anterior, posterior, and lateral fornices.

PREGNANCY, PLACENTA AND PARTURITION

Pregnancy is said to begin when an ovum is fertilized. It ends with the birth of the child. The process of childbirth is called **parturition**.

Fertilization takes place in the uterine tube. The fertilized ovum can now be called an **embryo**. After the embryo is three months old we call it a **fetus**.

The fertilized ovum undergoes repeated divisions. By the time the embryo reaches the uterus it is made up of several cells. It sticks to the endometrium. A special structure, the **placenta**, is formed partly by some cells of the embryo, and partly by cells from the endometrium (which is now called the **decidua**). The placenta is responsible for transport of nutrients and oxygen to the embryo, and for the removal of waste products. The essential elements of the placenta are **chorionic villi**. The villi are surrounded by maternal blood. Fetal blood circulates through capillaries in the villi. Maternal and fetal blood are separated by a very thin placental membrane. All substances passing from mother to fetus, or from fetus to mother pass through this membrane.

The enlarging fetus comes to be surrounded by the **amniotic cavity** that contains amniotic fluid. This fluid provides a cushion for the delicate fetus.

Towards the end of pregnancy the amniotic cavity fills the entire uterine cavity. When child birth sets in the membranes forming the wall of the amniotic cavity rupture and amniotic fluid is discharged from the uterus.

THE MAMMARY GLANDS

Although the mammary glands are present in both sexes they remain rudimentary in the male. In the female, they are well developed after puberty. Each breast is a soft rounded elevation present over the pectoral region. The skin over the centre of the elevation shows a darkly pigmented circular area called the *areola*. Overlying the central part of the areola there is a projection called the *nipple*.

Each mammary gland has an outer covering of skin deep to which there are several discrete masses of glandular tissue. These masses are separated (and covered) by considerable quantities of connective tissue and of adipose tissue.

The glandular tissue (or mammary gland proper) is made up of 15 to 20 lobes. Each lobe consists of a number of lobules. Each lobe drains into a *lactiferous duct* which opens at the summit of the nipple. Some distance from its termination each lactiferous duct shows a dilation called the *lactiferous sinus*.

The structure of the glandular elements of the mammary gland varies considerably at different periods of life as follows:

(**a**) Before the onset of puberty the glandular tissue consists entirely of ducts. The bulk of the breast consists of connective tissue and fat which widely separate the glandular elements.

(**b**) During pregnancy the ducts undergo marked proliferation and branching. Their terminal parts develop into proper alveoli. Each lobe is now a compound tubulo-alveolar gland. Towards the end of pregnancy the cells of the alveoli start secreting milk and the alveoli become distended.

The development of breast tissue during pregnancy takes place under the influence of hormones produced by the hypophysis cerebri.

18

Lymphoid Tissues and Immunity

Introductory Remarks

When circulating blood reaches the capillaries part of its fluid content passes into the surrounding tissues as tissue fluid. Most of this fluid re-enters the capillaries at their venous ends. Some of it is, however, returned to the circulation through a separate system of *lymphatic vessels* (usually called *lymphatics*). The fluid passing through the lymphatic vessels is called *lymph*. The smallest lymphatic (or lymph) vessels are lymphatic capillaries that join together to form larger lymphatic vessels. The largest lymphatic vessel in the body is the *thoracic duct*. It drains lymph from the greater part of the body. The thoracic duct ends by joining the left subclavian vein at its junction with the internal jugular vein. On the right side there is the *right lymphatic duct* that has a similar termination.

Scattered along the course of lymphatic vessels there are numerous small bean-shaped structures called *lymph nodes* that are usually present in groups. Lymph nodes are masses of lymphoid tissue described below. As a rule lymph from any part of the body passes through one or more lymph nodes before entering the blood stream. Lymph nodes act as filters removing bacteria and other particulate matter from lymph. Lymphocytes are added to lymph in these nodes.

Aggregations of lymphoid tissue are also found at various other sites. Two organs, the thymus and the spleen are almost entirely made up of lymphoid tissue. Prominent aggregations of lymphoid tissue are present in close relationship to the lining epithelium of the gut. Such aggregations present in the region of the pharynx constitute the *tonsils*. Isolated nodules of lymphoid tissue, and larger aggregations called *Peyer's patches* are present in the mucosa and submucosa of the small intestines (specially the ileum). The mucosa of the vermiform appendix contains abundant lymphoid tissue. Lymphoid tissue is seen in the mucosa of the large intestines. Collections of lymphoid tissue are also to be seen in the walls of the trachea and larger bronchi, and in relation to the urinary tract.

Lymph

Lymph is a transudate from blood and contains the same proteins as in plasma, but in smaller amounts, and in somewhat different proportions. Suspended in lymph there are cells that are chiefly lymphocytes. Large molecules of fat (chylomicrons) that are absorbed from the intestines enter lymph vessels. After a fatty meal these fat globules may be so numerous that lymph becomes milky (and is then called *chyle*).

LYMPHATIC VESSELS

Lymph capillaries (or lymphatic capillaries) begin blindly in tissues where they form a network (Fig. 13.1). The structure of lymph capillaries is basically similar to that of blood capillaries, but is adapted for much greater permeability. As compared to blood capillaries, much larger molecules can pass through the walls of lymph capillaries.

The structure of the thoracic duct and of other *larger lymph vessels* is similar to that of veins.

LYMPH NODES

Main groups of lymph nodes in the body

There are many groups of lymph nodes. From a clinical point poit of view the important ones are those that can be palpated through skin. (a) In the neck there are superficial and deep *cervical lymph nodes*. (b) In each axilla (armpit) there are *axillary lymph nodes*. (c) The *inguinal lymph nodes* lie on the front of the thigh just below the inguinal ligament.

Important groups of deep lying nodes are present in the thorax and in the abdomen.

Normal lymph nodes are not palpable. They become palpable when enlarged. They become tender when infected.

Structure of Lymph Nodes

Each lymph node consists of a connective tissue framework; and of numerous lymphocytes, and other cells, that fill the interstices of the network. The entire node is bean-shaped (Fig. 18.1).

When a section through a lymph node is examined (at low magnification) it is seen that the node has an outer zone that contains densely packed lymphocytes, and therefore stains darkly: this part is the *cortex*. Surrounded by the cortex, there is a lighter staining zone in which lymphocytes are fewer: this area is the *medulla* (Fig. 18.2).

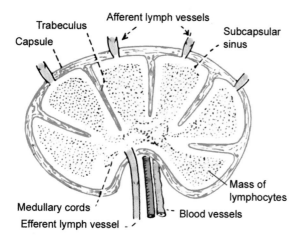

Fig. 18.1. Scheme to show some features of the structure of a lymph node.

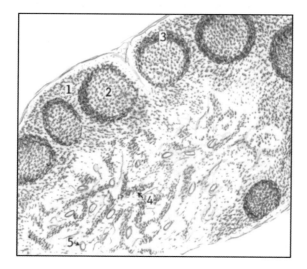

Fig.18.2. Section through a lymph node. 1-Cortex. 2, 3-Germinal center and outer zone of lymphatic follicle. 4-Medulla. 5-Blood vessel.

Within the cortex there are several rounded areas that are called *lymphatic follicles* or *lymphatic nodules*. Each nodule has a paler staining *germinal centre* surrounded by a zone of densely packed lymphocytes.

Within the medulla, the lymphocytes are arranged in the form of branching and anastomosing cords.

Each lymph node is covered by a *capsule*. A number of *septa* (or *trabeculae*) extend into the node from the capsule and divide the node into lobules. The remaining space within the node is filled by a delicate network of reticular fibres.

Summary of Functions of Lymph Nodes

Lymph nodes perform the following major functions.

1. They are centres of lymphocyte production. Both B-lymphocytes and T-lymphocytes are produced here by multiplication of preexisting lymphocytes. These lymphocytes pass into lymph and thus reach the blood stream.

2. Bacteria and other particulate matter are removed from lymph through phagocytosis by macrophages. Antigens thus carried into these cells are 'presented' to lymphocytes stimulating their proliferation. In this way lymph nodes play an important role in the immune response to antigens.

3. Plasma cells (representing fully mature B-lymphocytes) produce antibodies against invading antigens, while T-lymphocytes attack cells that are 'foreign' to the host body.

THE SPLEEN

The spleen is an important organ located in the upper part of the abdomen, on the left side (Fig. 18.3). It is in contact with the diaphragm, the stomach, and the left kidney. Its size is approximately that of a clenched fist. The spleen is supplied by the splenic artery (a branch of the coeliac trunk). The splenic vein joins the portal vein. It follows that all blood from the spleen has to pass through the liver.

Connective Tissue Basis

The spleen is the largest lymphoid organ of the body. The surface of the spleen is covered by peritoneum (referred to as the *serous coat*). Deep to the serous layer the organ has a *capsule*. *Trabeculae* arising from the capsule extend into the substance of the spleen.

The spaces between the trabeculae are pervaded by a network formed by reticular fibres. Fibroblasts (reticular cells) and macrophages are also present in relation to the reticulum. The interstices of the reticulum are

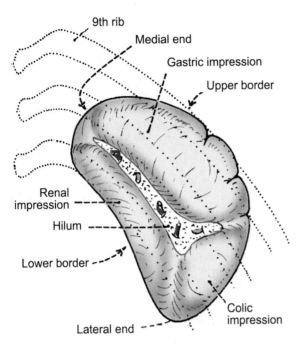

Fig. 18.3. The spleen.

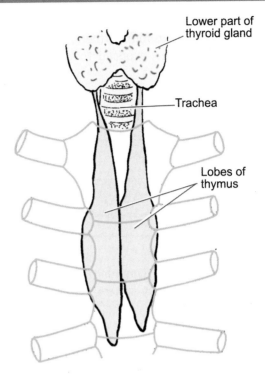

Fig. 18.4. The thymus.

pervaded by lymphocytes, blood vessels and blood cells, and by macrophages.

FUNCTIONS OF THE SPLEEN

1. Like other lymphoid tissues the spleen is a centre where both B-lymphocytes and T-lymphocytes multiply, and play an important role in immune responses.

2. The spleen contains the largest aggregations of macrophages of the mononuclear phagocyte system. In the spleen the main function of these cells is the destruction of red blood corpuscles that have completed their useful life. This is facilitated by the intimate contact of blood with the macrophages because of the presence of an open circulation. Macrophages also destroy worn out leucocytes, and bacteria.

3. In fetal life the spleen is a centre for production of *all* blood cells. In later life only lymphocytes are produced here.

THE THYMUS

The thymus lies in the thorax, behind the manubrium sterni, and in front of the heart. (This space is the anterior mediastinum). It consists of two lobes, right and left (Fig. 18.4). At birth the thymus weighs 10-15 g. The weight increases to 30-40 g at puberty. Subsequently, much of the organ is replaced by fat.

However, the thymus is believed to produce T-lymphocytes throughout life.

The right and left lobes that are joined together by fibrous tissue. Each lobe has a connective tissue capsule. Connective tissue septa passing inwards from the capsule incompletely subdivide the lobe into a large number of lobules.

Each lobule has an outer cortex and an inner medulla. Both the cortex and medulla contain cells of two distinct kinds of cells.

(a) *Epithelial Cells* (epitheliocytes) are flattened. They branch and form a network.

(b) *Lymphocytes* (also called *thymocytes*) fill the spaces in the reticulum (formed by epithelial cells).

Apart from epithelial cells and lymphocytes the thymus contains a fair number of *macrophages* (belonging to the mononuclear phagocyte system).

FUNCTIONS OF THE THYMUS

1. The role of the thymus in lymphopoiesis has been discussed in Chapter 12. Stem cells (from bone marrow) that reach the superficial part of the cortex divide repeatedly to form smaller lymphocytes. While in the thymus, lymphocytes acquire the ability to recognize a very large number of proteins (that are foreign to the body), and to react to them. Lymphocytes, that react only against proteins foreign to the body, are thrown into the circulation as circulating, immunologically competent T-lymphocytes. They lodge themselves in secondary lymph organs like lymph nodes, spleen etc., where they multiply to form further T-lymphocytes of their own type when exposed to the appropriate antigen.

Because of this important role, the thymus is regarded as a ***primary lymphoid organ*** (along with bone marrow).

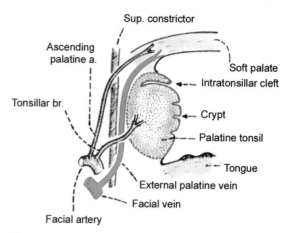

Fig. 18.6. Section through the palatine tonsil. Note its relationship to the palate and to the tongue.

MUCOSA ASSOCIATED LYMPHOID TISSUE

The aggregations of lymphoid tissue, present in relation to the alimentary system, are as follows.

(**a**) Near the junction of the oral cavity with the pharynx there are a number of collections of lymphoid tissue that are referred to as ***tonsils*** (Fig. 18.5).

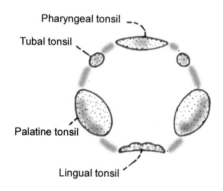

Fig. 18.5. Scheme to show various tonsils present near the junction of the oral cavity and the pharynx.

1. The largest of these are the right and left ***palatine tonsils*** (Fig. 18.6), present on either side of the communication between the mouth and the pharynx. (In common usage the word tonsils refers to the palatine tonsils).

2. Another midline collection of lymphoid tissue, the ***pharyngeal tonsil,*** is present on the posterior wall of the pharynx. In children the pharyngeal tonsil may hypertrophy and is then referred to as the ***adenoids***. The resulting swelling may be a cause of obstruction to normal breathing. The child tends to breathe through the mouth, and this may in turn lead to other abnormalities.

3. Smaller collections of lymphoid tissue are present on the dorsum of the posterior part of the tongue (***lingual tonsils***), and around the pharyngeal openings of the auditory tubes (***tubal tonsils***).

(**b**) Small collections of lymphoid tissue, similar in structure to the follicles of lymph nodes, may be present anywhere along the length of the gut. They are called ***solitary lymphatic follicles***. Larger aggregations of lymphoid tissue, each consisting of 10 to 200 follicles are also present in the small intestine. They are called ***aggregated lymphatic follicles*** or ***Peyer's patches***. These patches can be seen by naked eye.

DEFENCE MECHANISMS AND IMMUNITY

Defence Mechanisms
The animal body has to defend it self from infections, and other harmful agents. For this purpose it has developed a number of defence mechanisms. Some of these are non-specific and can take action against many substances. Others are specific and act against a specific harmful substance only.

Physical and Chemical Barriers
1. The skin and mucous membranes lining various cavities act as physical barriers to the passage of bacteria or viruses.
2. The eyelashes, hair in nostrils, wax in the external ear, and mucous over mucous membranes trap particulate matter.
3. Hydrochloric acid present in the stomach destroys most bacteria that are swallowed. Antibacterial substances are present in secretion of salivary and sebaceous glands, in saliva, in nasal secretions and in lacrimal fluid.

Once bacteria or other harmful substances enter the body other mechanisms come into play.

1. Phagocytes or macrophages have the ability to surround and destroy bacteria and other substances entering the body. These include some cells present in blood and in connections tissues.

2. Some proteins present in blood and in tissues are called **complement**. These proteins play a role in destruction of bacteria.

3. When organisms invade a tissue and damage it, an **inflammatory reaction** is set up. A similar reaction is also set up after physical injury to a part, or after injury by chemicals or other irritating substances.

Inflammatory Reaction

The main features of acute inflammation are:

1. Redness of the part.
2. Swelling.
3. Pain.
4. The part is warm.

Because of pain and swelling function may be lost (for example, in a finger).

Most of these features are a result of increased blood flow through the region, because the local capillaries dilate. Simultaneously permeability of capillaries increases. More fluid flows into the tissue and is the cause of swelling. White blood cells (leucocytes), particularly neutrophils, leave blood vessels to enter the tissue. Here they phagocytose unwanted matter. Later, many macrophages reach the site. They remove bacteria, dead cells and other damaged tissue.

Macrophages release a substance called **interleukin 1**. This stimulates the temperature regulating centre to raise body temperature. That is why inflammation anywhere in the body can cause fever.

In many cases destruction of tissue by inflammation leads to formation of pus (suppuration). Pus is made up of fluid in which there are cells including dead phagocytes, and bacteria, living or dead.

A small collection of pus deep to skin is called a **boil**. A larger collection is called an **abscess**. Generally, pus in boils tries to reach the surface of the skin. Here the boil ruptures and pus flows out. Sometimes an incision has to be given to drain out the pus. If pus does not drain out fully the abscess persists and small amounts of pus can keep flouring out of a narrow channel. This is called a **sinus**. Sometimes an abscess can drain into a cavity within the body, forming a **fistula**.

Usually, inflammation resolves after sometime and the tissue gradually returns to normal. However, if resolution is partial the inflammation becomes chronic. An area of chronic inflammation shows large number of lymphocytes. Sometimes the defense systems of the body are unable to kill off all bacteria. In that case they may try to wall of the areas. Nodular areas, called **granulomas** are thus formed. One example of an infection in which this happens is tuberculosis.

Lymphocytes and The Immune System

Numerous references have been made to the role of lymphocytes in protecting the body against foreign invaders. In this section we will briefly review their role.

Lymphocytes are an essential part of the **immune system** of the body that is responsible for defence against invasion by bacteria and other organisms. In contrast to granulocytes and monocytes which directly attack invading organisms, lymphocytes help to destroy them by producing substances called **antibodies**. These are protein molecules that have the ability to recognize a 'foreign' protein (i.e., a protein not normally present in the individual). The foreign protein is usually referred to as an **antigen**. An antigen may be part of an invading bacterium or other organism. It may be cellular (as when blood is transfused from one person to another, or when a tissue is transplanted from one person to another). It will be appreciated that there can be a very large number of such foreign proteins. The body itself also contains a very large number of proteins of its own. For any defence system to be effective it is necessary that lymphocytes should be able to distinguish between the proteins of the individual and those that are foreign to it. Every antigen can be neutralized only by a specific antibody. It follows that lymphocytes must be capable of producing a very wide range of antibodies; or rather that there must be a very wide variety of lymphocytes each variety programmed to recognize a specific antigen and to produce antibodies against it.

This function of antibody production is done by B-lymphocytes. When stimulated by the presence of antigen the cells enlarge and get converted to plasma cells. The plasma cells produce antibodies. T-lymphocytes are also concerned with immune responses, but their role is somewhat different from that of B-lymphocytes. T-lymphocytes specialize in recognizing cells that are foreign to the host body. These may be fungi, virus infected cells, tumour cells, or cells of another individual. T-lymphocytes have surface receptors which recognize specific antigens (there being many varieties of T-lymphocytes each type recognizing a specific antigen). When exposed to a suitable stimulus the T-lymphocytes multiply and form large cells which can destroy abnormal cells by direct contact, or by producing cytotoxic substances called **cytokines** or **lymphokines.** From the above it will be seen that while B-lymphocytes defend the body through blood borne antibodies, T-lymphocytes are responsible for cell mediated immune responses (**cellular immunity**). T-lymphocytes can also influence the immune responses of B-lymphocytes as well as those of other T-lymphocytes; and also those of non-lymphocytic cells.

Like B-lymphocytes some T-lymphocytes also retain a memory of antigens encountered by them, and they can respond more strongly when the same antigens are encountered again.

The destruction of foreign cells by T-lymphocytes is responsible for the 'rejection' of tissues or organs grafted from one person to another. Such rejection is one of the major problems in organ transplantation.

IMMUNITY

It is a well known fact that some persons are more prone, to being affected by infectious present in the environment, than others. The power to resist an infection (when exposed to it) is called immunity.

It is important to remember that many substances that cause disease e.g., bacteria, contain proteins. The body itself also contains a very large number of proteins of the own. Proteins not present in the body itself are foreign proteins. A foreign protein is called an antigen. When a foreign protein enters the body, it can set up reactions that are harmful. Hence, it is necessary for the body to recognise the antigen and to destroy it. The ability to do is the fundamental basis of immunity. The function of recognition and destruction of antigen is performed by lymphocytes.

Two distinct methods are used for this purpose.

(a) When a T- lymphocyte recognises a cell bearing an antigen the lymphocyte releases toxins that destroy the cell. As this is a cell to cell reaction, this type of immunity is called cell mediated immunity.

(b) When a β-lymphocyte recognises an antigen it converts itself into a plasma cell. The plasma cell produces **antibodies** that circulate in blood. The antibody binds with antigen. The complex formed by union of antigen and antibody is recognised by other cells (T-lymphocytes, macrophages) that destroy any cell bearing the antigen antibody complex. As antibodies circulate freely in blood, they can reach any part of the body. Immunity through antibodies is also called **humoral immunity**.

How immunity is acquired

The air we breathe, the water we drink and the foods we eat are often contaminated with disease-producing bacteria or viruses (which bear antigens). When a child encounters an antigen for the first time, lymphocytes produce some antibodies against them. Some lymphocytes are able to remember that such an antigen was encountered. Such lymphocytes multiply. When the same antigen invades the body again, the quantity of antibody produced is much greater than on the first exposure. Repeated exposures strengthen the response to the antigen. The result is that if a large dose of the antigen (bacteria) happens to enter the body, there is enough antibody to destroy them, and symptoms of disease do not develop. In other words, the person has acquired immunity against the particular organisms.

Similarly immunity can also be produced artificially. Bacteria can be grown in a laboratory. There are ways in which they can be killed or weakened so much that they can no longer produce disease. However, the antigens in them remain capable of stimulating antibody production. This is how vaccines are produced. If the vaccine is injected into a person antibodies are produced and the person acquires immunity against the organism from which the vaccine was prepared. Some common diseases for which vaccines are available are cholera, typhoid, tetanus, small pox, measles, diphtheria and whooping cough.

In some cases, antigens are repeatedly injected into an animal in gradually increasing doses. When concentration of antibodies reaches its maximum, the serum of the animal is taken and used as a vaccine. Immunity acquired in this way is called **passive immunity**. Vaccines against rabies and against snake venom are prepared in this way.

Allergy or Hypersensitivity

Many substances that are normally harmless can act as antigens, and antibodies can be produced against them. The first exposure to the antigen sensitises the individual to it. Subsequent exposure to the same antigen can produce a much stronger reaction, and this can lead to various symptoms. This is how allergic disorders are produced.

Exposure to dust, or to pollen of some plants can cause allergic rhinitis (leading to sneezing and running of nose). It can also lead to asthma. Similar reactions can be produced by some drugs (even by aspirin). In some cases the reaction can be so severe that it can result in death.

Substances (including cosmetics) applied to skin can cause symptoms which may be mild (redness, irritation), but sometimes there can be severe generalised reaction.

Autoimmune Diseases

We have seen that lymphocytes can distinguish between proteins present in the body, and those foreign to it. However, sometimes the lymphocytes may produce antibodies against one of the proteins present in the body. Lymphocytes then start attacking cells containing the protein destroying them. Some diseases caused in this way are rheumatoid arthritis, some diseases of the thyroid gland, and some disorders of blood.

AIDS (Acquired Immune Deficiency Syndrome)

This is a condition in which the immune system of the body becomes very weak. The person's ability to resist infections is lost and any infection can spread rapidly causing death.

AIDS is the result of infection by a virus (HIV or human immunodeficiency virus). The virus contains RNA. When the virus infects a cell this viral RNA produces new, (abnormal) DNA, which gets incorporated into the DNA of the cell. Because of the presence of this DNA the cell produces new copies of the virus. These spread into other cells of the body infecting them. The virus also infects blood, tissue fluids and secretions including semen. HIV infection spreads from one person to another through sexual intercourse. An infected mother passes the infection to offspring. A needle used for injection on an infected person can infect another person if reused. Transfusion of infected blood infects the recipient.

Because of easy spread, and the absence of effective drugs for cure, HIV infection is one of the most serious health problems facing the world today.

19

Endocrine Glands

Endocrine tissue is made up essentially of cells that produce secretions which are poured directly into blood. The secretions of endocrine cells are called **hormones**. Hormones travel through blood to target cells whose functioning they may influence profoundly. A hormone acts on cells that bear specific receptors for it. Some hormones act only on one organ or on one type of cell, while other hormones may have widespread effects. Along with the autonomic nervous system, the endocrine organs co-ordinate and control the metabolic activities and the internal environment of the body.

Endocrine cells are distributed in three different ways.

Some organs are entirely endocrine in function. They are referred to as **endocrine glands** (or **ductless glands**). Those traditionally included under this heading are the hypophysis cerebri (or pituitary gland), the pineal gland, the thyroid gland, the parathyroid glands, and the suprarenal (or adrenal) glands.

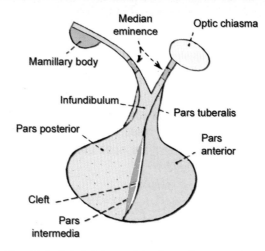

Fig. 19.1. Subdivisions of the hypophysis cerebri.

fibres. It is directly continuous with the central core of the infundibular stalk which is made up of nervous tissue. The pars posterior and the infundibular stalk are together referred to as the **neurohypophysis**.

The pars anterior (which is also called the **pars distalis**), and the pars intermedia, are both made up of cells having a direct secretory function. They are collectively referred to as the **adenohypophysis**.

ADENOHYPOPHYSIS

Pars Anterior

The cells of the pars anterior can be divided into **chromophil cells** that have brightly staining granules in their cytoplasm; and **chromophobe cells** in which granules are not prominent. Chromophil cells are further classified as **acidophil** when their granules stain with acid dyes (like eosin or orange G); or **basophil** when the granules stain with basic dyes (like haematoxylin). The acidophil cells are often called **alpha cells**, and the basophils are called **beta cells**.

Types of Acidophil Cells

(**1**) **Somatotrophs** produce the **somatropic hormone**, or **growth hormone [GH]**. This hormone controls body growth, specially before puberty.

THE HYPOPHYSIS CEREBRI

The hypophysis cerebri is also called the **pituitary gland**. It is suspended from the floor of the third ventricle (of the brain) by a narrow funnel-shaped stalk called the **infundibulum**, and lies in a depression on the upper surface of the sphenoid bone.

The hypophysis cerebri is one of the most important endocrine glands. It produces several hormones some of which profoundly influence the activities of other endocrine tissues. Its own activity is influenced by the hypothalamus, and by the pineal body.

Subdivisions of the Hypophysis Cerebri

The hypophysis cerebri has, in the past, been divided into an anterior part, the **pars anterior**; an intermediate part, the **pars intermedia**; and a posterior part the **pars posterior** (or **pars nervosa**) (Fig. 19.1). The pars posterior contains numerous nerve

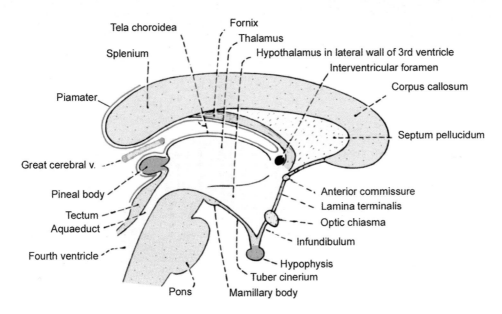

Fig. 19.2. Diagram to show the position of the hypophysis cerebri and of the pineal body relative to the third ventricle of the brain.

(2) *Mammotrophs* (or *lactotrophs*) produce the *mammotropic hormone* (also called *lactogenic hormone*, or LTH) which stimulates the growth and activity of the female mammary gland during pregnancy and lactation.

Types of Basophil Cells

(1) The *corticotrophs* produce the *corticotropic hormone* (also called *adreno-corticotropin* or ACTH). This hormone stimulates the secretion of some hormones of the adrenal cortex.

(2) *Thyrotrophs* produce the *thyrotropic hormone* (*thyrotropin* or TSH) which stimulates the activity of the thyroid gland.

(3) *Gonadotrophs* produce two types of hormones each type having a different action in the male and female.

(a) In the female, the first of these hormones stimulates the growth of ovarian follicles. It is, therefore, called the *follicle stimulating hormone* (FSH). It also stimulates the secretion of oestrogens by the ovaries. In the male the same hormone stimulates spermatogenesis.

(b) In the female, the second hormone stimulates the maturation of the corpus luteum, and the secretion by it of progesterone. It is called the *luteinizing hormone* (LH). In the male the same hormone stimulates the production of androgens by the interstitial cells of the testes, and is called the *interstitial cell stimulating hormone* (ICSH).

NEUROHYPOPHYSIS

Pars Posterior

The pars posterior of the hypophysis is associated with the release into the blood of two hormones. One of these is *vasopressin* (also called the *antidiuretic hormone* or ADH). This hormone controls reabsorption of water by kidney tubules. The second hormone is oxytocin. It controls the contraction of smooth muscle of the uterus.

It is now known that these two hormones are not produced in the hypophysis cerebri at all. They are synthesized in neurons located in the hypothalamus.

THE PINEAL GLAND

The pineal gland (or pineal body) is a small piriform structure present in relation to the posterior wall of the third ventricle of the brain (Fig. 19.2). It is also called the *epiphysis cerebri*. The pineal has for long been regarded as a vestigial organ of no functional importance. However, it is now known to be an endocrine gland of great importance.

The pineal body is made up mainly of cells called *pinealocytes*. The pinealocytes produce a number of hormones. These hormones have an important regulating influence on many other endocrine organs. The organs influenced include the adenohypophysis, the neurohypophysis, the thyroid, the parathyroids, the adrenal cortex and medulla, the gonads, and the pancreatic islets.

The best known hormone of the pineal gland is the amino acid **melatonin**.

THE THYROID GLAND

The thyroid gland is a very important endocrine organ. It is placed in the front of the neck, anterior to the larynx and trachea (Fig. 19.3).

Elementary Histology

The thyroid gland is covered by a fibrous capsule. Septa extending into the gland from the capsule divide it into lobules. On microscopic examination each lobule is seen to be made up of an aggregation of **follicles** (Fig. 19.4). Each follicle is lined by **follicular cells**. The follicle has a cavity which is filled by a material called.

Apart from follicular cells the thyroid gland contains C-cells (or **parafollicular cells**).

The Follicular Cells

1. The follicular cells secrete two hormones that influence the rate of metabolism. Iodine is an essential constituent of these hormones. One hormone

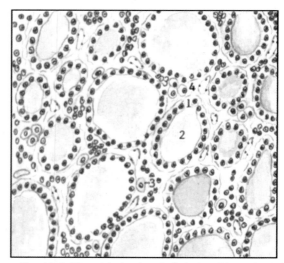

Fig. 19.4. Thyroid gland. 1-Follicle lined by cuboidal epithelium. 2-Colloid. 3-Parafollicular cells. 4-Connective tissue.

containing three atoms of iodine in each molecule is called **triiodothyronine** or T_3. The second hormone containing four atoms of iodine in each molecule is called tetraiodothyronine, T_4, or thyroxine. T_3 is much more active than T_4 (Fig. 19.5).

2. The activity of follicular cells is influenced by the thyroid stimulating hormone (TSH or thyrotropin) produced by the hypophysis cerebri.

The C-Cells (Parafollicular Cells)

They are also called **clear cells**, or **light cells**. C-cells secrete the hormone **thyro-calcitonin**. This hormone

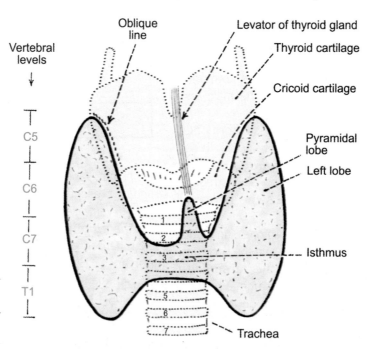

Fig. 19.3. Outline of the thyroid gland as seen from the front, and its relationship to the larynx and trachea.

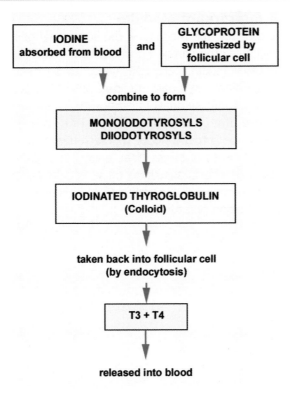

Fig. 19.5. Some steps in the formation of hormones by the thyroid gland.

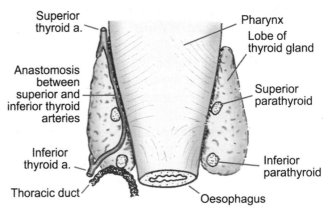

Fig. 19.6. Thyroid and parathyroid glands seen from behind.

has an action opposite to that of the parathyroid hormone on calcium metabolism. This hormone comes into play when serum calcium level is high. It tends to lower the calcium level by suppressing release of calcium ions from bone. This is achieved by suppressing bone resorption by osteoclasts.

THE PARATHYROID GLANDS

The parathyroid glands are so called because they lie in close relationship to the thyroid gland (Fig. 19.6). Normally, there are two parathyroid glands, one superior and one inferior, on either side; there being four glands in all.

The cells of the parathyroid glands are of two main types: *chief cells* (or *principal cells*), and *oxyphil cells* (or *eosinophil cells*).

The chief cells produce the *parathyroid hormone* (or *parathormone*). This hormone tends to increase the level of serum calcium by:

(**a**) increasing bone resorption through stimulation of osteoclastic activity;

(**b**) increasing calcium resorption from renal tubules (and inhibiting phosphate resorption);

(**c**) enhancing calcium absorption from the gut.

THE SUPRARENAL GLANDS

As implied by their name the right and left suprarenal glands lie in the abdomen, close to the upper poles of the corresponding kidneys. In many animals they do not occupy a 'supra' renal position, but lie near the kidneys (Fig. 19.7). They are, therefore, commonly called the *adrenal glands*.

The gland is made up of two functionally distinct parts: a superficial part called the *cortex*, and a deeper part called the *medulla*. The volume of the cortex is about ten times that of the medulla.

The Suprarenal Cortex

Layers of the Cortex

On the basis of the arrangement of its cells the cortex can be divided into three layers as follows.

(**a**) The outermost layer is called the *zona glomerulosa*.

(**b**) The next zone is called the *zona fasciculata*.

(**c**) The innermost layer of the cortex is called the *zona reticularis*.

D. Hormones produced by the Suprarenal Cortex

(**a**) The cells of the zona glomerulosa produce the hormones *aldosterone* and *deoxycorticosterone*. These hormones influence the electrolyte and water balance of the body. The secretion of aldosterone is influenced by renin secreted by juxta-glomerular cells of the kidney. The secretion of hormones by the zona glomerulosa appears to be largely independent of the hypophysis cerebri.

(**b**) The cells of the zona fasciculata produce the glucocorticoids **cortisone** and **cortisol** (**dihydrocortisone**). These hormones have widespread effects including those on carbohydrate metabolism and protein metabolism. They appear to decrease antibody responses and have an anti-inflammatory effect.

(**c**) The cells of the zona reticularis also produce some glucocorticoids; and sex hormones, both oestrogens and androgens.

The suprarenal cortex is essential for life. Removal or destruction leads to death unless the hormones produced by it are supplied artificially. Increase in secretion of corticosteroids causes dramatic reduction in number of lymphocytes.

The Suprarenal Medulla

Functionally, the medulla of the suprarenal gland is distinct from the cortex. Functionally, the cells of the suprarenal medulla are considered to be modified postganglionic sympathetic neurons. Like typical postganglionic sympathetic neurons they secrete noradrenalin (norepinephrine) and adrenalin (epinephrine) into the blood. This secretion takes place mainly at times of stress (fear, anger) and results in widespread effects similar to those of stimulation of the sympathetic nervous system (e.g., increase in heart rate and blood pressure).

20

The Nervous System

A brief introduction to the nervous system has been given in Chapter 3. The nervous system is made up of nervous tissue, and this has been described in Chapter 10. These sections must be read before studying this chapter.

CRANIAL CAVITY AND VERTEBRAL CANAL

The skull is divisible into a large upper and posterior part, the *cranial cavity*, and the *facial skeleton* forming the anterior and inferior part.

The cranial cavity is occupied by the brain, which is surrounded by three membranes (meninges) called the *duramater* (outermost), the *arachnoidmater* and the *piamater* (innermost). Between the arachnoidmater and the piamater there is the *subarachnoid space,* which is filled by *cerebrospinal fluid* (usually abbreviated to CSF). In addition to the brain, meninges, and CSF, the cranial cavity contains twelve pairs of cranial nerves that emerge from the brain and leave the cranial cavity through foramina in its walls. The cranial cavity also

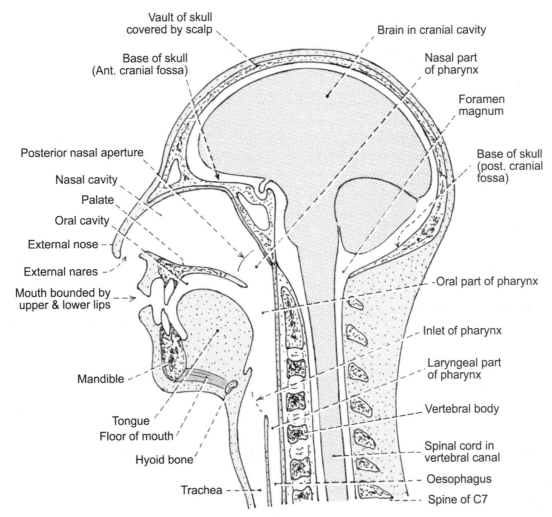

Fig. 20.1. Highly simplified presentation of some structures to be seen in a median section through the head and neck.

contains arteries that enter it from the neck to supply the brain and meninges. Venous blood drains into a series of *intracranial venous sinuses*.

The roof and side walls of the cranial cavity are formed by the vault of the skull. The skin and other soft tissues that cover the vault of the skull constitute the *scalp*. The floor of the cranial cavity is in the form of three large depressions. These are the *anterior, middle and posterior cranial fossae* (Fig. 20.1). Apart from the brain the cranial cavity contains two important endocrine glands. These are the hypophysis cerebri and the pineal gland.

Inferiorly, the cranial cavity has a large opening the *foramen magnum*, through which it communicates with the *vertebral canal*. The vertebral canal contains the spinal cord which is continuous with the lower end of the brain. Like the brain the spinal cord is surrounded by duramater, arachnoidmater and piamater. The subarachnoid space and CSF extend into it. The vertebral canal also contains blood vessels and roots of a series of spinal nerves that emerge from the spinal cord. The vertebral canal descends through the length of the vertebral column and reaches up to the sacrum. However, the spinal cord extends only up to the lower border of the first lumbar vertebra.

THE SPINAL CORD

The spinal cord is the most important content of the vertebral canal. The upper end of the spinal cord becomes continuous with the medulla oblongata at the level of the upper border of the first cervical vertebra. The lower end of the spinal cord generally lies at the level of the lower border of the first lumbar vertebra (Fig. 20.2).

When seen in transverse section the grey matter of the spinal cord forms an H-shaped mass (Fig. 20.3). In each half of the cord the grey matter is divisible into a larger ventral mass, the *anterior* (or *ventral*) *grey column*, and a narrow elongated *posterior (or dorsal) grey column*. In some parts of the spinal cord a small lateral projection of grey matter is seen between the ventral and dorsal grey columns. This is the *lateral grey column*. The grey matter of the right and left halves of the spinal cord is connected across the middle line by the *grey commissure*, that is traversed by the *central canal*.

The white matter of the spinal cord is divided into right and left halves, in front by a deep *anterior median fissure*, and behind by the *posterior median septum*. In each half of the cord the white matter medial to the dorsal grey column forms the *posterior funiculus* (or *posterior white column*).

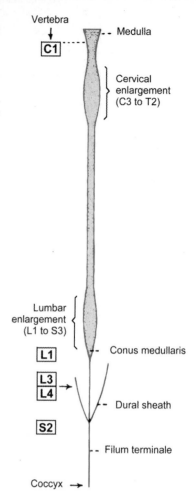

Fig. 20.2. Diagram showing some features of the spinal cord.

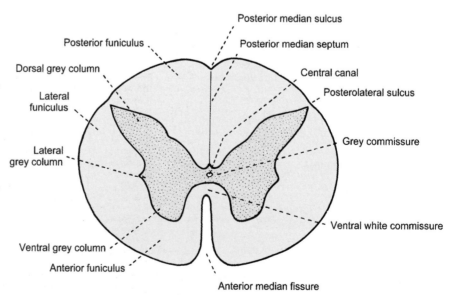

Fig. 20.3. Main features to be seen in a transverse section through the spinal cord.

The white matter medial and ventral to the anterior grey column forms the *anterior funiculus* (or *anterior white column*), while the white matter lateral to the anterior and posterior grey columns forms the *lateral funiculus*.

Spinal nerves and spinal segments

The spinal cord gives attachment, on either side, to a series of spinal nerves. Each spinal nerve arises by two roots, anterior (or ventral) and posterior (or dorsal) (Fig. 20.3). Each root is formed by aggregation of a number of rootlets that arise from the cord over a certain length (Fig. 20.4). The length of the spinal cord giving origin to the rootlets of one spinal nerve constitutes one *spinal segment*. The spinal cord is made up of thirty one segments: 8 cervical, 12 thoracic, 5 lumbar, 5 sacral and one coccygeal. [Note that in the cervical and coccygeal regions the number of spinal segments, and of spinal nerves, does not correspond to the number of vertebrae.

The ventral and dorsal nerve roots join each other to form a spinal nerve. Just proximal to their junction the dorsal root is marked by a swelling called the *dorsal nerve root ganglion*, or *spinal ganglion* (Fig. 20.5).

The spinal cord is not of uniform thickness. The spinal segments that contribute to the nerves of the upper limbs are enlarged to form the *cervical enlargement* of the cord. Similarly, the segments innervating the lower limbs forms the *lumbar enlargement* (Fig.20.2).

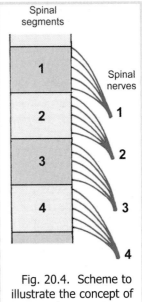

Fig. 20.4. Scheme to illustrate the concept of spinal segments.

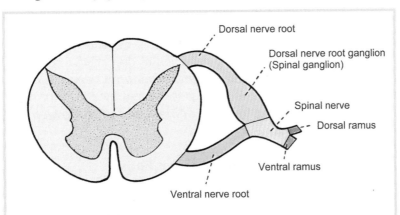

Fig. 20.5. Relationship of a spinal nerve to the spinal cord.

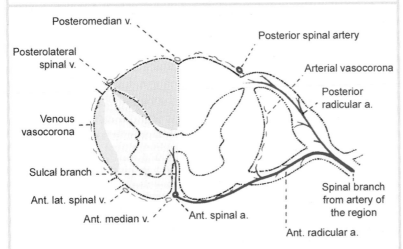

Fig. 20.6. Blood vessels supplying the spinal cord. In the left half of the figure, the area shaded green is supplied by the posterior spinal artery; the areas shaded pink is supplied by the arterial vasocorona; and the area shaded yellow is supplied by the anterior spinal artery.

Blood supply of the spinal cord

The spinal cord receives its blood supply from three longitudinal arterial channels that extend along the length of the spinal cord (Fig. 20.6). The *anterior spinal artery* is present in relation to the anterior median fissure. Two *posterior spinal arteries* (one on each side) run along the posterolateral sulcus (i.e., along the line of attachment of the dorsal nerve roots). In addition to these channels the pia mater covering the spinal cord has an arterial plexus (called the *arterial vasocorona*) which also sends branches into the substance of the cord.

The veins draining the spinal cord are arranged in the form of six longitudinal channels. These are *anteromedian* and *posteromedian* channels that lie in the midline; and *anterolateral* and *posterolateral* channels that are paired (Fig. 20.6). These channels are interconnected by a plexus of veins that form a *venous vasocorona.* The blood from these veins is drained into radicular veins that open into a venous plexus lying between the dura mater and the bony vertebral canal (*epidural* or *internal vertebral venous plexus*) and through it into various segmental veins.

GROSS ANATOMY OF THE BRAINSTEM

The brainstem consists (from above downwards) of the **midbrain**, the **pons** and the **medulla** (Fig. 20.7, 20.8). The midbrain is continuous, above, with the cerebral hemispheres. The medulla is continuous, below, with the spinal cord. Posteriorly, the pons and medulla are separated from the cerebellum by the fourth ventricle (Fig. 20.9). The ventricle is continuous, below, with the central canal, which traverses the lower part of the medulla, and becomes continuous with the central canal of the spinal cord. Cranially, the fourth ventricle is continuous with the aqueduct, which passes through the midbrain. The midbrain, pons and medulla are connected to the cerebellum by the superior, middle and inferior cerebellar peduncles, respectively.

A number of cranial nerves are attached to the brainstem. The third and fourth nerves emerge from the surface of the midbrain; and the fifth from the pons. The sixth, seventh and eighth nerves emerge at the junction of the pons and medulla. The ninth, tenth, eleventh and twelfth cranial nerves emerge from the surface of the medulla.

Gross Anatomy of the Medulla

The medulla is broad above, where it joins the pons; and narrows down below, where it becomes continuous with the spinal cord. The medulla is divided into a lower **closed part**, which surrounds the central canal; and an upper **open part**, which is related to the lower part of the fourth ventricle. The surface of the medulla is marked by a series of fissures or sulci that divide it into a number of regions. The **anterior median fissure** and the **posterior median sulcus** are upward continuations of the corresponding features seen on the spinal cord. On each side the **anterolateral sulcus** lies in line with the ventral roots of spinal nerves. The rootlets of the hypoglossal nerve emerge from this sulcus. The **posterolateral sulcus** lies in line with the dorsal nerve roots of spinal nerves, and gives attachment to rootlets of the glossopharyngeal, vagus and accessory nerves. The region between the anterior median sulcus and the anterolateral sulcus is occupied (on either side of the midline) by an elevation called the **pyramid.** The elevation is caused by a large bundle of fibres that descend from the cerebral cortex to the spinal cord. Some of these fibres cross from one side to the other in the lower part of the medulla, obliterating the anterior median fissure. These crossing fibres constitute the **decussation of the pyramids**. In the upper part of the medulla, the region between the anterolateral and posterolateral sulci shows a prominent, elongated, oval swelling named the **olive.** It is produced by a large mass of grey matter called the **inferior olivary nucleus.** The posterior part of the medulla, between the posterior median sulcus and the posterolateral sulcus, contains tracts that enter the medulla from the posterior funiculus of the spinal cord. These are the **fasciculus gracilis** lying medially, next to the middle line, and the **fasciculus cuneatus** lying laterally. These fasciculi end in rounded elevations called the **gracile** and **cuneate tubercles.** These tubercles are produced by masses of grey matter called the **nucleus gracilis** and the **nucleus cuneatus** respectively.

Just above these tubercles the posterior aspect of the medulla is occupied by a triangular fossa which forms the lower part of the floor of the fourth ventricle. This fossa is bounded on either side by the inferior cerebellar peduncle. The lower part of the medulla, immediately lateral to the fasciculus cuneatus, is marked by another longitudinal elevation called the **tuberculum cinereum.** This elevation is produced by an underlying collection of grey matter called the **spinal nucleus of the trigeminal nerve.** The grey matter of this nucleus is covered by a layer of nerve fibres that form the **spinal tract of the trigeminal nerve.**

Gross Anatomy of the Pons

The pons shows a convex **anterior surface**, marked by prominent transversely running fibres. Laterally, these fibres collect to form a bundle, the **middle cerebellar peduncle**. The trigeminal nerve emerges from the anterior surface, and the point of its emergence is taken as a landmark to define the plane of junction between the pons and the middle cerebellar peduncle. The anterior surface of the pons is marked, in the midline, by a shallow groove, the **sulcus basilaris,** which lodges the basilar artery. The line of junction between the pons and the medulla is marked by a groove through which a number of cranial nerves emerge. The abducent nerve emerges just above the pyramid and runs upwards in close relation to the anterior surface of the pons. The facial and vestibulocochlear nerves emerge in the interval between the olive and the pons. The posterior aspect of the pons forms the upper part of the floor of the fourth ventricle.

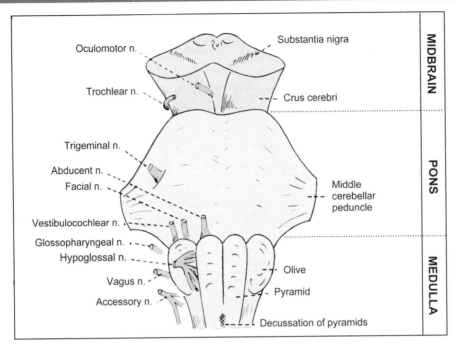

Fig. 20.7. Ventral aspect of the brainstem.

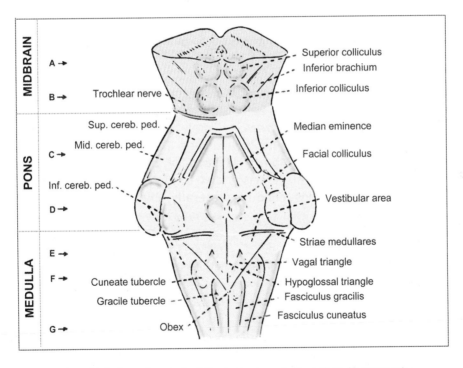

Fig. 20.8. Dorsal aspect of the brainstem. Letters G to A represent
levels at which transverse sections are shown in Figs. 20.10 to 20.16.

Gross Anatomy of the Midbrain

When the midbrain is viewed from the anterior aspect, we see two large bundles of fibres, one on each side of the middle line. These are the *crura* of the midbrain. The crura are separated by a deep fissure. Near the pons the fissure is narrow, but broadens as the crura diverge to enter the corresponding cerebral hemispheres. The oculomotor nerve emerges from the medial aspect of the crus (singular of crura) of the same side.

The posterior aspect of the midbrain is marked by four rounded swellings. These are the *colliculi,* one *superior* and one *inferior* on each side. Each colliculus is related laterally to a ridge called the *brachium.* The *superior brachium* connects the superior colliculus to the lateral geniculate body, while the *inferior*

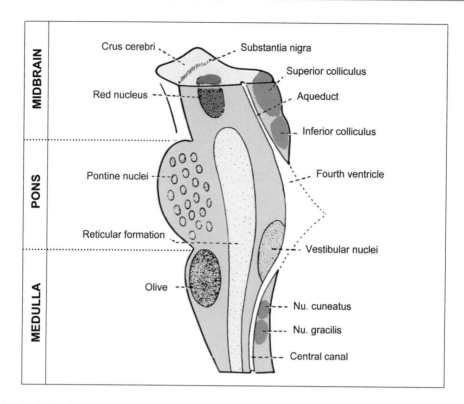

Fig. 20.9. Median section through the brainstem. Some important masses of grey matter are shown projected on to the median plane.

brachium connects the inferior colliculus to the medial geniculate body. Just below the colliculi, there is the uppermost part of a membrane, the **superior medullary velum,** which stretches between the two superior cerebellar peduncles, and helps to form the roof of the fourth ventricle. The trochlear nerve emerges from the velum, and then winds round the side of the midbrain to reach its ventral aspect.

INTERNAL STRUCTURE OF THE BRAINSTEM

The following description is confined to those features of internal structure that can be seen with the naked eye. The main features of the internal structure of the brainstem are most easily reviewed by examining transverse sections at various levels. These are illustrated in Figs. 20.10 to 20.14. The levels represented in these figures are indicated in Fig. 20.8.

Internal Structure of the Medulla

A section at the level of the pyramidal decussation (Fig. 20.10) shows some similarity to sections through the spinal cord. The central canal is surrounded by central grey matter. The ventral grey columns are present, but are separated from the central grey matter by decussating pyramidal fibres. The region behind the central grey matter is occupied by the fasciculus gracilis, medially; and by the fasciculus cuneatus laterally. Closely related to these fasciculi there are two tongue-shaped extensions of the central grey matter. The medial of these extensions is the **nucleus gracilis**, and the lateral is the **nucleus cuneatus**. More laterally, there is the **spinal nucleus of the trigeminal nerve**. The spinal nucleus of the trigeminal nerve is related superficially to the **spinal tract** of the nerve. The ventral part of the medulla is occupied, on either side of the middle line, by a prominent bundle of fibres: these fibres form the **pyramid**. The fibres of the pyramids are **corticospinal fibres** on their way from the cerebral cortex to the spinal cord. At this level in the medulla many of these fibres run backwards and medially to cross in the middle line. These crossing fibres constitute the **decussation of the pyramids**. Having crossed the middle line, the corticospinal fibres turn downwards to enter the lateral white column of the spinal cord. The anterolateral region of the medulla is continuous with the anterior and lateral funiculi of the spinal cord.

A section thorough the medulla at a somewhat higher level is shown in Fig. 20.11. The central canal surrounded by central grey matter, the nucleus gracilis, the nucleus cuneatus, the spinal nucleus of the trigeminal nerve, and the pyramids occupy the same

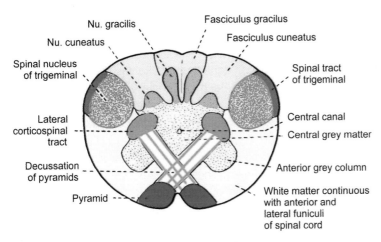

Fig. 20.10. Main features to be seen in a transverse section through the medulla at the level of the pyramidal decussation.

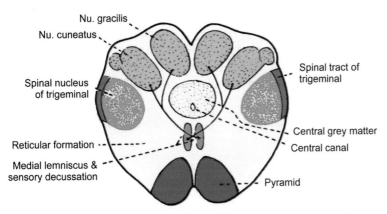

Fig. 20.11. Transverse section through the medulla to show the main features seen at the level of the sensory decussation.

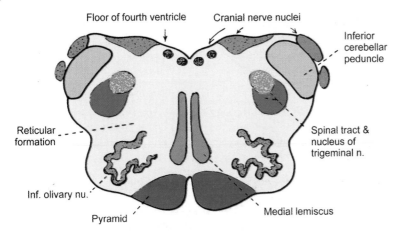

Fig. 20.12. Main features to be seen in a transverse section through the medulla at the level of the olive.

positions as at lower levels. The nucleus gracilis and the nucleus cuneatus are, however, much larger and are no longer continuous with the central grey matter. The fasciculus gracilis and the fasciculus cuneatus are less prominent. The region just behind the pyramids is occupied by a prominent bundle of fibres, the *medial lemniscus,* on either side of the middle line. The medial lemniscus is formed by

fibres arising in the nucleus gracilis and the nucleus cuneatus. These fibres cross the middle line and turn upwards in the lemniscus of the opposite side. Crossing fibres of the two sides constitute the *sensory decussation.* The region lateral to the medial lemniscus contains scattered neurons mixed with nerve fibres. This region is the *reticular formation*. More laterally there is a mass of white matter containing various tracts.

A section through the medulla at the level of the olive is shown in Fig. 20.12. The pyramids, the medial lemniscus, the spinal nucleus and tract of the trigeminal nerve, and the reticular formation are present in the same relative position as at lower levels. The medial lemniscus is, however, much more prominent and is somewhat expanded anteriorly. Lateral to the spinal nucleus (and tract) of the trigeminal nerve we see a large compact bundle of fibres. This is the *inferior cerebellar peduncle* that connects the medulla to the cerebellum. Posteriorly, the medulla forms the floor of the fourth ventricle. Here it is lined by a layer of grey matter in which are located several important cranial nerve nuclei. The *inferior olivary nucleus* forms a prominent feature in the anterolateral part of the medulla at this level. It is made up of a thin lamina of grey matter that is folded on itself like a crumpled purse. The nucleus has a hilum that is directed medially.

Internal Structure of the Pons

The pons is divisible into a ventral part and a dorsal part (Fig. 20.13).

The *ventral (or basilar) part* consists of transverse and vertical fibres. Amongst the fibres are groups of cells that constitute the *pontine nuclei*. When traced laterally the transverse fibres form the *middle cerebellar peduncle*. The vertical fibres are of two types. Some of them descend from the cerebral cortex to end in the pontine nuclei. Others are corticospinal fibres that descend through the pons into the medulla where they form the pyramids.

The ***dorsal part (or tegmentum)*** of the pons may be regarded as an upward continuation of the part of the medulla behind the pyramids. Superiorly, it is continuous with the tegmentum of the midbrain. It is bounded, posteriorly, by the fourth ventricle. Laterally, it is related to the ***superior cerebellar peduncles*** in its upper part (Fig. 20.13), and to the inferior cerebellar peduncles in its lower part (Fig. 20.14). The spinal nucleus and tract of the trigeminal nerve lie just medial to these peduncles. The medial lemniscus forms a transversely elongated band of fibres just behind the ventral part of the pons.

Internal Structure of the Midbrain

For convenience of description, the midbrain may be divided as follows (Fig. 20.15):

(1) The part lying behind a transverse line drawn through the cerebral aqueduct is called the ***tectum.*** It consists of the superior and inferior colliculi of the two sides.

(2) The part lying in front of the transverse line is made up of right and left halves called the ***cerebral peduncles.*** Each peduncle consists of three parts. From anterior to posterior side these are the ***crus cerebri*** (or ***basis pedunculi),*** the ***substantia nigra*** and the ***tegmentum.***

The ***crus cerebri*** consists of a large mass of vertically running fibres. These fibres descend from the cerebral cortex. Some of these pass through the midbrain to reach the pons, while others reach the spinal cord. The two crura are separated by a notch seen on the anterior aspect of the midbrain.

The ***substantia nigra*** is made up of pigmented grey matter and, therefore, appears dark in colour.

The ***tegmentum*** of the two sides is continuous across the middle line. It contains important masses of grey matter as well as fibre bundles. The largest of the nuclei is the ***red nucleus*** (Fig. 20.16) present in the upper half of the midbrain. The tegmentum also

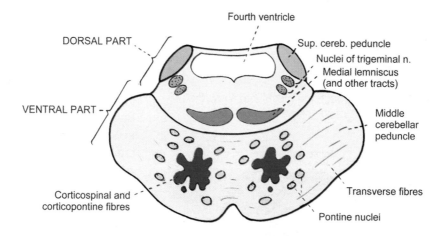

Fig. 20.13. Main features to be seen in a transverse section through the upper part of the pons.

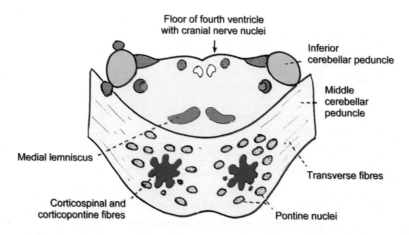

Fig. 20.14. Main features to be seen in a transverse section through the lower part of the pons.

contains the **reticular formation** which is continuous below with that of the pons and medulla. The fibre bundles of the tegmentum include the medial lemniscus which lies just behind the substantia nigra, lateral to the red nucleus. These are the fibres of the superior cerebellar peduncles that have their origin in the cerebellum and decussate before ending in the red nucleus (and in some other centres).

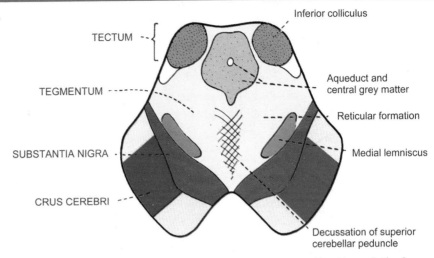

Fig. 20.15. Main features to be seen in a transverse section through the lower part of the midbrain.

GROSS ANATOMY OF THE CEREBELLUM

Subdivisions of the Cerebellum

The cerebellum lies in the posterior cranial fossa, behind the pons and the medulla. It is separated from the cerebrum by a fold of dura mater called the **tentorium cerebelli**.

The cerebellum consists of a part lying near the middle line called the **vermis,** and of two lateral **hemispheres.** It has two surfaces, **superior** and **inferior.** On the superior aspect, there is no line of distinction between vermis and hemispheres. On the inferior aspect, the two hemispheres are separated by a deep depression called the **vallecula.** The vermis lies in the depth of this depression. Anteriorly and posteriorly the hemispheres extend beyond the vermis and are separated by anterior and posterior **cerebellar notches.**

The surface of the cerebellum is marked by a series of fissures that run more or less parallel to one another. The fissures subdivide the surface of the cerebellum into

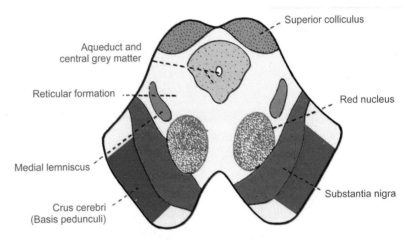

Fig. 20.16. Main features to be seen in a transverse section through the upper part of the midbrain.

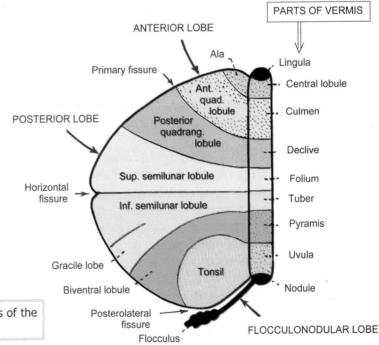

Fig. 20.17. Scheme to show the subdivisions of the cerebellum.

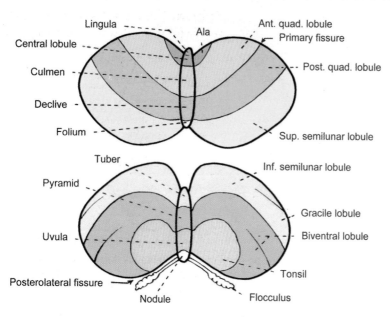

Fig. 20.18. Subdivisions of the cerebellum. A. As seen on the superior aspect. B. As seen on the inferior aspect.

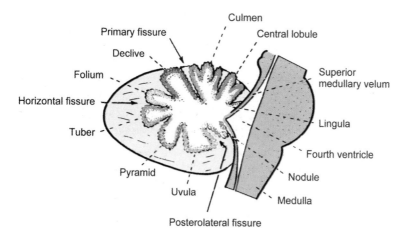

Fig. 20.19. Subdivisions of the vermis of the cerebellum as seen in a median section.

narrow leaf-like bands or **folia**. The long axis of the majority of folia is more or less transverse. Sections of the cerebellum cut at right angles to this axis have a characteristic tree-like appearance to which the term **arbor-vitae** (tree of life) is applied.

Some of the fissures on the surface of the cerebellum are deeper than others. They divide the cerebellum into **lobes** within which smaller **lobules** may be recognised. To show the various subdivisions of the cerebellum in a single illustration it is usual to represent the organ as if it has been 'opened out' so that the superior and inferior aspects can both be seen. Such an illustration is shown in Fig. 20.17. This should be compared with Figs. 20.18 A, B which are more realistic drawings of the superior and inferior surfaces, and with

Fig. 20.19 which is a middle line section showing the subdivisions of the vermis.

The deepest fissures in the cerebellum are (i) the **primary fissure** seen on the superior surface, and (ii) the **posterolateral fissure** seen on the inferior aspect. These fissures divide the cerebellum into three lobes. The part anterior to the primary fissure is the **anterior lobe.** The part between the two fissures is the **middle lobe** (sometimes called the **posterior lobe**). The remaining part is the **flocculonodular lobe.**

Cerebellar Peduncles

The fibres entering or leaving the cerebellum pass through three thick bundles called the cerebellar peduncles. The **inferior cerebellar peduncle** connects the posterolateral part of the medulla with the cerebellum. The **middle cerebellar peduncle** looks like a lateral continuation of the ventral part of the pons. It connects the pons to the cerebellum. The **superior cerebellar peduncle** is the main connection between the midbrain and the cerebellum.

Grey matter of the cerebellum

Most of the grey matter of the cerebellum is arranged as a thin layer covering the central core of white matter. This layer is the **cerebellar cortex**. Embedded within the central core of white matter there are masses of grey matter which constitute the **cerebellar nuclei.** These are as follows (Fig. 20.20):

(1) The **dentate nucleus** lies in the centre of each cerebellar hemisphere.

(2) The **emboliform nucleus** lies on the medial side of the dentate nucleus.

(3) The **globose nucleus** lies medial to the emboliform nucleus.

(4) The **fastigial nucleus** lies close to the middle line in the anterior part of the superior vermis.

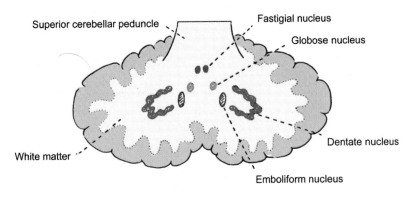

Fig. 20.20. Scheme to show the cerebellar nuclei.

GROSS ANATOMY OF THE CEREBRAL HEMISPHERES

EXTERIOR OF THE CEREBRAL HEMISPHERES

Poles, Surfaces, and Borders

The cerebrum consists of two cerebral hemispheres that are partially connected with each other. When viewed from the lateral aspect each cerebral hemisphere has the appearance shown in Fig. 20.21. Three somewhat pointed ends or **poles** can be recognised. These are the **frontal pole** anteriorly, the **occipital pole** posteriorly, and the **temporal pole** that lies between the frontal and occipital poles, and points forwards and somewhat downwards. A coronal section through the cerebral hemispheres (Fig. 20.22) shows that each hemisphere has three borders, **superomedial, inferolateral** and **inferomedial.** These borders divide the surface of the hemisphere into three large surfaces, **superolateral, medial** and

inferior. The inferior surface is further subdivided into an anterior **orbital** part and a posterior **tentorial** part (Fig. 20.23). The surfaces of the cerebral hemisphere are not smooth. They show a series of grooves or **sulci** which are separated by intervening areas that are called **gyri.**

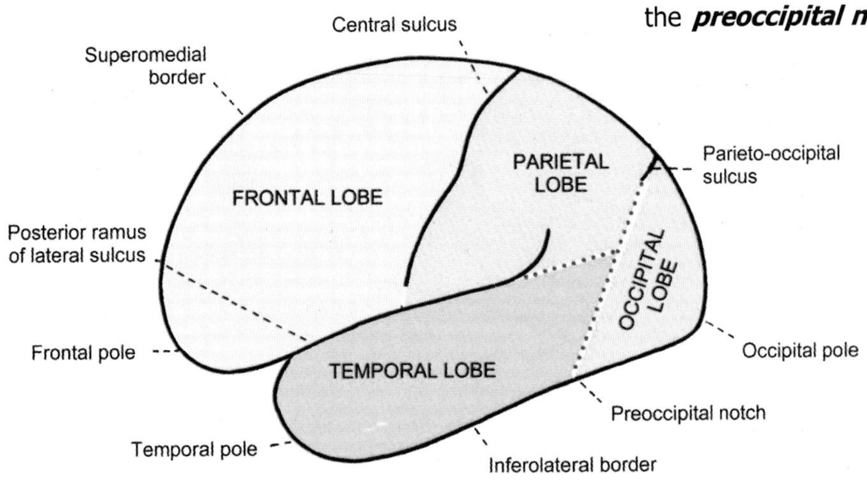

Lobes

For convenience of description each cerebral hemisphere is divided into four major subdivisions or **lobes.** To consider the boundaries of these lobes reference has to be made to some sulci and other features to be seen on each hemisphere (Fig. 20.21).

(1) On the superolateral surface of the hemisphere there are two prominent sulci. One of these is the **posterior ramus of the lateral sulcus** which begins near the temporal pole and runs backwards and slightly upwards. Its posteriormost part curves sharply upwards. The second sulcus that is used to delimit the lobes is the **central sulcus.** It begins on the superomedial margin a little behind the midpoint between the frontal and occipital poles, and runs downwards and forwards to end a little above the posterior ramus of the lateral sulcus.

(2) On the medial surface of the hemisphere, near the occipital pole, there is a sulcus called the **parieto-occipital sulcus** (Fig. 20.25). The upper end of this sulcus reaches the superomedial border and a small part of it can be seen on the superolateral surface (Fig. 20.21).

(3) A little anterior to the occipital pole the inferolateral border shows a slight indentation called the **preoccipital notch** (or **preoccipital incisure**).

To complete the subdivision of the hemisphere into lobes we now have to draw two imaginary lines. The first imaginary line connects the upper end of the parieto-occipital sulcus to the preoccipital notch. The second imaginary line is a backward continuation of the posterior ramus of the lateral sulcus (excluding the posterior upturned part) to meet the first line. We are now in a position to define the limits of the various lobes as follows:

Fig. 20.21. Lateral aspect of the cerebral hemisphere to show borders, poles and lobes.

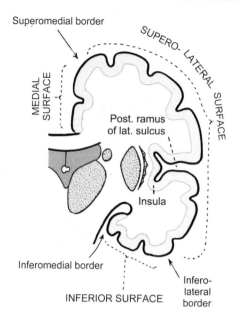

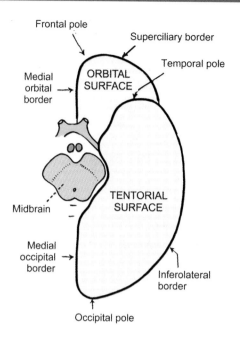

Fig. 20.22. Coronal section through a cerebral hemisphere to show its borders and surfaces.

Fig. 20.23. Inferior aspect of a cerebral hemisphere to show its borders, poles and surfaces.

(a) The ***frontal lobe*** lies anterior to the central sulcus, and above the posterior ramus of the lateral sulcus.

(b) The ***parietal lobe*** lies behind the central sulcus. It is bounded below by the posterior ramus of the lateral sulcus and by the second imaginary line; and behind by the upper part of the first imaginary line.

(c) The ***occipital lobe*** is the area lying behind the first imaginary line.

(d) The ***temporal lobe*** lies below the posterior ramus of the lateral sulcus and the second imaginary line. It is separated from the occipital lobe by the lower part of the first imaginary line.

Before going on to consider further subdivisions of each of the lobes named above, attention has to be directed to details of some structures already mentioned.

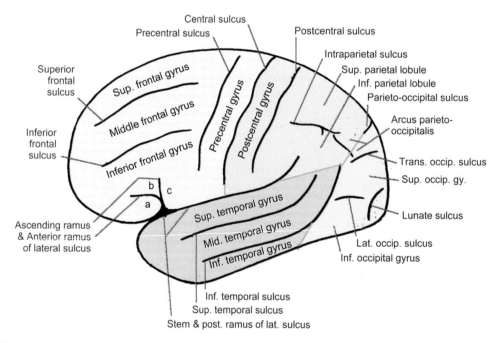

Fig. 20.24. Simplified presentation of sulci and gyri on the superolateral surface of the cerebral hemisphere.
a = pars orbitalis. b = pars triangularis. c = pars opercularis.

(a) The upper end of the central sulcus winds round the superomedial border to reach the medial surface. Here its end is surrounded by a gyrus called the **paracentral lobule** (Fig. 20.25). The lower end of the central sulcus is always separated by a small interval from the posterior ramus of the lateral sulcus (Fig. 20.21).

(b) The lateral sulcus begins on the inferior aspect of the cerebral hemisphere where it lies between the orbital surface and the anterior part of the temporal lobe (Fig. 20.27). It runs laterally to reach the superolateral surface. On reaching this surface it divides into three rami (branches). These rami are **anterior** (or **anterior horizontal**), **ascending** (or **anterior ascending**) and **posterior** (Fig. 20.24). The anterior and ascending rami are short and run into the frontal lobe in the directions indicated by their names. The posterior ramus has already been considered. Unlike most other sulci, the lateral sulcus is very deep. Its walls cover a fairly large area of the surface of the hemisphere called the **insula** (Fig. 20.23).

Further Subdivisions of the Superolateral Surface

Frontal Lobe

The frontal lobe is further subdivided as follows (Fig. 20.24). The **precentral sulcus** runs downwards and forwards parallel to and a little anterior to the central sulcus. The area between it and the central sulcus is the **precentral gyrus.** In the region anterior to the precentral gyrus there are two sulci that run in an anteroposterior direction. These are the **superior** and **inferior frontal sulci.** They divide this region into **superior, middle** and **inferior frontal gyri.**

Temporal Lobe

The temporal lobe has two sulci that run parallel to the posterior ramus of the lateral sulcus. They are termed the **superior and inferior temporal sulci.** They divide the superolateral surface of this lobe into **superior, middle and inferior temporal gyri.**

Parietal Lobe

The parietal lobe shows the following subdivisions:

The **postcentral sulcus** runs downwards and forwards parallel to and a little behind the central sulcus. The area between these two sulci is the **postcentral gyrus.** The rest of the parietal lobe is divided into a **superior parietal lobule** and an **inferior parietal lobule** by the **intraparietal sulcus.** Some other sulci are shown in Fig. 20.24.

Occipital Lobe

The occipital lobe shows three rather short sulci. One of these, the **lateral occipital sulcus** lies horizontally and divides the lobe into **superior and inferior occipital gyri.** The **lunate sulcus** runs downwards and slightly forwards just in front of the occipital pole. The upper end of the parieto-occipital sulcus (which just reaches the superolateral surface from the medial surface) is surrounded by the **arcus parieto-occipitalis.**

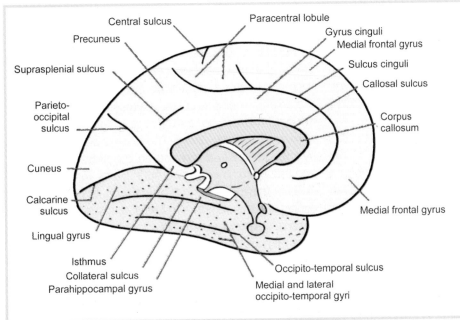

Fig. 20.25. Simplified presentation of sulci and gyri on the cerebral hemisphere as seen from the medial aspect. The medial surface and the tentorial surface (shaded in dots) are seen. The corpus callosum and some other median structures have been cut across.

Labels: Central sulcus, Paracentral lobule, Precuneus, Gyrus cinguli, Medial frontal gyrus, Suprasplenial sulcus, Sulcus cinguli, Callosal sulcus, Parieto-occipital sulcus, Corpus callosum, Cuneus, Calcarine sulcus, Medial frontal gyrus, Lingual gyrus, Isthmus, Collateral sulcus, Parahippocampal gyrus, Medial and lateral occipito-temporal gyri, Occipito-temporal sulcus

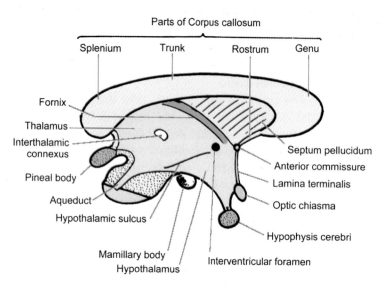

Fig. 20.26. Enlarged view of part of Fig. 20.25 to show some structures to be seen on the medial aspect of the cerebral hemisphere.

Medial Surface of Cerebral Hemisphere

When the two cerebral hemispheres are separated from each other by a cut in the middle line the appearances seen are shown in Figs. 20.25 and 20.26. The structures seen are as follows:

The **corpus callosum** is a prominent arched structure consisting of commissural fibres passing from one hemisphere to the other (Fig. 20.26). It consists of a central part called the **trunk,** a posterior end or **splenium,** and an anterior end or **genu.** A little below the corpus callosum we see the third ventricle of the brain. A number of structures can be identified in relation to this ventricle. The **interventricular foramen** through which the third ventricle communicates with the lateral ventricle can be seen in the upper and anterior part. Posteroinferiorly, the ventricle is continuous with the **cerebral aqueduct.** The lateral wall of the ventricle is formed in greater part by a large mass of grey matter called the **thalamus.** The anteroinferior part of the lateral wall of the third ventricle is formed by a collection of grey matter that constitutes the **hypothalamus.**

Above the thalamus there is a bundle of fibres called the **fornix.** Posteriorly, the fornix is attached to the undersurface of the corpus callosum, but anteriorly it disappears from view just in front of the interventricular foramen. Extending between the fornix and the corpus callosum there is a thin lamina called the **septum pellucidum** (or **septum lucidum**), which separates the right and left lateral ventricles from each other. Removal of the septum pellucidum brings the interior of the lateral ventricle into view.

In the anterior wall of the third ventricle there are the **anterior commissure** and the **lamina terminalis.** Posteriorly, the third ventricle is related to the **pineal gland** and inferiorly to the **hypophysis cerebri.**

Above the corpus callosum (and also in front of and behind it) we see the sulci and gyri of the medial surface of the hemisphere (Fig. 20.25). The most prominent of the sulci is the **cingulate sulcus** which follows a curved course parallel to the upper convex margin of the corpus callosum. The part of the medial surface of the hemisphere between the cingulate sulcus and the superomedial border consists of two parts. The smaller posterior part which is wound around the end of the central sulcus is called the **paracentral lobule.** The large anterior part is called the **medial frontal gyrus.**

The part of the medial surface behind the paracentral lobule and the gyrus cinguli shows two major sulci that cut off a triangular area called the **cuneus.** The triangle is bounded anteriorly and above by the **parieto-occipital sulcus;** inferiorly by the **calcarine sulcus;** and posteriorly by the superomedial border of the hemisphere. The calcarine sulcus extends forwards beyond its junction with the parieto-occipital sulcus and ends a little below the splenium of the corpus callosum. Between the parieto-occipital sulcus and the paracentral lobule there is a quadrilateral area called the **precuneus.**

Inferior Surface of Cerebrum

When the cerebrum is separated from the hindbrain by cutting across the midbrain, and is viewed from below, the appearances seen are shown in Fig. 20.27. Posterior to the midbrain we see the undersurface of the splenium of the corpus callosum. Anterior to the midbrain there is a depressed area called the **interpeduncular fossa.** The fossa is bounded in front by the **optic chiasma** and on the sides by the right and left **optic tracts.** The optic tracts wind round the sides of the midbrain to terminate on its posterolateral aspect. In this region two swellings, the **medial and lateral geniculate bodies,** can be seen.

Certain structures are seen within the interpeduncular fossa. These are closely related to the floor of the third ventricle (see also Fig. 20.26). Anterior and medial to the crura of the midbrain there are two rounded swellings called the **mamillary bodies.** Anterior to these bodies there is a median elevation called the **tuber cinereum,** to which the infundibulum of the hypophysis cerebri is attached. The triangular interval between the mamillary bodies and the midbrain is pierced by numerous small blood vessels and is called the **posterior perforated substance.** A similar area lying on each side of the optic chiasma is called the **anterior perforated substance**.

In addition to these structures we see the sulci and gyri on the orbital and tentorial parts of the inferior surface of the each cerebral hemisphere (described below). The orbital and tentorial parts of the inferior surface are separated from each other by the stem of the lateral sulcus.

Orbital Surface

Close to the medial border of the orbital surface there is an anteroposterior sulcus: it is called the **olfactory sulcus** because the olfactory bulb and tract lie superficial to it. The area medial to this sulcus is called the **gyrus rectus**. The rest of the orbital surface is divided by an H-shaped **orbital sulcus** into **anterior, posterior, medial** and **lateral orbital gyri.**

Tentorial Surface

The tentorial surface is marked by two major sulci that run in an anteroposterior direction. These are the **collateral sulcus** medially, and the **occipitotemporal sulcus** laterally. The posterior part of the collateral sulcus runs parallel to the calcarine sulcus: the area between them is the **lingual gyrus.** Anteriorly, the lingual gyrus becomes continuous with the **parahippocampal gyrus** which is related medially to the midbrain and to the interpeduncular fossa. The anterior end of the parahippocampal gyrus is cut off from the curved temporal pole of the hemisphere by a curved **rhinal sulcus.** This part of the parahippocampal gyrus forms a hook-like structure called the **uncus.** Posteriorly, the parahippocampal gyrus becomes continuous with the gyrus cinguli through the isthmus (Fig. 20.25). The area between the collateral sulcus and the rhinal sulcus medially, and the occipitotemporal sulcus laterally, is the **medial occipitotemporal gyrus.** The area lateral to the occipitotemporal sulcus is called the **lateral occipitotemporal gyrus.** This gyrus is continuous (around the inferolateral margin of the cerebral hemisphere) with the inferior temporal gyrus.

SOME STRUCTURES WITHIN THE CEREBRAL HEMISPHERES

For a proper understanding of the structure of the cerebrum, brief reference to the development of the brain is necessary. At an early stage of development the brain is made up of three hollow vesicles. These are the **prosen-cephalon**, the **mesen-cephalon** and the **rhombencephalon** (in craniocaudal sequence) (Fig. 20.28). The mesen-cephalon gives rise to the midbrain, while the rhombencephalon forms the hindbrain (i.e., the pons, the medulla, and the cerebellum). The cerebrum develops from the prosencephalon which soon shows a subdivision into a median part, the **diencephalon,** and two lateral eva-ginations (the **telen-cephalic vesicles**) which together constitute the **telencephalon.** In subsequent development, the telencephalic vesicles

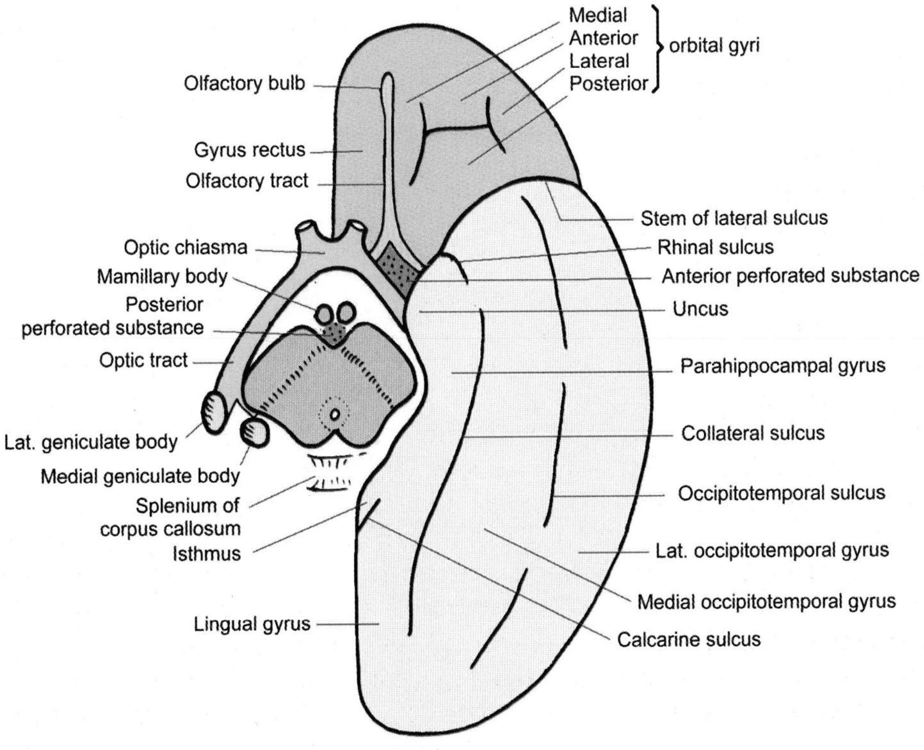

Fig. 20.27. Structures to be seen on the inferior aspect of the cerebral hemisphere.

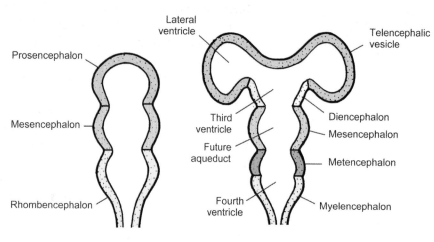

Fig. 20.28. Two stages in the development of the brain.

grow much faster than the diencephalon. As they enlarge they eventually overlap the diencephalon and fuse with its lateral aspect. One telencephalic vesicle, along with the corresponding half of the diencephalon constitutes one cerebral hemisphere. From what has been said above it will be clear that the diencephalic part of the hemisphere lies medially and inferiorly relative to the part derived from the telencephalon.

The developing brain has a series of cavities within it. The cavity of each telencephalic vesicle becomes one *lateral ventricle.* The *third ventricle* may be regarded as the cavity of the diencephalon. The interventricular foramina connecting the lateral ventricles to the third ventricle represent the sites of the original telencephalic evaginations.

Keeping these facts in mind we may now examine the basic structure of the cerebral hemispheres as seen in a coronal section (Fig. 20.29).

The surface of the cerebral hemisphere is covered by a thin layer of grey matter called the *cerebral cortex*. The cortex follows the irregular contour of the sulci and gyri of the hemisphere and extends into the depths of the sulci. As a result of this folding of the cerebral surface, the cerebral cortex acquires a much larger surface area than the size of the hemispheres would otherwise allow.

The greater part of the cerebral hemisphere deep to the cortex is occupied by white matter within which are embedded certain important masses of grey matter. Immediately lateral to the third ventricle there are the *thalamus* and *hypothalamus* (and certain smaller masses) derived from the diencephalon. More laterally there is the *corpus striatum* which is derived from the telecephalon. It consists of two masses of grey matter, the *caudate nucleus* and the *lentiform nucleus*. A little lateral to the lentiform nucleus we see the cerebral cortex in the region of the insula. Between the lentiform nucleus and the insula there is a thin layer of grey matter called the *claustrum.* The caudate nucleus, the lentiform nucleus, the claustrum and some other masses of grey matter (all of telencephalic origin) are referred to as *basal ganglia.*

The white matter that occupies the interval between the thalamus and caudate nucleus medially, and the lentiform nucleus laterally, is called the *internal capsule.* It is a region of considerable importance as major ascending and descending tracts pass through it. The white matter that radiates from the upper end of the internal capsule to the cortex is called the *corona radiata.*

The two cerebral hemispheres are interconnected by fibres passing from one to the other. These fibres constitute the *commissures* of the cerebrum. The largest of these the *corpus callosum* which is seen just above the lateral ventricles in Fig. 20.29.

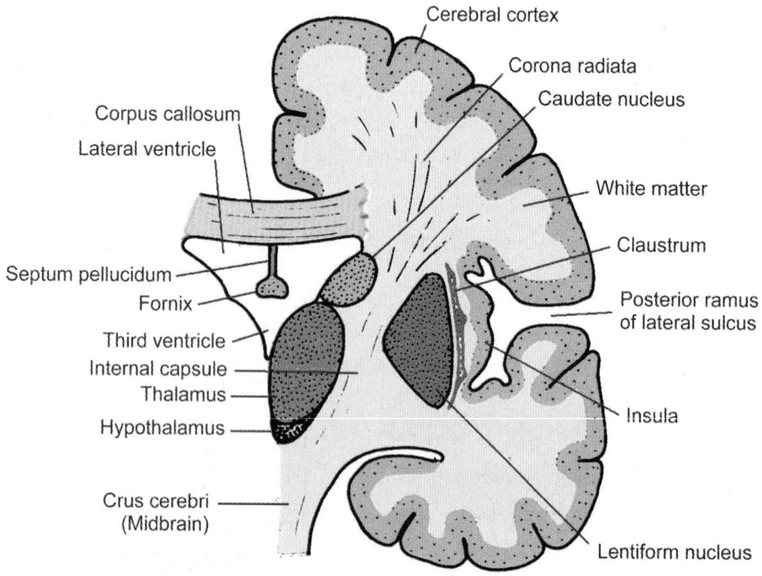

Fig. 20.29. Coronal section through a cerebral hemisphere to show some important masses of grey matter, and some other structures, within it.

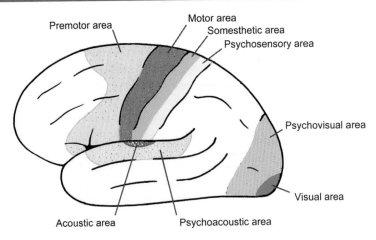

Fig. 20.30. Functional areas on the superolateral aspect of the cerebral hemisphere.

IMPORTANT FUNCTIONAL AREAS OF THE CEREBRAL CORTEX

Some areas of the cerebral cortex can be assigned specific functions. These areas can be defined in terms of sulci and gyri described in preceding pages.

Motor area

The motor area is located in the precentral gyrus on the superolateral surface of the hemisphere (Fig. 20.30), and in the anterior part of the paracentral lobule on the medial surface.

Specific regions within the area are responsible for movements in specific parts of the body. Stimulation of the paracentral lobule produces movement in the lower limbs. The trunk and upper limb are represented in the upper part of the precentral gyrus, while the face and head are represented in the lower part of the gyrus.

Premotor area

The premotor area is located just anterior to the motor area. It occupies the posterior parts of the superior, middle and inferior frontal gyri (Fig. 20.30).

Stimulation of the premotor area results in movements, but these are somewhat more intricate than those produced by stimulation of the motor area.

Motor Speech Area

The motor speech area of Broca lies in the inferior frontal gyrus). Injury to this region results in inability to speak (*aphasia*) even though the muscles concerned are not paralysed. These effects occur only if damage occurs in the left hemisphere in right handed persons; and in the right hemisphere in left handed persons. In other words motor control of speech is confined to one hemisphere: that which controls the dominant upper limb.

Sensory Area

The sensory area of classical description is located in the postcentral gyrus (Fig. 20.30). It also extends on to the medial surface of the hemisphere where it lies in the posterior part of the paracentral lobule. Responses can be recorded from the sensory area when individual parts of the body are stimulated. A definite representation of various parts of the body can be mapped out in the sensory area. It corresponds to that in the motor area in that the body is represented upside down.

Visual Areas

The areas concerned with vision are located in the occipital lobe, mainly on the medial surface, both above and below the calcarine sulcus.

Acoustic Area

The acoustic area, or the area for hearing, is situated in the temporal lobe. It lies in that part of the superior temporal gyrus which forms the inferior wall of the posterior ramus of the lateral sulcus.

The Internal Capsule

We have seen that a large number of nerve fibres interconnect the cerebral cortex with centres in the brainstem and spinal cord, and with the thalamus. Most of these fibres pass through the interval between the thalamus and caudate nucleus medially, and the lentiform nucleus laterally. This region is called the *internal capsule.* Superiorly, the internal capsule is continuous with the corona radiata; and, below, with the crus cerebri (of the midbrain). The internal capsule may be divided into the following parts (Fig. 20.31).

(a) The *anterior limb* lies between the caudate nucleus medially, and the anterior part of the lentiform nucleus laterally.

(b) The *posterior limb* lies between the thalamus medially, and the posterior part of the lentiform nucleus on the lateral side.

(c) In transverse sections through the cerebral hemisphere the anterior and posterior limbs of the internal capsule are seen to meet at an angle open outwards. This angle is called the *genu* (genu = bend).

(d) Some fibres of the internal capsule lie behind the posterior end of the lentiform nucleus. They constitute its *retrolentiform part.*

(e) Some other fibres pass below the lentiform nucleus (and not medial to it). These fibres constitute the *sublentiform part* of the internal capsule.

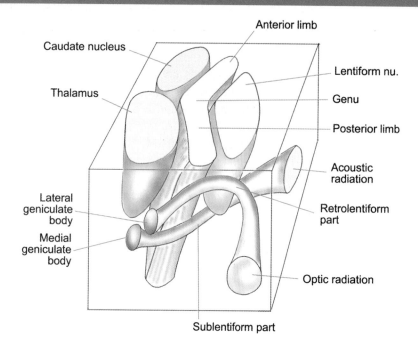

Fig. 20.31. Scheme to show the subdivisions of the internal capsule.

Corpus Callosum

The corpus callosum is made up of a large mass of nerve fibres that connect the two cerebral hemispheres (Fig. 20.26). It is subdivided into a central part or **trunk,** an anterior end that is bent on itself to form the **genu,** and an enlarged posterior end called the **splenium.** A thin lamina of nerve fibres connects the genu to the upper end of the lamina terminalis. These fibres form the **rostrum** of the corpus callosum. The corpus callosum is intimately related to the lateral ventricles. Its undersurface gives attachment to the septum pellucidum (Figs. 20.26).

The fibres of the corpus callosum interconnect the corresponding regions of almost all parts of the cerebral cortex of the two hemispheres.

SOME IMPORTANT TRACTS

We have seen that a collection of nerve fibres within the central nervous system, that connects two masses of grey matter, is called a tract. Tracts may be ascending or descending. They are usually named after the masses of grey matter connected by them. Thus a tract beginning in the cerebral cortex and descending to the spinal cord is called the corticospinal tract, while a tract ascending from the spinal cord to the thalamus is called the spinothalamic tract. We have noted that

tracts are sometimes referred to as fasciculi or lemnisci. The major tracts passing through the spinal cord and brainstem are shown schematically in Fig. 20.32. The position of the tracts in a transverse section of the spinal cord is shown in Fig. 20.33A.

DESCENDING TRACTS ENDING IN THE SPINAL CORD

Corticospinal tract

The corticospinal tract is made up, predominantly, of axons of cells lying in the motor area of the cerebral cortex. From this origin fibres pass through the corona radiata to enter the internal capsule where they lie in the posterior limb (Figs. 20.34). After passing through the internal capsule the fibres enter the crus cerebri (of the midbrain): they occupy the middle two-thirds of the crus. The fibres then descend through the ventral part of the pons to enter the pyramids in the upper part of the medulla. Near the lower end of the medulla about 80 per cent of the fibres cross to the opposite side. (The crossing fibres of the two sides constitute the **decussation of the pyramids**.)

The fibres that have crossed in the medulla enter the lateral funiculus of the spinal cord and descend as the **lateral corticospinal tract** (Fig. 20.33). The fibres of this tract terminate in grey matter at various levels of the spinal cord. The fibres end by synapsing with cells in the ventral grey column (directly or through intervening neurons).

The corticospinal fibres that do not cross in the pyramidal decussation enter the anterior funiculus of the spinal cord to form the **anterior corticospinal tract.** On reaching the appropriate level of the spinal cord the fibres of this tract cross the middle line to reach grey matter on the opposite side of the cord. Their manner of termination is similar to that of fibres of the lateral corticospinal tract. In this way the corticospinal fibres of both the lateral and anterior tracts ultimately connect the cerebral cortex of one side with ventral column neurons in the opposite half of the spinal cord.

The cerebral cortex controls voluntary movement through this tract. Interruption of the tract anywhere in its course leads to paralysis of the muscles concerned. As the fibres are closely packed in their course through the internal capsule and brainstem small lesions here can cause widespread paralysis.

The neurons that give origin to the fibres of the corticospinal tracts are often referred to as **upper motor neurons** in distinction to the ventral column neurons and their processes which constitute the **lower motor neurons.** Interruption of either of these neurons leads to paralysis, but the nature of the paralysis is distinctive in each case.

Some other descending tracts that reach the spinal cord

These are (Fig. 20.32):

1. The **rubrospinal tract** (from red nucleus in the midbrain to spinal cord.

2. The **tectospinal tract** (from superior colliculus to spinal cord).

3. The **vestibulospinal tract** (from vestibular nuclei to spinal cord).

4. The **olivospinal tract** (from olive to spinal cord).

5. **Reticulospinal tracts** (from reticular formation of brainstem to spinal cord).

Significance of Descending tracts

The various descending tracts mentioned above, that end in relation to ventral column neurons, influence their activity, and thereby have an effect on contraction and tone of skeletal muscle.

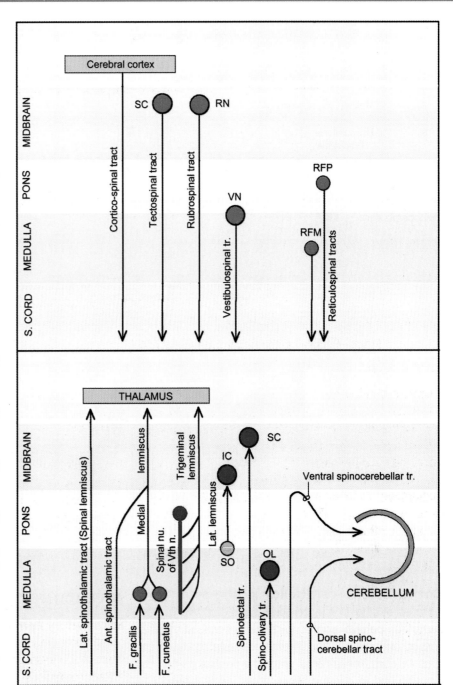

Fig. 20.32. 1. Scheme to show the various tracts passing through the brainstem. SC = superior colliculus; RN = red nucleus; VN = vestibular nuclei; OL = inferior olivary nucleus. RFP = reticular formation of pons. RFM = reticular formation of medulla; IC = inferior collicus; SO = superior olivary nucleus.

DESCENDING TRACTS ENDING IN THE BRAINSTEM

Corticonuclear tracts

The nuclei of cranial nerves that supply skeletal muscle are functionally equivalent to ventral column neurons of the spinal cord. They are under cortical control through fibres that are closely related in their origin and course to corticospinal fibres. At various levels of the brainstem these fibres cross to the opposite side to end by synapsing with cells in cranial nerve nuclei.

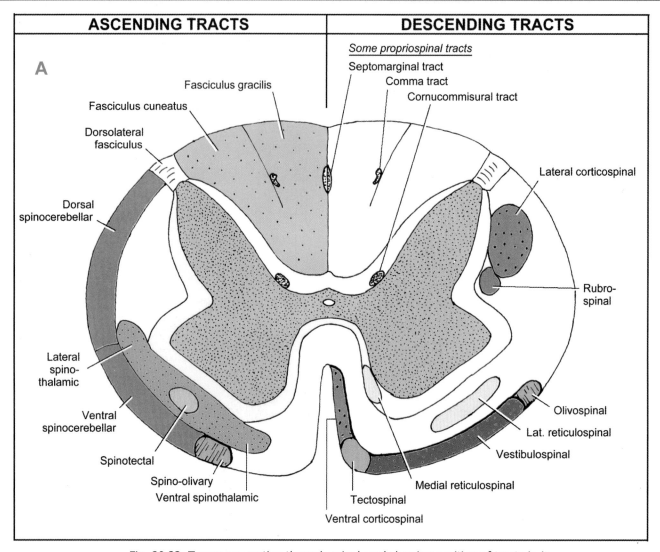

ASCENDING TRACTS	DESCENDING TRACTS

A

Fasciculus gracilis

Fasciculus cuneatus

Dorsolateral fasciculus

Dorsal spinocerebellar

Lateral spino-thalamic

Ventral spinocerebellar

Spinotectal

Spino-olivary

Ventral spinothalamic

Some propriospinal tracts

Septomarginal tract

Comma tract

Cornucommisural tract

Lateral corticospinal

Rubro-spinal

Olivospinal

Lat. reticulospinal

Vestibulospinal

Medial reticulospinal

Tectospinal

Ventral corticospinal

Fig. 20.33. Transverse section through spinal cord showing position of tracts in it.

Cortico-ponto-cerebellar pathway

Fibres arising in the cerebral cortex of the frontal, temporal, parietal and occipital lobes descend through the corona radiata and internal capsule to reach the crus cerebri. These fibres enter the ventral part of the pons to end in pontine nuclei of the same side.

Axons of neurons in the pontine nuclei form the transverse fibres of the pons. These fibres cross the middle line and pass into the middle cerebellar peduncle of the opposite side. The fibres of this peduncle reach the cerebellar cortex.

The cortico-ponto-cerebellar pathway forms the anatomical basis for control of cerebellar activity by the cerebral cortex.

ASCENDING TRACTS

Introductory Remarks

The ascending tracts of the spinal cord and brainstem represent one stage of multineuron pathways by which afferent impulses arising in various parts of the body are conveyed to different parts of the brain. The *first order neurons* of these pathways are usually located in spinal (dorsal nerve root) ganglia. We have seen that the neurons in these ganglia are unipolar. Each neuron gives off a peripheral process and a central process. The peripheral processes of the neurons form the afferent fibres of peripheral nerves. They end in relation to sensory end organs (receptors) situated in various tissues. The central processes of these neurons enter the spinal cord through the dorsal nerve roots. Having entered the cord the central processes, as a rule, terminate by synapsing with cells in spinal grey matter. Some of them may run upwards in the white

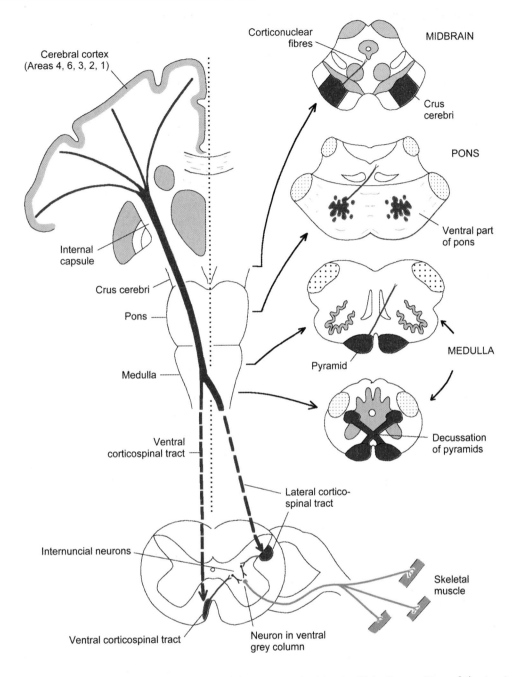

Fig. 20.34. Scheme to show the course of the corticospinal tracts. Note the position of the tracts at various levels of the brainstem.

matter of the cord to form ascending tracts (Fig. 20.35). The majority of ascending tracts are, however, formed by axons of cells in spinal grey matter. These are **second order** sensory neurons (Fig. 20.37). In the case of pathways that convey sensory information to the cerebral cortex the second order neurons end by synapsing with neurons in the thalamus. **Third order** sensory neurons located in the thalamus carry the sensations to the cerebral cortex.

The Posterior Column — Medial Lemniscus Pathway

Fasciculus gracilis and fasciculus cuneatus:

These tracts occupy the posterior funiculus of the spinal cord and are, therefore, often referred to as the **posterior column tracts** (Fig. 20.33). They are formed predominantly by central processes of neurons located in dorsal nerve root ganglia i.e., by first order sensory neurons (Fig. 20.35). The fibres of these fasciculi extend upwards as far as the lower part of the medulla. Here the fibres of the gracile and cuneate fasciculi terminate by synapsing with neurons in the nucleus gracilis and nucleus cuneatus respectively.

Medial Lemniscus

The neurons of the gracile and cuneate nuclei are second order sensory neurons. Their axons run forwards and medially (as **internal arcuate fibres**) to cross the middle line. The crossing fibres of the two sides constitute the **sensory decussation.** Having crossed the middle line, the fibres turn upwards to form a prominent bundle called the **medial lemniscus**

(Fig. 20.35). The medial lemniscus runs upwards through the medulla, pons and midbrain to end in the thalamus (ventral posterolateral nucleus).

(c) Third order sensory neurons located in the thalamus give off axons that pass through the internal capsule and the corona radiata to reach the somatosensory areas of the cerebral cortex.

The pathway described above carries:

(1) Some components of the sense of touch. These include deep touch and pressure, the ability to localise exactly the part touched (tactile localisation), the ability to recognise as separate two points on the skin that

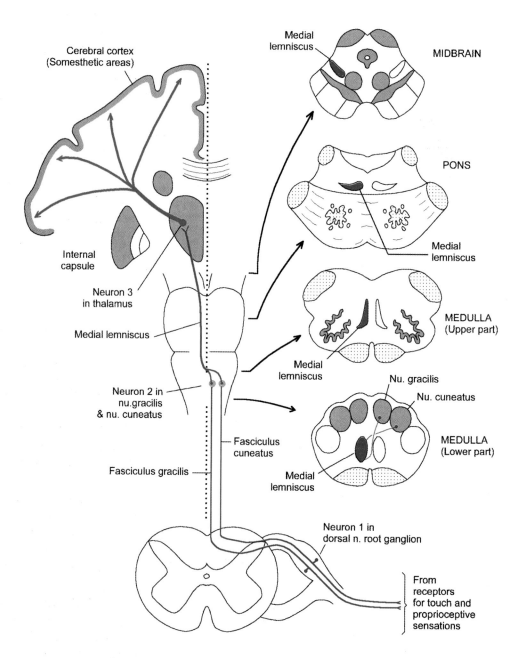

Fig. 20.35. Scheme to show the main features of the posterior column - medial lemniscus pathway. Note the position of the medial lemniscus at various levels of the brainstem.

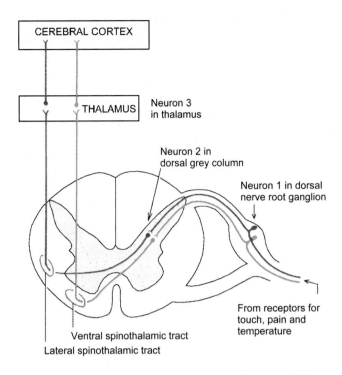

Fig. 20.36. Scheme to illustrate the main features of the spinothalamic tracts.

are touched simultaneously (tactile discrimination), and the ability to recognise the shape of an object held in the hand (stereognosis).

(2) Proprioceptive impulses that convey the sense of position and of movement of different parts of the body.

(3) The sense of vibration.

Spinothalamic Pathway

(a) The first order neurons of this pathway are located in spinal ganglia. The central processes of these neurons enter the spinal cord and terminate in relation to spinal grey matter (Fig. 20.36).

(b) The second order neurons of this pathway are located in the spinal grey matter. The axons of these neurons constitute the anterior and lateral spinothalamic tracts. They ascend through the medulla, pons and midbrain to end in the thalamus.

SPINOCEREBELLAR PATHWAYS

These pathways carry proprioceptive impulses arising in muscles and tendons to the cerebellum.

(a) The first order neurons of these pathways are located in dorsal nerve root ganglia. They end in spinal grey matter.

(b) The second order neurons of the pathway begin in spinal grey matter. They run up the spinal cord as spinocerebellar tracts (ventral and dorsal).

The *dorsal spinocerebellar tract* passes through the inferior cerebellar peduncle to reach the cerebellum (Fig. 20.37). The *ventral (anterior) spinocerebellar tract* ascends to the pons. Here it enters the superior cerebellar peduncle to reach the cerebellum.

SOME IMPORTANT MASSES OF GREY MATTER

1. The most important grey matter in the brain is the *cerebral cortex* which has already been considered.

2. The *thalamus* is a large mass of grey matter. Its position is seen in Fig. 20.38. The thalami of the right and left sides are separated only by the cavity of the third ventricle. The upper surface of the thalamus lies in the floor of the lateral ventricle. Lateral to the thalamus we see the internal capsule.

The thalamus receives the terminations of major sensory pathways ascending from the spinal cord and brainstem. These include the medial lemniscus, and

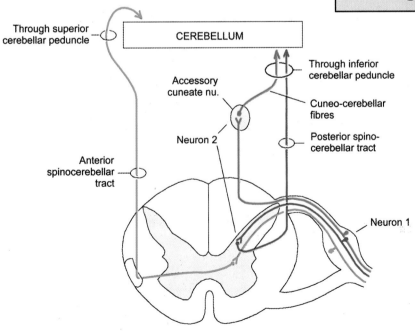

Fig. 20.37. Scheme to illustrate the main features of spinocerebellar pathways.

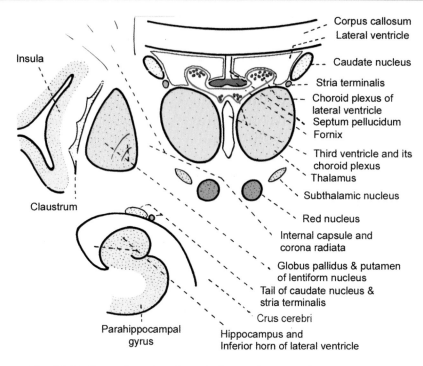

Fig. 20.38. Coronal section through the cerebrum to show structures related to the thalamus.

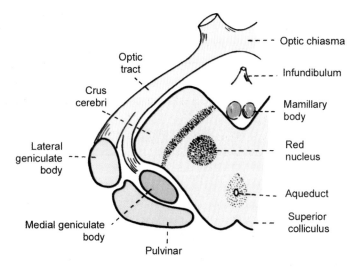

Fig. 20.39. Diagram to show the location of the medial and lateral geniculate bodies.

the spinothalamic tracts. The sensations are relayed to the sensory areas of the cerebral cortex.

3. The *hypothalamus* lies immediately below the thalamus. It is concerned with visceral functions. These include eating and drinking behaviour, regulation of sexual activity, control of the autonomic nervous system, control of endocrine glands, temperature regulation and emotional behaviour.

4. Lying below the posterior part of the thalamus there are the medial and lateral geniculate bodies. The *medial geniculate body* is a relay station on the pathway of hearing.

The *lateral geniculate body* is a relay station on the pathway of vision (Fig. 20.39).

5. The *caudate nucleus* and the *lentiform nucleus* are closely related to the internal capsule and the thalamus (Figs. 20.40, 20.41). They are also closely related to the lateral ventricle. The two nuclei together form the *corpus striatum*. The corpus striatum plays an important role in control of motor activity. Degenerative changes in the corpus striatum lead to *Parkinsonism*, in which the body becomes rigid and movements become very difficult.

THE VENTRICLES OF THE BRAIN

The interior of the brain contains a series of cavities (Fig. 20.42). The cerebrum contains a median cavity, the *third ventricle*, and two *lateral ventricles*, one in each cerebral hemisphere (right or left) (Fig. 20.43). The lateral ventricle has a complex shape. It has a central part, and three horns: anterior, posterior and inferior. Each lateral ventricle opens into the thirds ventricle through an interventricular foramen. The third ventricle is continuous caudally with the cerebral aqueduct (Fig. 20.44), which passes through the midbrain, and opens into the fourth ventricle. The fourth ventricle is situated dorsal to the pons and medulla, and ventral to the cerebellum (Fig. 20.45). It communicates, inferiorly, with the central canal, which passes through the lower part of the medulla and the spinal cord. The ventricular system is filled with the cerebrospinal fluid (CSF). Some additional details about the ventricles can be seen in Figs. 20.43, 20.44 and 20.45.

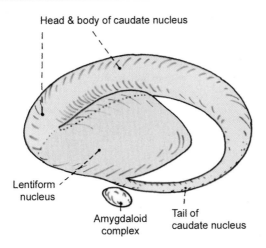

Fig. 20.40. The corpus striatum viewed from the lateral aspect.

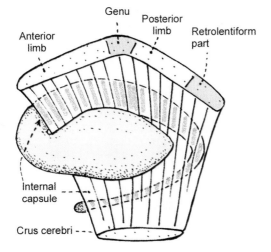

Fig. 20.41. Relationship of the corpus striatum to the internal capsule (viewed from the lateral side).

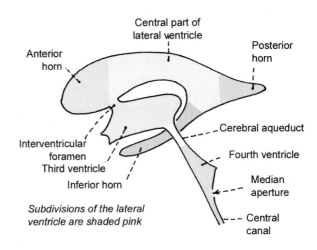

Subdivisions of the lateral ventricle are shaded pink

Fig. 20.42. The ventricular system of the brain. Lateral view.

Cerebrospinal fluid

In addition to the ventricular system, cerebrospinal fluid fills the subarachnoid space which surrounds the brain. The CSF provides a fluid cushion which protects the brain from injury. It also helps to carry nutrition and remove waste products.

CSF is formed in ***choroids plexuses*** present in the ventricles. These are bunches of capillaries. The fluid formed in each lateral ventricle flows into the third ventricle through the interventricular foramen. From the third ventricle it passes through the aqueduct into the fourth ventricle. Here it passes through apertures in the roof of the fourth ventricle to enter the subarachnoid space. CSF is reabsorbed into the

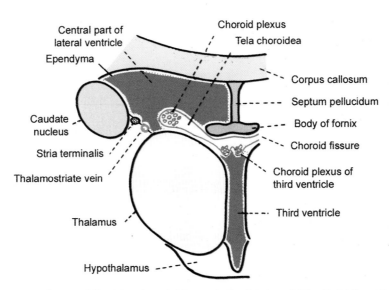

Fig. 20.43. Central part of the lateral ventricle and the third ventricle. Note the structures forming the walls of the ventricles. Note also the relationship of the tela choroidea and choroid plexuses to these ventricles.

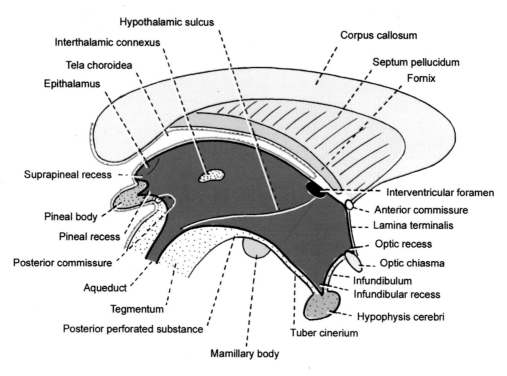

Fig. 20.44. Boundaries and recesses of the third ventricle. Note the mode of formation of the tela choroidea that lies in the roof of the ventricle.

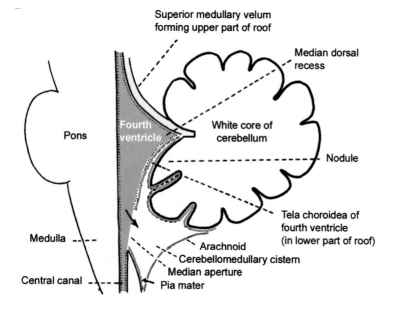

Fig. 20.45. Mid-sagittal section through the fourth ventricle and related structures. The piamater is shown in green.

circulation through **arachnoid villi** present in intracranial venous sinuses.

CSF can be obtained for examination by introducing a needle into the subarachnoid space in the lumbar region. This procedure is called **lumbar puncture.**

21

The Special Senses

THE EYE AND SOME RELATED STRUCTURES

THE EYELIDS AND CONJUNCTIVA

The part of the eye seen on the face consists of a part that is white, and a circular area in front that looks dark. The 'white of the eye' is formed by the outermost coat of the eyeball which is called the **sclera**. The sclera is lined by a thin transparent membrane the **ocular conjunctiva**. The circular dark part in the centre is the **iris** which we see through a transparent disc like structure the **cornea** which covers it. At the centre of the iris there is an aperture called the **pupil**. The pupil appears black because the interior of the eye (which we see through the pupil) is dark. When we view the 'eyes' we see only a small part of the eyeball in the interval between the upper and lower eyelids. This interval is called the **palpebral fissure** (Fig. 21.2).

The upper and lower eyelids (or palpebrae) protect the eyeball, specially the cornea, from injury in several ways.

Firstly, they provide protection against mechanical injury by reflex closure when any object suddenly approaches the eye. The same happens when the cornea is touched (**corneal reflex**).

Secondly, they help to keep the cornea moist as follows: When the eyelids are closed (i.e., when the upper and lower eyelids meet) a capillary space separates the posterior surfaces of the lids from the cornea and the anterior part of the sclera. This space is the **conjunctival sac** (Fig. 21.1). It contains a thin film of lacrimal fluid, which keeps the cornea and conjunctiva moist.

With the 'eyes' open the cornea has a tendency to dry up, but this is prevented by periodic, unconscious closure of the lids (blinking). Every time this happens the film of lacrimal fluid over the cornea is replenished. Thirdly, lids protect the eyes from sudden exposure to

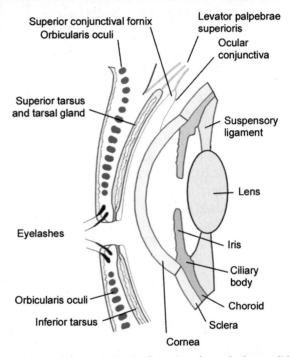

Fig. 21.1. Schematic sagittal section through the eyelids and anterior part of the eyeball.

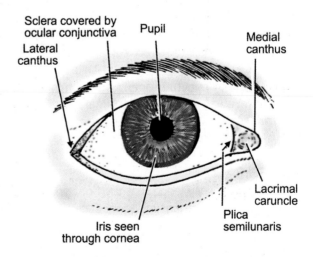

Fig. 21.2. Some features of the eye as seen on the face. The eyelashes are omitted. The interval between the two eyelids is the palpebral fissure.

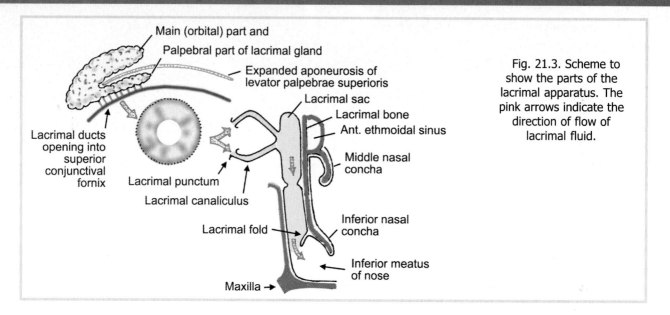

Fig. 21.3. Scheme to show the parts of the lacrimal apparatus. The pink arrows indicate the direction of flow of lacrimal fluid.

bright light by reflex closure. In bright light partial closure of the lids may assist the pupils in regulating the light falling on the retina.

We have seen above that the space separating the upper and lower eyelids is called the palpebral fissure. The medial and lateral ends of the fissure are called the **angles** of the eye. Each angle is also called the **canthus** (Fig. 21.2). The lateral canthus is in contact with the sclera. At the medial canthus the upper and lower lids are separated by a triangular interval called the **lacus lacrimalis**. In the floor of this area there is a rounded pink elevation called the **lacrimal caruncle**. Just lateral to the caruncle there is a fold of conjunctiva called the **plica semilunaris**. Each eyelid has a free edge to which eyelashes are attached. Just lateral to the lacrimal caruncle each lid margin has a slight elevation called the **lacrimal papilla**. On the summit of the papilla there is a small aperture called the **lacrimal punctum**. It is important to note that the punctum is normally in direct contact with the ocular conjunctiva.

Each lacrimal punctum opens into a minute canal that drain away excessive lacrimal fluid into the **lacrimal sac**. From here the fluid passes into a duct that opens into the nose (Fig. 21.3).

THE EYEBALL

It is common knowledge that the right and left eyes are the peripheral organs of vision. Each eyeball is like a camera. It has a **lens** which produces images of objects that we see. The images fall on a membrane called the **retina**. Cells in the retina convert the light images into nervous impulses which pass through the optic nerves and other parts of the visual pathway to

reach visual areas of the cerebral cortex. It is in the cortex that vision is actually perceived.

The greater part of the eyeball (posterior five sixths) is shaped like a sphere and has a diameter of about 24 mm. The anterior one sixth is much more convex than the posterior part. It represents part of a sphere having a diameter of about 15 mm. The outer wall of the posterior five sixths of the eyeball is formed by a thick white opaque membrane called the **sclera**. The wall of the anterior one sixth is transparent and is called the **cornea**.

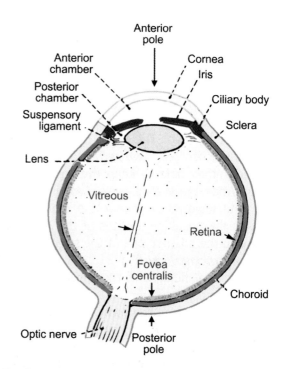

Fig. 21.4. Horizontal section across the eyeball to show the main features of its structure.

A horizontal section across an eyeball is shown in Fig. 21.4. Note the following features:

The wall of the eyeball is made up of three main layers.

(1) The outermost layer is called the **fibrous coat**. It is formed posteriorly by the sclera; and anteriorly by the cornea.

(2) The next layer is the **vascular coat**. It has the following subdivisions. The part lining the inner surface of most of the sclera is thin and is called the **choroid**. Near the junction of the sclera with the cornea the vascular coat is thick and forms the **ciliary body**. The ciliary body is continuous with the **iris** which lies a short distance behind the cornea.

The space between the iris and the cornea is called the **anterior chamber**. The space between the iris and the front of the lens is called the **posterior chamber**.

(3) The innermost layer of the wall of the eyeball is called the **retina.**

Light falling on the retina has to pass through a number of **refracting media** before reaching the retina and forming an image on it. These are (a) the cornea; (b) a fluid, the **aqueous humour**, which fills the anterior and posterior chambers; (c) the lens; and (d) a jelly like **vitreous body** which fills the eyeball posterior to the lens.

The centre of the cornea is called the **anterior pole** of the eyeball. The opposite end is called the **posterior pole**. The **visual axis** of the eye passes from the anterior pole to the posterior pole.

Muscles of the orbit

The muscles of the orbit include the **extraocular muscles** which are the four recti (superior, inferior, medial and lateral), two oblique muscles (superior and inferior), and the levator palpebrae superioris. They are responsible for movements of the eyeball. Two muscles (made up of smooth muscle), the **sphincter pupillae** and the **dilator pupillae** change the size of the pupil and control the amount of light entering the eye.

The Visual Pathway

The peripheral receptors for light are situated in the retina. These are called rods and cones. Impulses received by them pass through other cells present in the retina. Nerve fibres arising in the retina constitute the optic nerves. The two optic nerves join to form the optic chiasma in which many of their fibres cross to the opposite side. The uncrossed fibres of the optic nerve, along with the fibres that have crossed over from the opposite side form the **optic tract** (Fig. 21.5). The optic tract terminates predominantly in the **lateral geniculate body**. Fresh fibres arising in the lateral geniculate body form the **geniculocalcarine tract** (or optic radiation) which ends in the **visual areas** of the cerebral cortex. Vision is actually perceived in the cerebral cortex.

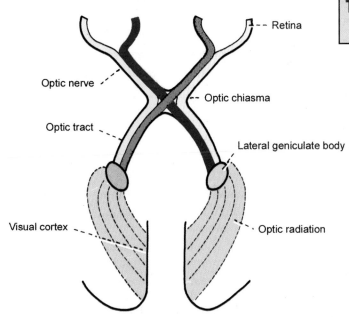

Fig. 21.5. The optic pathway. Note that the fibres from the medial (or nasal) half of each retina cross to the optic tract of the opposite side.

THE EAR AND SOME RELATED STRUCTURES

Anatomically speaking, the ear is made up of three main parts called the **external ear**, the **middle ear** and the **internal ear**. The external ear and the middle ear are concerned exclusively with hearing. The internal ear has a **cochlear part** concerned with hearing; and a **vestibular part** which provides information to the brain regarding the position and movements of the head.

The main parts of the ear are shown in Fig. 21.6. The part of the ear that is seen on the surface of the body (i.e., the part that the lay person calls the ear) is anatomically speaking the **auricle** or **pinna**. Leading inwards from the auricle there is a tube called the **external acoustic meatus**. The auricle and external acoustic meatus together form the external ear. The inner end of the external acoustic meatus

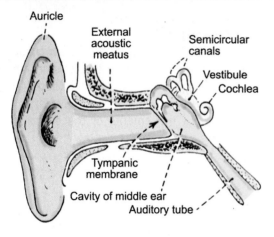

Fig. 21.6. Scheme to show the main parts of the ear.

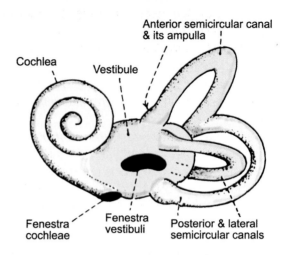

Fig. 21.7. Bony labyrinth seen from the lateral side.

is closed by a thin membranous diaphragm called the **tympanic membrane**. This membrane separates the external acoustic meatus from the middle ear.

The middle ear is a small space placed deep within the temporal bone. It is also called the **tympanum** (from which we get the adjective tympanic applied to structures connected with the middle ear). Medially the middle ear is closely related to parts of the internal ear. The cavity of the middle ear is continuous with that of the nasopharynx through a passage called the **auditory tube**. Within the cavity of the middle ear there are three small bones that are collectively called the **ossicles** of the ear. The ossicles are called **malleus** (= like a hammer); the **incus** (= like an anvil, used by blacksmiths); and the **stapes** (= like a stirrup in which the foot of a horse rider fits). The three ossicles form a chain that is attached on one side to the tympanic membrane and at the other to a part of the internal ear.

The internal ear is in the form of a cavity within the petrous temporal bone having a very complex shape. This bony cavity (or **bony labyrinth**) has a central part called the **vestibule**. Continuous with the front of the vestibule there is a spiral shaped cavity, the bony **cochlea**. Posteriorly, the vestibule is continuous with three **semicircular canals**.

Sound waves travelling through air reach the ears. In many lower animals in which the auricle is large and mobile it may help in directing the sound waves into the external acoustic meatus. The auricle is of doubtful functional significance in man. Waves striking the tympanic membrane produce vibrations in it. These vibrations are transmitted through the chain of ossicles present in the middle ear to reach the internal ear. Specialised end organs in the cochlea act as transducers which convert the mechanical vibrations into nervous impulses. These impulses travel through the cochlear

part of the vestibulocochlear nerve to reach the brain. Actual perception of sound takes place in the auditory (or acoustic) areas in the cerebral cortex.

The Auricle

The auricle is made up of a skeleton of elastic cartilage and fibrous tissue, which is covered on both sides by a layer of thin skin.

EXTERNAL ACOUSTIC MEATUS

We have seen that the external acoustic meatus is a tube passing medially from the bottom of the concha of the auricle. It is closed medially by the tympanic membrane (Fig. 21.6).

The cartilage or bone is lined by a layer of thin skin which is continuous with that over the concha. The wall of the bony part of the meatus is formed by the temporal bone.

The skin lining the external acoustic meatus contains numerous **ceruminous glands**. These are modified sweat glands that produce the wax of the ear, or **cerumen**.

THE MIDDLE EAR

The middle ear is also called the **tympanic cavity** or **tympanum** (Fig. 21.6). It is a space lying in the petrous temporal bone. We have seen that the middle ear is separated from the external acoustic meatus by the tympanic membrane. From Fig. 21.6 it will be seen that part of the tympanic cavity lies above the level of the tympanic membrane: this part is called the **epitympanic recess.** We have also seen that three ossicles, the malleus, the incus and the stapes lie within the middle ear. The tympanic cavity communicates with the cavity of the nasopharynx through the **auditory tube**. It also communicates with a large space in the petrous part of the temporal bone, called the **mastoid antrum;** and with smaller spaces within the mastoid process called the **mastoid air cells**. These spaces, the tympanic cavity itself, and the auditory tube are all lined by mucous membrane. Because of their communication with the nasopharynx these spaces are filled with air.

THE INTERNAL EAR

We have seen that the internal ear is in the form of a complex system of cavities within the petrous temporal bone. Because of the complex shape of these intercommunicating cavities the internal ear is referred to as the **labyrinth**.

The wall of the **bony labyrinth** is made up of dense bone. Lying within the bony labyrinth there is a system of ducts which constitute the **membranous labyrinth**. The space within the membranous labyrinth is filled by a fluid called the **endolymph.** The space between the membranous labyrinth and the bony labyrinth is filled by another fluid called the **perilymph.**

The **parts of the bony labyrinth** are shown in Fig. 21.7. These are as follows.

(a) In the central part of the bony labyrinth there is a cavity called the **vestibule**.

(b) Anterior to the vestibule we see the **bony cochlea**. The cavity of the bony cochlea is divided into two parts. One part, called the **scala vestibuli**, is continuous posteriorly with the cavity of the vestibule. The second part is called the **scala tympani**. The scala tympani opens into the middle ear at the fenestra cochleae.

(c) Posteriorly, the cavity of the vestibule is continuous with the three **semicircular canals** (Fig. 21.7).

The **parts of the membranous labyrinth** are shown in Fig. 21.8. Within each semicircular canal the membranous labyrinth is represented by a **semicircular duct** [It is important to distinguish carefully between the terms semicircular canal, and semicircular duct]. The part of the membranous labyrinth in the cochlea is called the **duct of the cochlea**. In the vestibule the membranous labyrinth is represented by two distinct membranous sacs called the **saccule** and the **utricle.**

Pathway of hearing

The first neurons of the pathway of hearing are located in the spiral ganglion which lies within a bony tunnel running

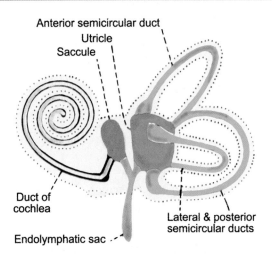

Fig. 21.8. Scheme to show the parts of the membranous labyrinth. Note the ampullated ends of the semicircular ducts.

along the cochlea. These neurons are bipolar. Peripheral processes of neurons lying in this ganglion innervate the hair cells of the **spiral organ** (organ of Corti) (Fig. 21.9). The central processes of the neurons form the cochlear nerve. The fibres of the cochlear nerve terminate in the **cochlear nuclei** present in the pons.

Fibres arising from the cochlear nuclei terminate in the superior olivary complex. Third order neurons arising in this complex form an important ascending bundle called the **lateral lemniscus**.

The fibres of the lateral lemniscus ascend to the midbrain and terminate in the **inferior colliculus**.

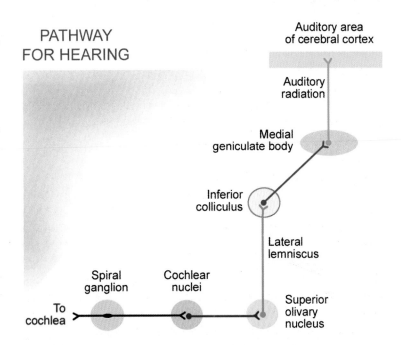

Fig. 21.9. Simplified scheme to show the pathway for hearing.

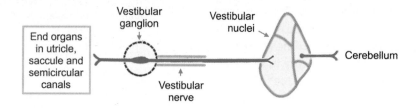

Fig. 21.10. Vestibular pathway.

Fibres arising in the colliculus reach the ***medial geniculate body***. Fibres arising in the medial geniculate body form the ***acoustic radiation*** which ends in the acoustic area of the cerebral cortex.

Vestibular pathway

The vestibular apparatus provides very important information to the brain which helps in the control of posture. The apparatus consists of the utricle, the saccule, and the semicircular ducts. The utricle and saccule contain specialised end organs called ***maculae***. The semicircular ducts contain end organs called ***ampullary crests*** or ***cristae***.

The maculae of the utricle and saccule provide information about the position of the head. The ampullary crests give information about movements of the head.

These end organs are innervated by peripheral processes arising from the ***vestibular ganglion*** (Fig. 21.10). The central processes arising from the ganglion form the ***vestibular nerve***. The nerve ends in ***vestibular nuclei*** (present at the junction of the medulla and pons). Fibres arising from the vestibular nuclei reach the cerebellum. Posture is controlled by tracts arising from vestibular nuclei and indirectly through the cerebellum.

Pathway for taste

End organs for taste are ***taste buds*** present on the tongue (and also on the palate and epiglottis). Nerve fibres from taste buds travel through the facial, glossopharyngeal and vagus nerves. The fibres end in the medulla (in the upper part of the ***nucleus of the solitary tract***, also called the ***gustatory nucleus***). Tracts beginning in this nucleus carry the sensations to the cerebral cortex, and to some other centres in the brain.

Olfactory pathway

Receptors for the sense of smell are located in the olfactory mucosa present in the upper part of the nose. Fibres arising from the receptors form the olfacatory nerve. The fibres of this nerve end in the olfactory bulb (lying in relation to the brain). From the olfactory bulb new fibres travel through the olfactory tract and end in olfactory areas present in relation to the inferior surface of the cerebral hemisphere.

PART FOUR

THE
UPPER
EXTREMITY

22

Bones of the Upper Extremity

An introduction to the various bones present in the upper extremity has been given in Chapter 2. Beginners are advised to read this introduction.

THE CLAVICLE

The clavicle is a long bone having a shaft, and two ends (Figs.22.1, 22.2). The medial end is much thicker than the shaft and is easily distinguished from the lateral end which is flattened. The anterior and posterior aspects of the bone can be distinguished by the fact that the shaft (which has a gentle S-shaped curve) is convex forwards in the medial two thirds, and concave forwards in its lateral one third. The inferior aspect of the bone is distinguished by the presence of a shallow groove on the shaft, and by the presence of a rough area near its medial end. The side to which a clavicle belongs can be determined with the information given above.

For purposes of description it is convenient to divide the clavicle into the lateral one third which is flattened, and the medial two thirds which are cylindrical.

The *lateral one third* has two surfaces, superior and inferior. These surfaces are separated by two borders, anterior and posterior. The anterior border is concave and shows a small thickened area called the *deltoid tubercle*. The lower surface (of the lateral one third) shows a prominent thickening near the posterior border; this is the *conoid tubercle*. Lateral to the tubercle there is a rough ridge that runs obliquely up to the lateral end of the bone, and is called the *trapezoid line*.

The *medial two thirds* of the shaft has four surfaces: anterior, posterior, superior and inferior, that are not clearly marked off from each other. The large rough area present on the inferior aspect of the bone near the medial end forms part of the inferior surface.

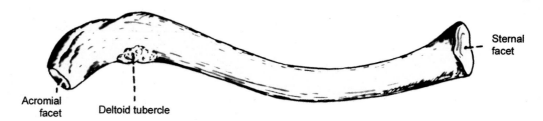

Fig. 22.1. Right clavicle seen from above.

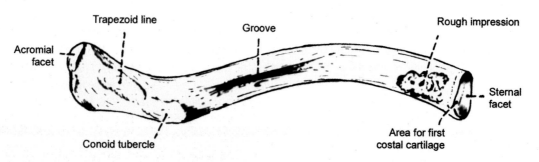

Fig. 22.2. Right clavicle seen from below.

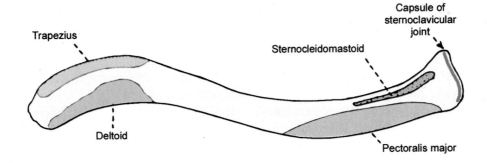

Fig. 22.3. Right clavicle showing attachments, seen from above.

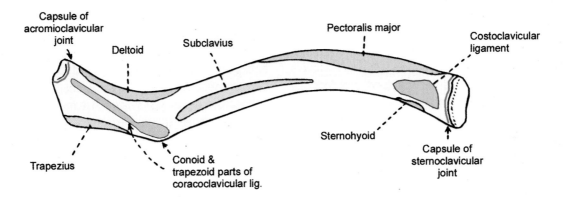

Fig. 22.4. Right clavicle showing attachments, seen from below.

The middle third of the inferior aspect shows a longitudinal groove.

The *lateral or acromial end* of the clavicle bears a smooth facet which articulates with the acromion of the scapula to form the acromioclavicular joint.

The *medial or sternal end* of the clavicle articulates with the manubrium sterni, and also with the first costal cartilage. The articular area extends on to the inferior surface of the bone. The uppermost part of the sternal surface is rough for ligamentous attachments.

Some Attachments on the Clavicle

1. The pectoralis major (clavicular head) arises from the anterior surface of the medial half of the shaft.

2. The deltoid arises from the anterior border of the lateral one third of the shaft.

3. The sternocleidomastoid (clavicular head) arises from the medial part of the upper surface.

4. The sternohyoid (lateral part) arises from the lower part of the posterior surface just near the sternal end.

5. The trapezius is inserted into the posterior border of the lateral one third of the shaft.

6. The subclavius is inserted into the groove on the inferior surface of the shaft.

THE SCAPULA

The greater part of the scapula consists of a flat triangular plate of bone called the *body* (Figs. 22.5 to 22.7). The upper part of the body is broad, representing the base of the triangle. The inferior end is pointed and represents the apex. The body has anterior (or costal) and posterior (or dorsal) surfaces which can be distinguished by the fact that the anterior surface is smooth, but the upper part of the posterior surface gives off a large projection called the *spine*. At its lateral angle the bone is enlarged and bears a large shallow oval depression called the *glenoid cavity* which articulates with the head of the humerus. The side to which a given scapula belongs can be determined from the information given above.

In addition to its costal and dorsal surfaces the body has three angles: superior, inferior and lateral; and three borders: medial, lateral and superior. Arising from the body there are three processes. In addition to the spine already mentioned there is an acromion process and a coracoid process.

The *lateral border* runs from the glenoid cavity to the inferior angle. The *medial border* extends from the superior angle to the inferior angle. The *superior border* passes laterally from the superior angle, but is separated from the glenoid cavity (representing the lateral angle) by the root of the coracoid process. A deep *suprascapular notch* is seen at the lateral end of the superior border.

The *costal surface* lies against the posterolateral part of the chest wall. It is somewhat concave from above downwards. The *dorsal surface* gives attachment to the spine. The part above the spine forms the *supraspinous fossa*, along with the upper surface of the spine. The area below the spine forms the *infraspinous fossa* (along with the lower surface of the spine). The supraspinous and infraspinous fossae communicate with each other through the *spinoglenoid notch* that lies on the lateral side of the spine.

The *glenoid cavity* is pear shaped and forms the shoulder joint along with the head of the humerus. Just below the cavity the lateral border shows a rough raised area called the *infraglenoid tubercle*. Immediately above the glenoid cavity there is a rough area called the *supraglenoid tubercle*. The region of the glenoid cavity is often regarded as the head of the scapula. Immediately medial to it there is a constriction which constitutes the *neck*.

The *spine* of the scapula is triangular in form. Its anterior border is attached to the dorsal surface of the body. Its posterior border is free: it is greatly thickened and forms the *crest of the spine*. The medial end of the spine lies near the medial border of the scapula: this part is referred to as the *root of the spine*. The lateral border of the spine is free and forms the medial boundary of the *spino-glenoid notch*.

The *acromion* is continuous with the lateral end of the spine. It forms a projection that is directed forwards and partly overhangs the glenoid cavity. The lateral border meets the crest of the spine at a sharp angle termed the *acromial angle*. The medial border of the acromion shows the presence of a small oval facet for articulation with the lateral end of the clavicle.

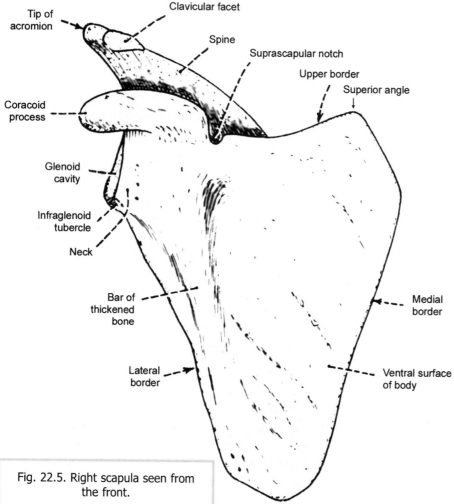

Fig. 22.5. Right scapula seen from the front.

The *coracoid process* is shaped like a bent finger. The root of the process is attached to the body of the scapula just above the glenoid cavity. The lower part of the root is marked by the supraglenoid tubercle. The tip of the coracoid process is directed straight forwards.

Some Attachments on the Scapula
(Figs. 22.7, 22.8)

1. The deltoid takes origin from the lower border of the crest of the spine; and from the lateral margin, tip and upper surface of the acromion.

2. The trapezius is inserted into the upper border of the crest of the spine, and into the medial border of the acromion.

3. The short head of the biceps brachii arises from the (lateral part of the) tip of the coracoid process; and the

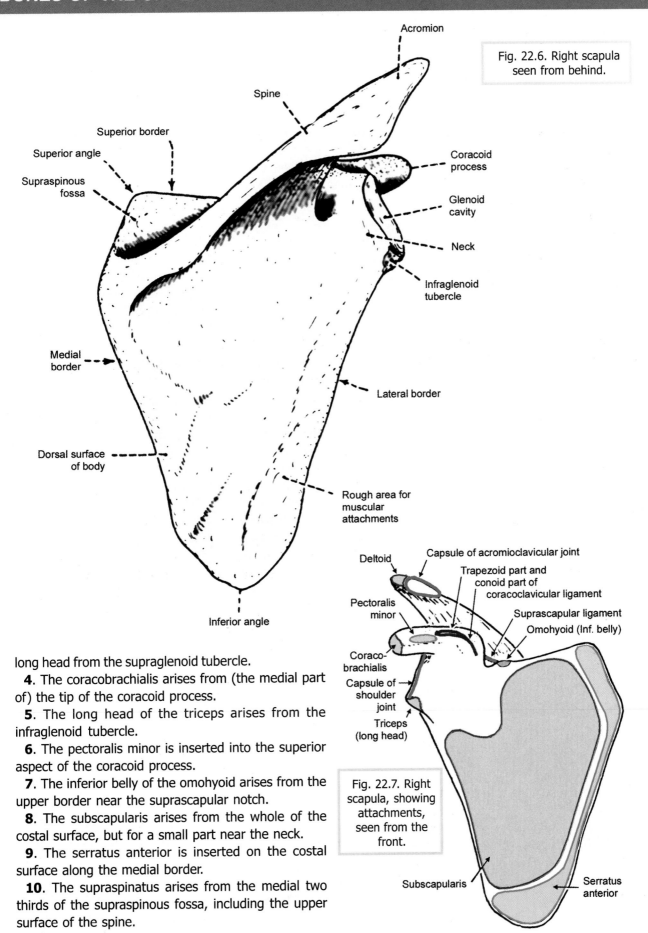

Acromion

Spine

Superior border

Superior angle

Supraspinous fossa

Coracoid process

Glenoid cavity

Neck

Infraglenoid tubercle

Medial border

Lateral border

Dorsal surface of body

Rough area for muscular attachments

Inferior angle

Fig. 22.6. Right scapula seen from behind.

Deltoid

Capsule of acromioclavicular joint

Trapezoid part and conoid part of coracoclavicular ligament

Suprascapular ligament

Omohyoid (Inf. belly)

Pectoralis minor

Coraco-brachialis

Capsule of shoulder joint

Triceps (long head)

Fig. 22.7. Right scapula, showing attachments, seen from the front.

Subscapularis

Serratus anterior

long head from the supraglenoid tubercle.

4. The coracobrachialis arises from (the medial part of) the tip of the coracoid process.

5. The long head of the triceps arises from the infraglenoid tubercle.

6. The pectoralis minor is inserted into the superior aspect of the coracoid process.

7. The inferior belly of the omohyoid arises from the upper border near the suprascapular notch.

8. The subscapularis arises from the whole of the costal surface, but for a small part near the neck.

9. The serratus anterior is inserted on the costal surface along the medial border.

10. The supraspinatus arises from the medial two thirds of the supraspinous fossa, including the upper surface of the spine.

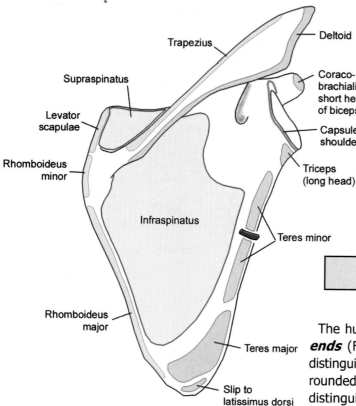

Trapezius

Deltoid

Supraspinatus

Coraco-brachialis & short head of biceps

Levator scapulae

Capsule of shoulder joint

Rhomboideus minor

Triceps (long head)

Infraspinatus

Teres minor

Rhomboideus major

Teres major

Slip to latissimus dorsi

Fig. 22.8. Right scapula, showing attachments, seen from behind.

11. The infraspinatus arises from the greater part of the infraspinous fossa, but for a part near the lateral border and a part near the neck.

12. The teres minor arises from the upper two thirds of the rough strip on the dorsal surface, near the lateral border.

13. The teres major arises from the lower one third of the rough strip along the dorsal aspect of the lateral border

14. The levator scapulae is inserted into a narrow strip along the dorsal aspect of the medial border, extending from the superior angle to the level of the root of the spine.

15. The rhomboideus minor is inserted into the dorsal aspect of the medial border, opposite the root of the spine.

16. The rhomboideus major is inserted into the dorsal aspect of the medial border, from the root of the spine to the inferior angle.

17. The capsule of the shoulder joint and the glenoidal labrum are attached to the margins of the glenoid cavity. In its upper part the attachment of the capsule extends above the supraglenoid tubercle so that the origin of the long head of the biceps is within the capsule.

THE HUMERUS

The humerus has a **shaft**, and **upper and lower ends** (Figs. 22.9, 22.10). The upper end is easily distinguished from the lower by the presence of a large rounded head. The medial and lateral sides can be distinguished by the fact that the head is directed medially. The anterior aspect of the upper end shows a prominent vertical groove called the **intertubercular sulcus**. The side to which a given bone belongs can be determined from the information given above.

The **head** is rounded and has a smooth convex articular surface. It is directed medially, and also somewhat backwards and upwards. It forms the shoulder joint along with the glenoid cavity of the scapula. It may be noted that the articular area of the head is much greater than that of the glenoid cavity.

In addition to the head, the upper end of the humerus shows two prominences called **the greater and lesser tubercles** (or tuberosities). These two tubercles are separated by the **intertubercular sulcus**.

The **lesser tubercle** lies on the anterior aspect of the bone medial to the sulcus, between it and the head.

The **greater tubercle** is placed on the lateral aspect of the upper. The tubercle shows three areas (or impressions) where muscles are attached (Fig.22.13).

The junction of the head with the rest of the upper end is called the **anatomical neck**, while the junction of the upper end with the shaft is called the **surgical neck**.

The **shaft** of the humerus has three borders: anterior, medial and lateral. These are easily distinguished in the lower part of the bone. When traced upwards the **anterior border** becomes continuous with the anterior margin of the greater tubercle. The **medial border**

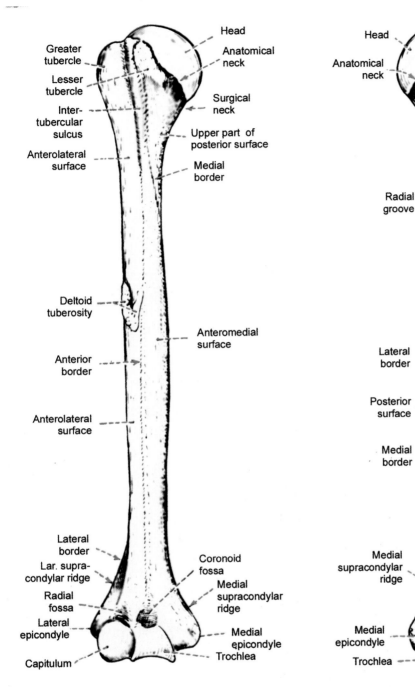

Fig. 22.9. Right humerus seen from the front.

Fig. 22.10. Right humerus seen from behind.

reaches the lesser tubercle. The lower part of the *lateral border* can be seen from the front, but its upper part runs upwards on the posterior aspect of the bone.

The three borders divide the shaft into three surfaces. The *anterolateral surface* lies between the anterior and lateral borders; the *anteromedial surface* between the anterior and medial borders, and the *posterior surface* between the medial and lateral borders.

We may now note certain additional features of the shaft. The anterolateral surface has a V-shaped rough

area called the *deltoid tuberosity* which is present near the middle of this surface. When the shaft is observed from behind we see that its upper part is crossed by a broad and shallow *radial groove* which runs downwards and laterally across the posterior and anterolateral surfaces.

The lower end of the humerus is irregular in shape and is also called the condyle. The lowest parts of the medial and lateral borders of the humerus form sharp ridges that are called the *medial and lateral supracondylar ridges* respectively. Their lower ends

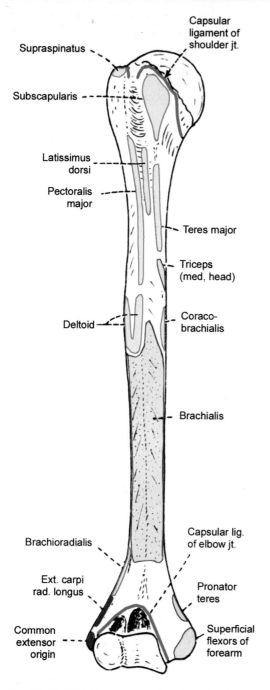

Fig. 22.11. Right humerus , showing attachments, seen from the front.

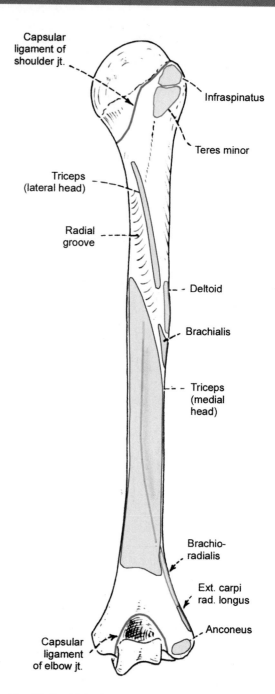

Fig. 22.12. Right humerus , showing attachments, seen from behind.

terminate in two prominences called the ***medial and lateral epicondyles***. Between the two epicondyles the lower end presents an irregular shaped articular surface which is divisible into medial and lateral parts. The lateral part is rounded and is called the ***capitulum***. It articulates with the head of the radius. The medial part of the articular surface is shaped like a pulley and is called the ***trochlea***. The trochlea articulates with the upper end (***trochlear notch***) of the ulna. The anterior aspect of the lower end of the humerus shows

two depressions: one just above the capitulum and another above the trochlea. The depression above the capitulum is called the ***radial fossa*** and that above the trochlea is called the ***coronoid fossa*** (Fig. 22.9). Another depression is seen above the trochlea on the posterior aspect of the lower end (Fig. 22.10). This depression is called the ***olecranon fossa***.

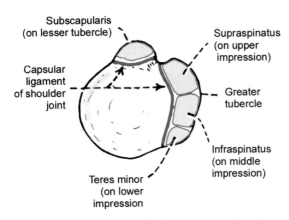

Fig. 22.13. Upper end of right humerus, showing attachments, seen from above.

Some Attachments on the Humerus

(Figs. 22.11, 22.12)

1. The *supraspinatus* is inserted into the upper impression on the greater tubercle.

2. The *infraspinatus* is inserted into the middle impression on the greater tubercle.

3. The *teres minor* is inserted into the lower impression on the greater tubercle.

4. The *subscapularis* is inserted into the lesser tubercle.

5. The *pectoralis major* is inserted into the lateral lip of the intertubercular sulcus.

6. The *latissimus dorsi* is inserted into the floor of the intertubercular sulcus.

7. The *teres major* is inserted into the medial lip of the intertubercular sulcus.

Of the three insertions into the intertubercular sulcus that of the pectoralis major is the most extensive, and that of the latissimus dorsi is the shortest.

8. The *deltoid* is inserted into the deltoid tuberosity.

9. The *coracobrachialis* is inserted into the rough area on the middle of the medial border.

10. The *brachialis* arises from the lower halves of the anteromedial and anterolateral surfaces of the shaft. Part of the area of origin extends onto the posterior aspect.

11. The *pronator teres* (humeral head) arises from the anteromedial surface, near the lower end of the medial supracondylar ridge.

12. The *brachioradialis* arises from the upper two thirds of the lateral supracondylar ridge.

13. The *extensor carpi radialis longus* arises from the lower one third of the lateral supracondylar ridge.

14. The superficial flexor muscles of the forearm arise from the anterior aspect of the medial epicondyle. This origin is called the *common flexor origin*.

15. The *common extensor origin* for the superficial extensor muscles of the forearm is located on the anterior aspect of the lateral condyle.

16. The lateral head of the *triceps* arises from the oblique ridge on the upper part of the posterior surface, just above the radial groove. The medial head of the muscle arises from the posterior surface below the radial groove. The upper end of the area of origin extends on to the anterior aspect of the shaft.

17. The *anconeus* arises from the posterior surface of the lateral epicondyle.

18. The *capsular ligament of the shoulder joint* is attached on the anatomical neck except on the medial side where the line of attachment dips down by about a centimetre to include a small area of the shaft within the joint cavity.

19. The *capsular ligament of the elbow joint* is attached to the lower end of the bone.

Important relations

1. The intertubercular sulcus lodges the tendon of the long head of the biceps brachii.

2. The surgical neck of the bone is related to the axillary nerve and to the anterior and posterior circumflex humeral vessels.

3. The radial nerve and the profunda brachii vessels lie in the radial groove between the attachments of the lateral and medial heads of the triceps.

4. The ulnar nerve crosses behind the medial epicondyle.

THE RADIUS

The radius is a long bone having a shaft and two ends (Figs. 22.14, 22.15). The upper end bears a disc shaped head. In contrast the lower end is much enlarged. The lateral and medial sides of the bone can be distinguished by examining the shaft which is convex laterally and has a sharp medial (or interosseous) border. The anterior and posterior aspects of the bone may be identified by looking at the lower end: it is smooth anteriorly, but the posterior aspect is marked by a number of ridges and grooves. The side to which a given radius belongs can be determined from the information given above.

The *upper end* of the bone consists of a head, a neck and a tuberosity. The *head* is disc shaped. Its upper surface is slightly concave and articulates with the capitulum of the humerus. The circumference of the head (representing the edge of the disc) articulates with a notch on the ulna to form the **superior radioulnar joint**.

The region just below the head is constricted to form the **neck**. Just below the medial part of the neck there is an elevation called the **radial tuberosity**.

The shaft of the radius has three borders (anterior, posterior, and interosseous) and three surfaces (anterior, posterior and lateral).

The **interosseous or medial border** forms a sharp ridge which extends from just below the tuberosity to the lower end of the shaft. The **anterior border** begins at the radial tuberosity and runs downwards and laterally across the anterior aspect of the shaft. This part of the anterior border is called the **anterior oblique line**. It then runs downwards and forms the lateral boundary of the smooth anterior aspect of the lower part of the shaft. The upper part of the **posterior border** runs downwards and laterally from the posterior part of the tuberosity. The lower part of the posterior border runs downwards along the middle of the posterior aspect of the shaft to the lower end. The **anterior surface** lies between the interosseous and anterior borders; the **posterior surface** between the interosseous and posterior borders; and the **lateral surface** between the anterior and posterior borders.

The lower end of the radius has anterior, lateral and posterior surfaces continuous with the corresponding surfaces of the shaft. In addition it has a medial surface and an inferior surface. The lateral surface is prolonged downwards as a projection called the **styloid process**. The medial aspect of the lower end has an articular area called the **ulnar notch**. It articulates with the lower end of the ulna to form the **inferior radioulnar**

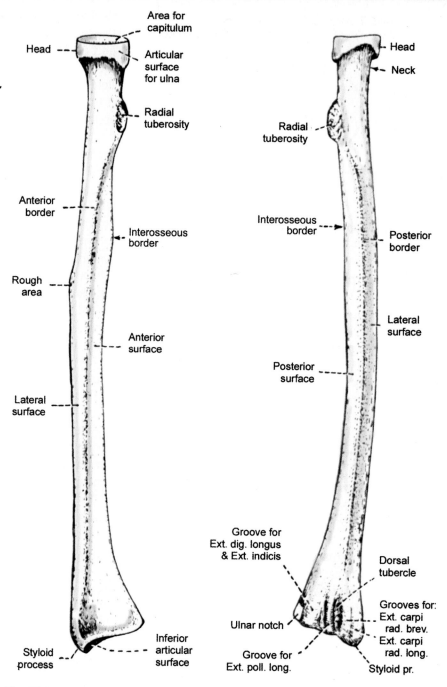

Fig. 22.14. Right radius seen from the front.

Fig. 22.15. Right radius seen from behind.

joint. The posterior aspect of the lower end is marked by a number of vertical grooves separated by ridges. The most prominent ridge is called the **dorsal tubercle**. The inferior surface of the lower end takes part in forming the wrist joint.

Attachments on the Radius

A. *The following muscles are inserted into the radius (Figs. 22.16, 22.17).*

1. The **biceps brachii** is inserted into the rough posterior part of the radial tuberosity.

2. The **supinator** is inserted into the upper part of the lateral surface. The area of insertion extends on to the anterior and posterior aspects of the shaft.

3. The **pronator teres** is inserted into the rough area on the middle of the lateral surface, at the point of maximum convexity of the shaft.

4. The **brachioradialis** is inserted into the lowest part of the lateral surface just above the styloid process.

5. The **pronator quadratus** is inserted into the lower part of the anterior surface, and into the triangular area on the medial side of the lower end.

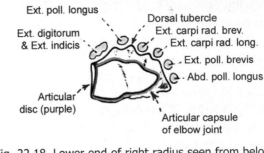

Fig. 22.18. Lower end of right radius seen from below. The related tendons are shown.

B. The following muscles take origin from the radius.

1. The **flexor digitorum superficialis** (radial head) arises from the upper part of the anterior border (oblique line).

2. The **flexor pollicis longus** arises from the upper two thirds of the anterior surface.

3. The **abductor pollicis longus** arises from the upper part of the posterior surface.

4. The **extensor pollicis brevis** arises from a small area on the posterior surface below the area for the abductor pollicis longus.

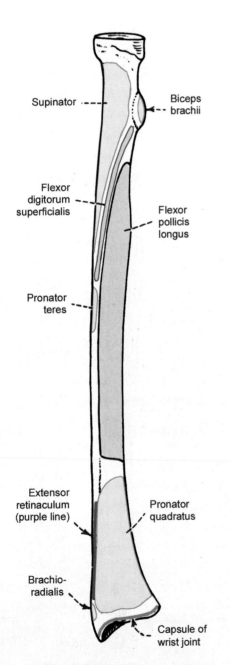

Fig. 22.16. Right radius, showing attachments, seen from the front.

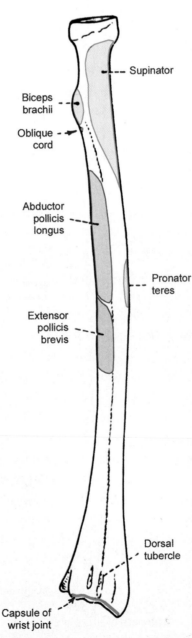

Fig. 22.17. Right radius, showing attachments, seen from behind.

THE ULNA

The ulna has a **shaft**, an **upper end** and a **lower end** (Figs. 22.19, 22.20). The upper end is large, while the lower end is small. The upper end has a large **trochlear notch** on its anterior aspect. The medial and lateral sides of the bone can be distinguished by examining the shaft: its lateral margin is sharp and thin, while its medial side is rounded. The side to which an ulna belongs can be determined from these facts.

The **upper end** of the ulna consists of two prominent projections called the **olecranon process** and the **coronoid process**. The olecranon process forms the uppermost part of the ulna. The coronoid process projects forwards from the anterior aspect of the ulna just below the olecranon process. The trochlear notch covers the anterior aspect of the olecranon process and the superior aspect of the coronoid process. It takes part in forming the elbow joint and articulates with the trochlea of the humerus.

The coronoid process has an upper surface which forms the lower part of the trochlear notch. In addition it has anterior, medial and lateral surfaces. The lower part of the anterior surface shows a rough projection called the *tuberosity* of the ulna. The upper part of the lateral surface of the coronoid process shows a concave articular facet called the *radial notch*. The radial notch articulates with the head of the radius forming the *superior radio-ulnar joint*. The bone shows a depression just below the radial notch. The posterior border of this depression is formed by a ridge called the *supinator crest*.

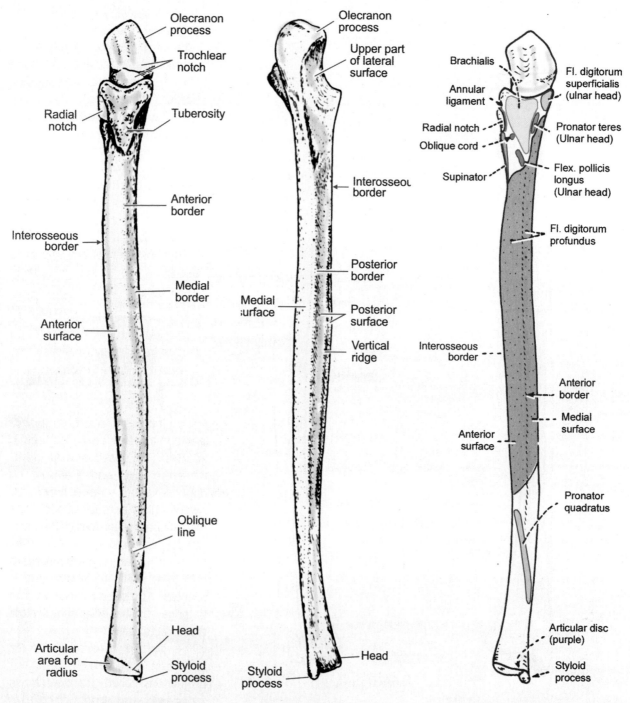

Fig. 22.19. Right ulna seen from the front.

Fig. 22.20. Right ulna seen from behind.

Fig. 22.21. Right ulna , showing attachments, seen from the front.

The lower end of the ulna consists of a disc-like **head** and a **styloid process**. The head has a circular inferior surface. This surface is separated from the cavity of the wrist joint by an articular disc. The head has another convex articular surface on its lateral side: this surface articulates with the ulnar notch of the radius to form the **inferior radioulnar joint**. The styloid process is a small downward projection that lies on the posteromedial aspect of the head. The tip of the styloid process of the ulna lies at a higher level than the styloid process of the radius.

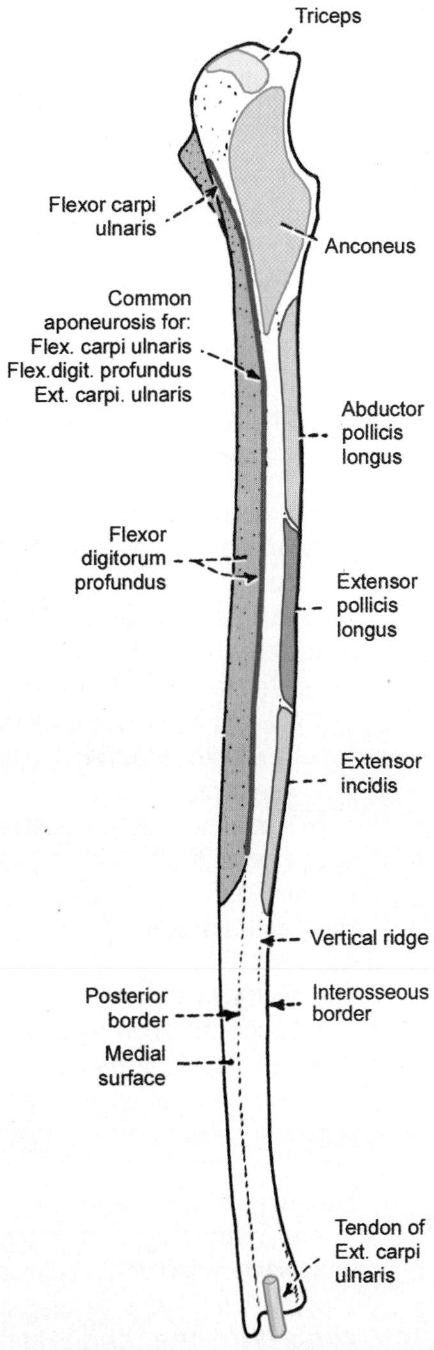

The shaft of the ulna has a sharp lateral or interosseous border, and less prominent anterior and posterior borders. It has anterior, posterior and medial surfaces. The upper part of the **interosseous border** is continuous with the supinator crest mentioned above. The **anterior border** begins at the tuberosity of the ulna. Its lower end lies in front of the styloid process. The **posterior border** begins on the posterior aspect of the olecranon process and ends at the styloid process. The **anterior surface** of the ulna lies between the interosseous and anterior borders The **medial surface** lies between the anterior and posterior borders. The **posterior surface** is bounded by the interosseous and posterior borders.

Important Attachments on the Ulna
(Figs. 22.21, 22.22)

1. The **brachialis** is inserted into the anterior surface of the coronoid process including the tuberosity.

2. The **triceps** is inserted into the posterior part of the superior surface of the olecranon process.

3. The **flexor digitorum profundus** arises from the upper three fourths of the anterior and medial surfaces.

4. The **supinator** arises from the supinator crest and from the triangular area in front of it.

5. The **flexor pollicis longus** (occasional ulnar head) arises from the lateral border of the coronoid process.

6. The **flexor digitorum superficialis** (ulnar head) arises from the tubercle at the upper end of the medial margin of the coronoid process.

7. The **pronator teres** (ulnar head) arises from the medial margin of the coronoid process.

8. The **pronator quadratus** arises from the oblique ridge on the lower part of the anterior surface of the shaft.

9. The **flexor carpi ulnaris** (ulnar head) arises from the medial side of the olecranon process, and from the upper two thirds of the posterior border through an aponeurosis common to it, the extensor carpi ulnaris and the flexor digitorum profundus.

10. The **extensor carpi ulnaris** (ulnar head) arises from the posterior border by an aponeurosis common to it, the flexor carpi ulnaris and the flexor digitorum profundus.

11. The posterior surface of the ulna is divided into medial and lateral parts by a vertical ridge. The lateral part lies between the vertical ridge and the interosseous border. This part of the posterior surface may be divided into four parts.

a) The uppermost part gives origin to the **abductor pollicis longus**.

b) The next part gives origin to the **extensor pollicis longus**.

c) The third part gives origin to the **extensor indicis**

d) The lowest part is devoid of attachments.

Fig. 22.22. Right ulna , showing attachments, seen from behind.

THE SKELETON OF THE HAND

The skeleton of the hand consists of the bones of the wrist, the palm, and of the digits.

The skeleton of the wrist consists of eight, small, roughly cuboidal carpal bones. The skeleton of the palm is made up of five metacarpal bones. These are miniature 'long' bones. The skeleton of the fingers is made up of the phalanges. There are three phalanges (proximal, middle and distal) in each digit except the thumb which has only two phalanges (proximal and distal).

THE CARPAL BONES

The carpal bones are arranged in two rows, proximal and distal (Fig. 22.23). The proximal row is made up (from lateral to medial side) of the *scaphoid*, *lunate*, *triquetral* and *pisiform* bones. The distal row is made up (from lateral to medial side) of the *trapezium*, *trapezoid*, *capitate* and *hamate* bones.

The carpal bones of the proximal row (except the pisiform) take part in forming the wrist joint. The distal row of carpal bones articulate with the metacarpal bones. Each carpal bone articulates with neighbouring carpal bones to form intercarpal joints.

The Scaphoid Bone

The scaphoid bone can be distinguished because of its distinctive boat-like shape. The proximal part of the bone is covered by a large, convex, articular surface for the radius. Distally and laterally the palmar surface of the bone bears a projection called the *tubercle*.

The medial surface of the scaphoid articulates with the lunate bone (proximally) and with the capitate (distally). The distal surface of the scaphoid articulates with the trapezium (laterally) and with the trapezoid bone (medially).

The Lunate Bone

The lunate bone can be distinguished because it is shaped like a lunar crescent.

Proximally, the bone has a convex articular facet that takes part in forming the wrist joint. The bone articulates laterally with the scaphoid; medially with the triquetral; and distally with the capitate. Between the areas for the capitate and for the triquetral the lunate may articulate with the hamate bone.

The Triquetral Bone

The triquetral bone is a small and roughly cuboidal. The distal part of its palmar surface articulates with the pisiform bone. It takes part in forming the wrist joint: it comes into contact with the articular disc of the inferior radioulnar joint.

Its lateral surface articulates with the hamate bone. The proximal surface articulates with the lunate bone.

The Pisiform Bone

This bone is shaped like a pea. Its dorsal aspect bears a single facet for articulation with the triquetral bone.

The Trapezium

This bone bears a thick prominent *ridge* on its palmar aspect. This ridge is called the *tubercle*. The trapezium articulates proximally and medially with the scaphoid;

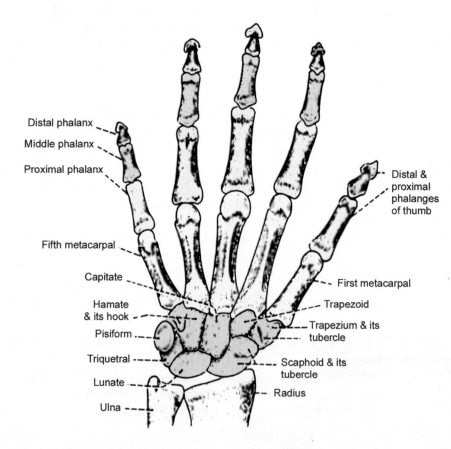

Distal phalanx

Middle phalanx

Proximal phalanx

Distal & proximal phalanges of thumb

Fifth metacarpal

Capitate

First metacarpal

Hamate & its hook

Trapezoid

Pisiform

Trapezium & its tubercle

Triquetral

Scaphoid & its tubercle

Lunate

Radius

Ulna

Fig. 22.23. Skeleton of the hand seen from the front.

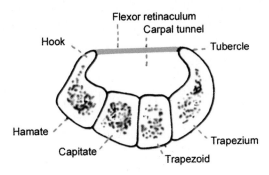

Fig. 22.24. Schematic section across the distal row of carpal bones.

distally and laterally with the first metacarpal bone; medially with the trapezoid bone; and distally and medially with the base of the second metacarpal bone.

The Trapezoid Bone

This bone is of small size and is irregular shape. It articulates distally with the base of the 2nd metacarpal bone, laterally with the trapezium, medially with the capitate, and proximally with the scaphoid.

The Capitate Bone

The capitate bone is the largest carpal bone, and bears a rounded *head* at one end.

The capitate lies right in the middle of the carpus. Proximally, it articulates with the lunate bone.. Distally the capitate bone articulates mainly with the third metacarpal bone, but it also articulates with the second and fourth metacarpal bones.

Its lateral aspect articulates with the scaphoid (proximally) and with the trapezoid (distally). Medially, it articulates with the hamate bone.

The Hamate Bone

The hamate has a prominent hook-like process attached to its palmar aspect. The hamate is triangular in shape, the apex of the triangle being directed proximally. The apex may articulate with the lunate bone. Distally the hamate articulates with the 4th and 5th metacarpal bones. Medially and proximally the hamate articulates with the triquetral bone, and laterally with the capitate.

The Carpal Tunnel

The carpal bones are so arranged that the dorsal, medial and lateral surfaces of the carpus form one convex surface. On the other hand the palmar surface is deeply concave with overhanging medial and lateral projections. This concavity is converted into the carpal tunnel by a band of fascia called the *flexor retinaculum* (Fig. 22.24).

The retinaculum is attached, medially to the pisiform bone and to the hook of the hamate; and laterally to the tubercle of the scaphoid and to the tubercle of the trapezium.

THE METACARPAL BONES

The hand has five metacarpal bones. They are numbered from lateral to medial side so that the bone related to the thumb is the first metacarpal, and that related to the little finger is the fifth. Each metacarpal is a miniature long bone having a shaft, a distal end and a proximal end.

The distal end forms a rounded head. It bears a large convex articular surface for articulation with the proximal phalanx of the corresponding digit. The shaft is triangular in cross section and has medial, lateral and dorsal surfaces. The bases (or proximal ends) of the metacarpal bones are irregular in shape. They articulate with the distal row of carpal bones. The first metacarpal articulates with the trapezium; the second mainly with the trapezoid; the third mainly with the capitate; the fourth and fifth with the hamate bone. Numerous other smaller articulations exist.

The bases of the second and third, third and fourth, and fourth and fifth metacarpal bones also articulate with each other.

THE PHALANGES OF THE HAND

Each digit of the hand, except the thumb, has three phalanges: proximal, middle and distal. The thumb has only two phalanges, proximal and distal. Each phalanx has a distal end or head, a proximal end or base, and an intervening shaft or body.

Attachments on the Skeleton of the Hand

The skeleton of the hand gives attachment to numerous muscles and other structures. Details of these will be mentioned when we study these structures.

23

Joints of the Upper Extremity

JOINTS CONNECTING THE SCAPULA & CLAVICLE

The Acromioclavicular Joint

This is a plane synovial joint. It is formed by articulation of small facets at the lateral end of the clavicle and the medial margin of the acromion. Movements at this joint accompany those at the sternoclavicular joint. These movements are necessary for allowing various movements of the scapula associated with movements of the arm at the shoulder joint.

Coracoclavicular ligament

The main bond of union between the scapula and clavicle is through the coracoclavicular ligament. The ligament consists of two parts, conoid and trapezoid. The trapezoid part is attached, below, to the upper surface of the coracoid process of the scapula; and, above, to the trapezoid line on the inferior surface of the clavicle. The conoid part is attached, below, to the root of the coracoid process just lateral to the scapular notch. It is attached, above, to the inferior surface of the clavicle on the conoid tubercle.

Coracoacromial ligament

The coracoacromial ligament connects the coracoid and acromial processes of the scapula, and along with them forms the coracoacromial arch. It is triangular. Its apex is attached to the medial aspect of the tip of the acromion. Its base is attached to the lateral border of the coracoid process. The coracoacromial arch protects the head of the humerus and prevents its upward dislocation.

THE STERNOCLAVICULAR JOINT

The sternoclavicular joint is synovial. There are three elements taking part in it; namely the medial end of the clavicle, the clavicular notch of the manubrium sterni, and the upper surface of the first costal cartilage. Its cavity is subdivided into two parts by an intra-articular disc. The articular surfaces of the clavicle and sternum are concavo-convex.

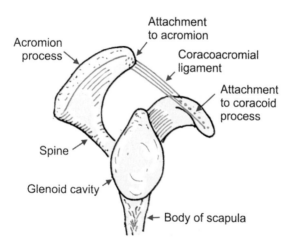

Fig. 23.1. Upper part of scapula, lateral view, to show attachments of coracoacromial ligament.

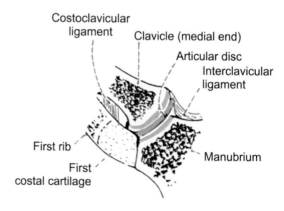

Fig. 23.2. Sternoclavicular joint as seen in coronal section.

The capsular ligament is attached laterally to the margins of the clavicular articular surface; and medially to the margins of the articular areas on the sternum and on the first costal cartilage. It is strong anteriorly and posteriorly where it constitutes the anterior and posterior sternoclavicular ligaments. However, the main bond of union at this joint is the articular disc. The disc is attached laterally to the clavicle on a rough area above and posterior to the area for the sternum. Inferiorly, the disc is attached to the sternum and to the first costal cartilage at their junction. Anteriorly and posteriorly the disc fuses with the capsule.

There are two other ligaments associated with this joint.

The interclavicular ligament passes between the sternal ends of the right and left clavicles (Fig. 23.2). The costoclavicular ligament is attached above to the rough area on the inferior aspect of the medial end of the clavicle. Inferiorly, it is attached to the first costal cartilage and to the first rib.

The movements occurring at this joint are secondary to movements of the scapula, which are in turn secondary to movements of the arm. Simultaneous movements also occur at the acromioclavicular joint.

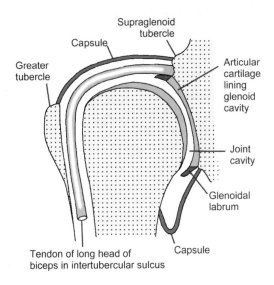

Fig. 23.3. Schematic coronal section through the shoulder joint.

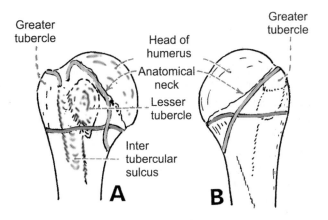

Fig. 23.4. Upper end of humerus seen from: A. the front; B. from behind, to show the attachment of the capsular ligament.

THE SHOULDER JOINT

The shoulder joint is a synovial joint of the ball and socket variety. The joint is formed by the head of the humerus and the glenoid cavity of the scapula.

The articular surface of the head of the humerus is rounded like a hemisphere (Fig. 23.4). It is directed medially, backwards and upwards. It is covered by a layer of hyaline articular cartilage which is thickest in the centre and thinnest at the periphery thus increasing the convexity. The glenoid cavity is directed laterally and forwards. It is much smaller than the head of the humerus (Fig. 23.3). The cavity is shallow. The depth of the cavity is increased somewhat by the articular cartilage lining it; the cartilage is thinnest in the centre and thickest at the periphery. The depth of the cavity is also increased by the presence of a rim of fibrocartilage attached to the margin of the glenoid cavity: this is the glenoidal labrum (Fig. 23.3).

The capsular ligament is attached, medially, to the margins of the glenoid cavity beyond the glenoidal labrum. Superiorly, the line of attachment extends above the origin of the long head of the biceps from the supraglenoid tubercle. On the lateral side the capsule is attached to the head of the humerus just beyond the articular surface i.e., to the anatomical neck; however, on the medial side the line of attachment extends downwards on to the shaft so that part of it is within the joint cavity. The capsule is strengthened by the following ligaments.

a) The glenohumeral ligaments, superior, middle and inferior, are attached medially to the upper part of the anteromedial margin of the glenoid cavity. Laterally the superior ligament reaches the upper part of the lesser tubercle of the humerus. The middle ligament is attached to the lower part of the lesser tubercle, and the inferior ligament on the anatomical neck (Fig. 23.5).

b) The coraco-humeral ligament is attached, medially to the root of the coracoid process (above the supraglenoid tubercle), and laterally to the greater tubercle of the humerus.

c) The transverse humeral ligament stretches between the greater and lesser tubercles. It converts the inter-tubercular sulcus into a canal through which the tendon of the long head of the biceps leaves the joint cavity.

The shoulder joint is surrounded by a number of muscles that support it. These are the supraspinatus (superiorly), the subscapularis (in front), the infraspinatus and teres minor (behind) and the long head of the triceps (below). With the exception of the long head of the triceps, the tendons of these muscles blend with the capsule forming what is called the rotator cuff. The long head of the triceps is some distance away from the capsule: as a result the inferior part of the capsule is least supported and is the weakest part.

The joint is surrounded by a number of bursae. They facilitate movements between structures surrounding the joint.

The synovial membrane lines the inside of the capsular ligament, both sides of the glenoidal labrum and the non-articular parts of the humerus enclosed within the capsule. The tendon of the long head of the biceps is enclosed in a tubular sheath of synovial membrane: this sheath is prolonged, for some distance, into the intertubercular sulcus.

The shoulder joint is supplied by the anterior and posterior circumflex humeral, and the suprascapular

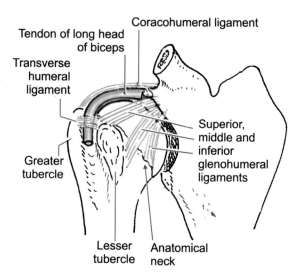

Fig. 23.5. Some ligaments of the shoulder joint.

arteries; and by the suprascapular, axillary and lateral pectoral nerves.

Movements at the shoulder joint

Movements of the arm take place at the shoulder joint. These are described with reference to the plane of the scapula. Note that the scapula is placed obliquely (behind the thorax) and that the glenoid cavity faces forwards and laterally.

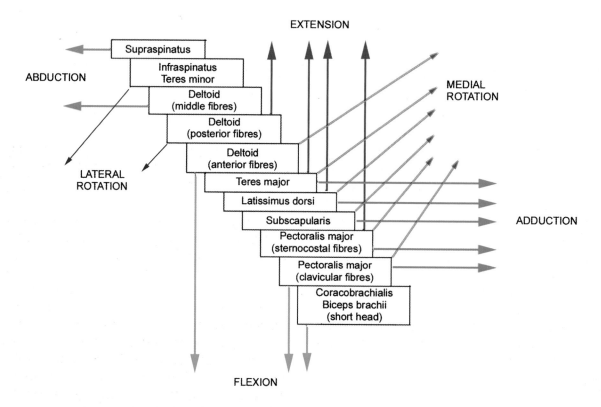

Fig. 23.6. Scheme to show muscles producing movements at the shoulder joint

1. The movements of abduction and adduction take place in the plane of the scapula. In abduction the arm moves laterally and somewhat forwards. In adduction the arm returns to the side of the body. Abduction and adduction take place partly at the shoulder joint, and partly by rotation of the scapula.

2. Flexion and extension take place at right angles to the plane of the scapula. In flexion the arm moves forwards and somewhat medially. Reversal of this movement is extension.

3. Medial and lateral rotation of the humerus takes place around an imaginary axis passing vertically through the bone. In medial rotation the anterior aspect of the humerus rotates to face medially. The reverse takes place in lateral rotation.

THE ELBOW JOINT

This is a synovial joint of the hinge variety. Three bones take part in forming it. These are the lower end of the humerus and the upper ends of the radius and ulna. The capitulum of the humerus articulates with the concave upper surface of the head of the radius (humero-radial joint); and the trochlear of the humerus articulates with the trochlear notch at the upper end of the ulna (humero-ulnar joint). The cavity of the joint is continuous with that of the superior radio-ulnar joint.

The line of attachment of the articular capsule to the humerus is shown in Figs. 23.7A, B. Note that the coronoid fossa, the radial fossa and the olecranon fossa lie within the joint cavity. Inferiorly, the capsule is attached to the coronoid and olecranon processes of the ulna around the margins of the articular surface. On the lateral side it is not attached directly to the radius, but to the annular ligament of the superior radioulnar joint, which encircles the head of the bone.

The capsular ligament is thickened on the medial and lateral sides to form the ulnar and radial collateral ligaments.

The ulnar collateral ligament is triangular in form. Its apex is attached to the medial epicondyle of the humerus, and its base to the ulna. Some details are shown in Fig. 23.8.

The radial collateral ligament is attached at its upper end to the lateral epicondyle of the humerus and below to the annular ligament of the superior radioulnar joint (Fig. 23.9).

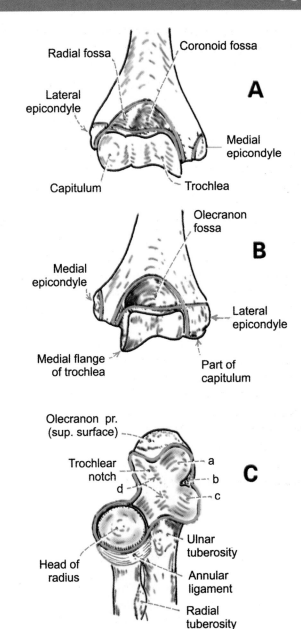

Fig. 23.7. Attachment of the capsular ligament of the elbow joint to the humerus. A. Anterior aspect. B. Posterior aspect. Epiphyseal lines are also shown. C. Lower articular surfaces of elbow joint, and capsular attachment.

The synovial membrane of the joint covers all non-articular areas of bone enclosed within the capsule. These include the radial, coronoid and olecranon fossae.

The elbow joint receives its blood supply from the arterial anastomoses around it. It receives its nerve supply from nerves that cross it: mainly the musculocutaneous and the radial, but also from the ulnar, the median and the anterior interosseus nerves.

The movements allowed at the elbow joint are flexion and extension. When the joint is extended the supinated forearm passes somewhat laterally (relative to the arm). The lateral angle between the arm and forearm is about 160 degrees and is called the carrying angle.

The muscles responsible for producing flexion at the elbow joint are the brachialis, the biceps brachii and the brachioradialis. Extension is produced by the triceps. The anconeus plays a minor role in extension.

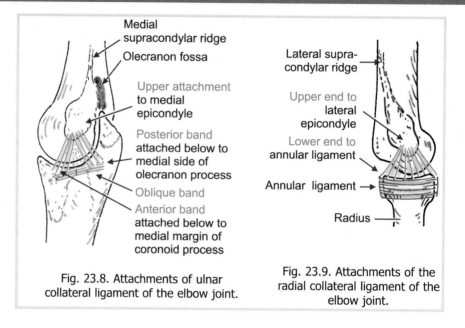

Fig. 23.8. Attachments of ulnar collateral ligament of the elbow joint.

Fig. 23.9. Attachments of the radial collateral ligament of the elbow joint.

THE RADIOULNAR JOINTS

The upper and lower ends of the radius and ulna are joined to each other at the superior and inferior radioulnar joints. The shafts of the two bones are united by the interosseus membrane (sometimes called the middle radioulnar joint). The superior and inferior joints are both synovial and of the pivot variety.

At the superior radioulnar joint the head of the radius rotates within a ring formed by the radial notch of the ulna and the annular ligament (Fig. 23.7C). The annular ligament surrounds the circumference of the head of the radius and is attached anteriorly and posteriorly to margins of the radial notch of the ulna. We have seen that the annular ligament is continuous above with the capsular ligament of the elbow joint. The cavity of the superior radioulnar joint is continuous with that of the elbow joint.

The inferior radioulnar joint is formed by articulation of the convex articular surface on the lateral side of the head of the ulna with the ulnar notch of the radius. The chief bond of union between the two bones is through an articular disc. The disc is triangular. Its apex (directed medially) is attached to the ulna on a depression just lateral to the styloid process. Its base is attached to the radius on the lower margin of the ulnar notch. Its upper surface forms part of the inferior radioulnar joint and articulates with the inferior surface of the head of the ulna. Its lower surface (Fig. 23.10) forms part of the proximal articular surface of the wrist

joint. The cavities of these two joints are completely separated by the disc.

Supination And Pronation Of Forearm:

These are rotary movements that take place at the superior and inferior radioulnar joints. When the forearm is held so that the palm faces forwards, the radius and ulna lie parallel to each other: this is the position of supination. In pronation the forearm rotates (along with the hand) so that the radius crosses in front of the ulna and its lower end comes to lie medial to that of the ulna.

The muscles responsible for supination are the supinator and the biceps brachii. The latter can act only after the forearm has been semi-flexed. Pronation is produced by the pronator quadratus and the pronator teres.

The role of the brachioradialis in supination and pronation is controversial.

THE WRIST JOINT

The wrist joint is a synovial joint of the ellipsoid variety. It has a concave proximal articular surface formed by the distal end of the radius, and by the inferior surface of the articular disc of the inferior radioulnar joint. The distal articular surface is convex. It is formed by the proximal surfaces of the scaphoid, lunate and triquetral bones. The articular capsule is attached to the margins

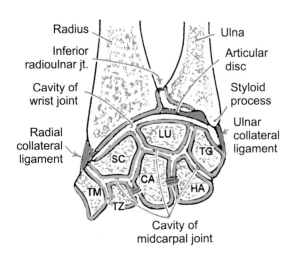

Fig. 23.10. Schematic coronal section through the wrist to show the formation of the articular surfaces of the inferior radioulnar, wrist and midcarpal joints.

proximally to the styloid process of the radius and distally to the lateral side of the scaphoid bone.

The movements at the wrist joint are flexion, extension, adduction and abduction.. The muscles responsible for the movements are shown in Fig. 23.11.

OTHER JOINTS OF THE UPPER LIMB

of the proximal and distal articular surfaces. Parts of it are thickened to form several ligaments. The anterior part of the capsule is thickened in its lateral part to form the palmar radiocarpal ligament; and in its medial part to form the **palmar ulnocarpal ligament**. The posterior part of the capsule is thickened in its lateral part to form the **dorsal radiocarpal ligament**. The strongest bonds of union are, however, the ulnar and radial collateral ligaments.

The **ulnar collateral ligament** is attached proximally to the styloid process of the ulna; and distally to the medial side of the triquetral and pisiform bones (Fig. 23.10). The radial collateral ligament is attached

The **midcarpal joint** is present between the proximal and distal row of carpal bones. It allows the same movements as the wrist joint, extending their range considerably.

The **carpometacarpal joint of the thumb** is a synovial joint. It is a typical example of a saddle joint. The bones taking part are the distal surface of the trapezium, and the proximal surface of the first metacarpal. The surface of the metacarpal is convex from side to side and concave from front to back. The surface on the trapezium shows reciprocal curvatures.

Compared to other carpometacarpal joints this joint has considerable mobility. The movements of the thumb differ from those of other digits as the thumb is rotated through 90° on its long axis, relative to the other digits. As a result its ventral surface faces medially (not anteriorly) and its dorsal surface faces laterally (not posteriorly as in other digits). Therefore, flexion and extension of the thumb take place in a plane parallel

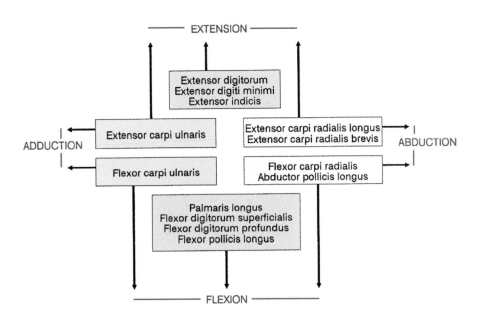

Fig. 23.11. Scheme to show the muscles responsible for movements at the wrist joint.

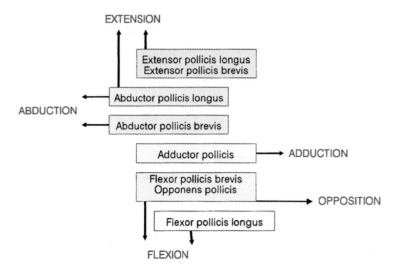

Fig. 23.12. Scheme to show the muscles responsible for movements at the carpometacarpal joint of the thumb. Note that flexion is associated with a certain amount of medial rotation, and extension with lateral rotation.

to that of the palm while abduction and adduction of the thumb take place in a plane at right angles to that for the other digits (i.e., at right angles to the plane of the palm).

The muscles producing movements of the thumb are shown in Fig. 23.12.

The remaining *intercarpal*, *carpo-metacarpal*, and *intermetacarpal joints* are all plane joints and permit slight gliding movements only. These movements confer considerable resilience to the region of the wrist.

The *metacarpophalangeal joints* are typical ellipsoid joints allowing flexion, extension, abduction and adduction of the fingers. Rotation is not permitted.

The *interphalangeal joints* are typical hinge joints of the condylar variety. The thumb has only one such joint. Each finger has two joints, proximal and distal. Movements at these joints are important in gripping and other uses of the fingers.

24

Muscles of the Upper Extremity

MUSCLES OF THE PECTORAL REGION

Pectoralis Major

Origin:

The pectoralis major takes origin from the following (Fig. 24.1):

a) Medial half of the anterior surface of the clavicle.

b) The anterior surface of the sternum.

c) The medial parts of the upper seven costal cartilages.

d) The aponeurosis of the external oblique muscle.

Insertion:

The fibres of the muscle converge towards the anterior aspect of the upper end of the humerus. They are inserted into the lateral lip of the intertubercular sulcus ('e' in figure). The tendon of insertion is bilaminar, and consists of an anterior and a posterior lamina. The anterior lamina receives the clavicular and upper sternocostal fibres. The posterior lamina receives the fibres from the lower costal cartilages and from the aponeurosis of the external oblique muscle.

Nerve Supply:

Lateral and medial pectoral nerves (C 5, 6, 7, 8 T1).

Actions:

The muscle is an adductor, medial rotator and flexor of the arm.

Pectoralis Minor

Origin (Fig. 24.2):

The pectoralis minor takes origin mainly by slips from the 3rd, 4th and 5th ribs (near their junctions with the costal cartilages).

Insertion:

The muscle ends in a tendon which is inserted into the coracoid process of the scapula.

Nerve Supply:

Medial and lateral pectoral nerves (C6, 7, 8).

Actions:

a) The muscle helps the serratus anterior in moving the scapula forwards around the chest wall (in protracting the arm).

b) The muscle helps the levator scapulae and the rhomboids to rotate the scapula backwards.

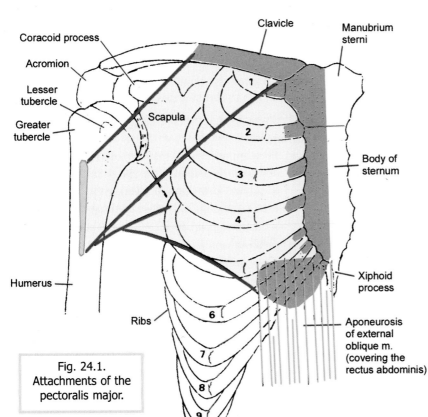

Fig. 24.1. Attachments of the pectoralis major.

Coracoid process — Acromion — Lesser tubercle — Greater tubercle — Scapula — Humerus — Ribs — Clavicle — Manubrium sterni — Body of sternum — Xiphoid process — Aponeurosis of external oblique m. (covering the rectus abdominis)

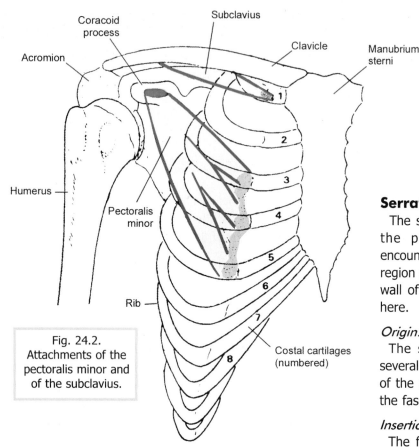

Fig. 24.2.
Attachments of the pectoralis minor and of the subclavius.

The muscle lies in front of the axillary artery and is used to divide the artery into its first, second and third parts.

Subclavius

Origin:
The subclavius arises from the junction of the first rib with its costal cartilage (Fig. 24.2).

Insertion:
The muscle is inserted into a groove on middle one third of the inferior surface of the clavicle.

Nerve Supply:
The nerve to the subclavius (C5, 6) arises from the upper trunk of the brachial plexus (Erb's point).

Actions:
The subclavius depresses the clavicle.

Clavipectoral fascia

This fascia fills the gap between the clavicle (above) and the medial edge of the pectoralis minor (below). Near its upper end the fascia splits to enclose the subclavius. At the medial edge of the pectoralis minor its splits to enclose the pectoralis minor. At the lower (lateral) edge of the pectoralis minor the fascia

becomes continuous with the axillary fascia (forming the floor of the axilla). The clavipectoral fascia is pierced by the thoracoacromial artery and vein, the cephalic vein, and the lateral pectoral nerve. Some lymphatics of the breast and pectoral region passing to the apical lymph nodes of the axilla also pass through it.

Serratus Anterior

The serratus anterior does not belong to the pectoral region. However, it is encountered in the lateral part of the pectoral region and takes part in forming the medial wall of the axilla. It is therefore described here.

Origin:
The serratus anterior takes origin, by several digitations from the outer surfaces of the upper eight (or nine) ribs, and from the fascia covering the intercostal muscles.

Insertion:
The fibres of the muscle run backwards round the wall of the thorax. They pass deep to the scapula to reach its medial border. The entire muscle is inserted into the costal surface of the scapula along its medial border.

Nerve Supply:
The nerve to the serratus anterior is a branch of the branchial plexus and arises from the roots C5, 6, 7.

Actions:
(a) The muscle pulls the scapula forwards around the chest wall to protract the upper limb.
(b) It rotates the scapula (alongwith the trapezius) so that the glenoid cavity is turned upwards.

THE AXILLA

The axilla is the region of the arm pit. The boundaries of the axilla are as follows.

The **anterior wall** is formed by the pectoralis major, the pectoralis minor and the clavipectoral fascia. The **posterior wall** is formed by muscles lying in front of the scapula. In the upper part there is the subscapularis, and lower down there are the teres major and the latissimus dorsi. The latissimus dorsi winds round the lower margin of the teres major, the two together forming the thick posterior fold of the axilla. The **medial wall** is formed by the upper few ribs and intercostal spaces. They are covered by the upper part of a large muscle called the serratus anterior. The *lateral wall* is formed by the humerus in the region of the intertubercular sulcus. The sulcus is occupied by the tendon of the long head of the biceps brachii. The short head of the same muscle, and the coracobrachialis lie just medial to it. The *floor* of the axilla is formed by axillary fascia, covered by skin. The axillary fascia has an aperture through which the axillary tail of the breast enters the axilla. The *apex* of the axilla faces upwards and somewhat medially and lies at the level of the outer border of the first rib. Behind the apex there is the upper border of the scapula, and in front of it there is the clavicle. These three structures form the boundaries of an opening through which the axillary vessels and the brachial plexus pass from the neck into the axilla. The opening is, therefore, called the *cervicoaxillary canal*.

The *contents of the axilla* are the axillary artery and vein, and the axillary lymph nodes.

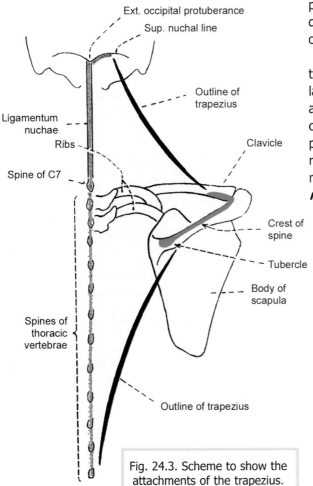

Fig. 24.3. Scheme to show the attachments of the trapezius.

MUSCLES OF THE UPPER LIMB SEEN ON THE BACK

The muscles of the upper limb, to be seen on the back, are concerned with movements of the scapula. It is important to understand these as they, in turn, affect movements of the arm.

Movements of the scapula

The scapula is held in position by muscles attached to it and its position depends upon the relative degree of contraction of different muscles. In *protraction* the entire bone slides forwards over the chest wall. Reversal of this movement is *retraction*. In *elevation* the entire bone moves upwards (as in shrugging the shoulders); and the opposite movement is called *depression*.

In addition to these simple movements the scapula can undergo rotation. To understand rotation imagine that the scapula is transfixed by an imaginary nail passing through the centre of its body. Rotation is described in terms of movement of the inferior angle of the scapula.

In *forward rotation* (also called *lateral rotation*) the inferior angle passes forwards and somewhat laterally. Simultaneously, the superior angle and the acromion pass backwards and medially. The glenoid cavity comes to face upwards. This movement takes place during abduction of the arm, and is essential for raising the arm above the head. Reversal of this movement constitutes *backward (or medial) rotation*.

The muscles of the upper limb present on the back are the trapezius, the latissimus dorsi, the levator scapulae, the rhomboideus major and the rhomboideus minor.

Trapezius (Fig. 24.3)

Origin:

The muscles has a long linear origin from the following structures.

1. Medial one-third of superior nuchal line.

2. External occipital protuberance.

3. Ligamentum nuchae.

4. Spine of 7th cervical vertebra.

5. Spines of all thoracic vertebrae and intervening supraspinous ligaments.

Insertion:

The muscle is inserted into:

1. The posterior border of the lateral one-third of the clavicle.

2. The medial margin of the acromion.

3. The spine of the scapula.

Nerve Supply:

The muscle is supplied by the spinal part of the accessory nerve and by branches from the third and fourth cervical nerves.

Actions:

The trapezius takes part in performing the following movements:

1. Forward rotation of the scapula, along with the serratus anterior.

2. Elevation of the scapula, along with the levator scapulae.

3. Retraction of the scapula, along with rhomboids.

4. The muscles of the two sides acting together draw the head backwards. Each muscle acting alone draws the head backwards and laterally to its own side.

Latissimus Dorsi (Fig. 24.4)

Origin:

The latissimus dorsi has a long origin from the following:

1) The spines of the lower six thoracic vertebrae and the intervening supraspinous ligaments.

2) The lumbar fascia.

3) The iliac crest.

The fibres of the muscle converge towards the axilla. Here the muscle winds round the lower border of the teres major to reach its anterior aspect. The two muscles together form the posterior fold of the axilla.

Insertion:

The muscle ends in a tendon which is inserted into the **anterior** aspect of the upper end of the humerus, in the floor of the intertubercular sulcus.

Nerve Supply:

The muscle is supplied by the thoracodorsal nerve (C6, C7, C8).

Actions:

1. Adduction of the arm.

2. Medial rotation of the arm.

3. Extension of the arm.

Levator Scapulae

Origin:

From the transverse processes of the upper four cervical vertebrae.

Insertion:

Medial margin of the scapula from the superior angle to the root of the spine.

Nerve Supply:

Branches from spinal nerves C3 & C4 and from the dorsal scapula nerve (C5).

Actions:

See under rhomboideus major.

Rhomboideus minor

Origin:

From lowest part of ligamentum nuchae and from the spines of vertebrae C7 & T1.

Insertion:

Medial margin of the scapula opposite the root of the spine.

Nerve supply:

Dorsal scapular nerve.

Actions: See under rhomboideus major

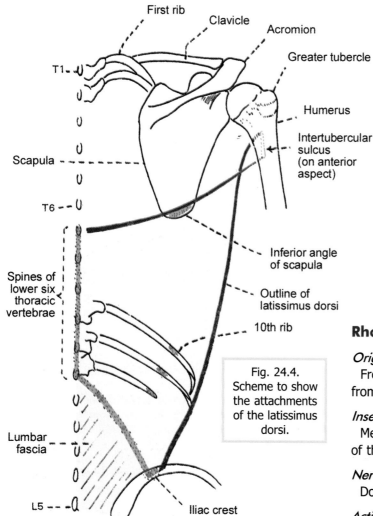

First rib
Clavicle
Acromion
Greater tubercle
T1
Humerus
Intertubercular sulcus (on anterior aspect)
Scapula
T6
Inferior angle of scapula
Spines of lower six thoracic vertebrae
Outline of latissimus dorsi
10th rib
Lumbar fascia
L5
Iliac crest

Fig. 24.4. Scheme to show the attachments of the latissimus dorsi.

Rhomboideus major

Origin:

From spines of vertebrae T2 to T5.

Insertion:

Into medial margin of scapula (from the level of the root of the spine to the inferior angle).

Nerve supply: Dorsal scapular nerve (C5).

Actions of levator scapula and rhomboideus muscles:

The levator scapulae elevates the scapula, while the rhomboideus muscles retract it. Acting together they steady the scapula during movements of the upper limb. They also produce backward rotation of the scapula.

MUSCLES OF THE SCAPULAR REGION

In the scapular region we see several muscles that take origin from the scapula and gain insertion into the humerus. These are the deltoid, the supraspinatus, the infraspinatus, the teres major, the teres minor, and the subscapularis.

Deltoid (Fig. 24.5)

Origin:

The deltoid has one continuous origin from:

1) Upper surface and anterior border of the lateral one third of the clavicle.

2) Lateral margin and upper surface of the acromion.

3) Lower lip of crest of spine of scapula.

Insertion:

Deltoid tuberosity on the lateral aspect of the shaft of the humerus.

Nerve Supply:

By the axillary nerve (C5, C6).

Actions:

1) The anterior fibres cause flexion and medial rotation of the humerus.

2) The posterior fibres cause extension and lateral rotation.

3) The acromial part of the muscle produces abduction of the arm at the shoulder joint (See below).

Mechanism of abduction of the arm:

Abduction of the arm is a complicated movement and the deltoid is one of the most important muscles for it. Abduction of the arm takes place partly at the shoulder joint, and partly by rotation of the scapula. The first few degrees of abduction at the shoulder joint are produced by the supraspinatus. Abduction up to 90 degrees is produced by the deltoid. Further abduction is produced by forward rotation of the scapula produced by the serratus anterior and the trapezius acting together.

Supraspinatus

This muscle covers the posterior aspect of the scapula above the spine, and passes to the uppermost part of the humerus.

Origin:

From medial two-thirds of supraspinous fossa of scapula.

Insertion:

Into uppermost impression on greater tubercle of humerus.

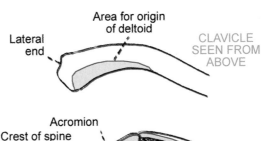

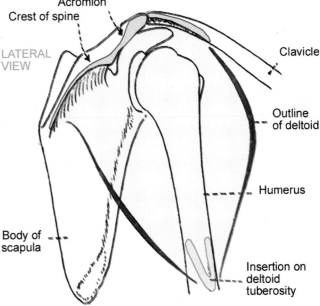

Fig. 24.5. Attachments of the deltoid muscle.

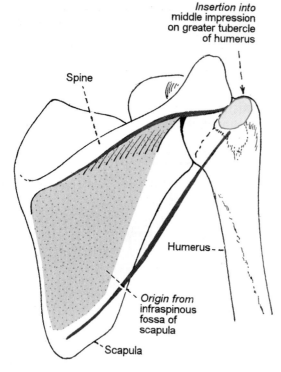

Fig. 24.6. Attachments of the infraspinatus.

Actions:

1. The supraspinatus, acting along with other muscles, around the shoulder joint, stabilises it.

2. It is an abductor of the arm.

Infraspinatus (Fig. 24.6)

Origin:

From medial two-thirds of the infraspinous fossa, of the scapula.

Insertion:

Into middle impression on greater tubercle of humerus .

Actions:

These are described along with those of the teres minor.

Nerve Supply:

Suprascapular nerve (C4, 5, 6).

Teres Minor

Origin:

From dorsal surface of scapula along the upper two-thirds of the lateral border.

Insertion:

Into lowest impression on greater tubercle of humerus.

Nerve supply: Axillary nerve.

Actions common to infraspinatus and teres minor:

1. These muscles are adductors and lateral rotators of the humerus.

2. They stabilize the shoulder joint and strengthen the posterior part of its capsule.

3. During abduction of the arm (by the deltoid and the supraspinatus) their downward pull prevents the head of the humerus from getting stuck under the coraco-acromial arch. This allows abduction to take place smoothly.

Teres Major (Fig. 24.7)

Origin:

From dorsal surface of scapula; the area of origin overlies the inferior angle and the lower one third of the lateral border.

Insertion:

On ***anterior*** aspect of humerus, into the medial lip of intertubercular sulcus.

Nerve supply:

Lower subscapular nerve (C6, 7).

Actions:

These are described along with those of the subscapularis.

Subscapularis (Fig. 24.7)

Origin:

Medial two-thirds of the subscapular fossa (on costal surface of scapula).

Insertion

Lesser tubercle of humerus.

Nerve supply:

Upper and lower subscapular nerves (C5, 6, 7).

Actions of teres major and subscapularis:

Both the teres major and the subscapularis are adductors and medial rotators of the arm. In addition the teres major can extend the arm.

Along with other muscles surrounding the shoulder joint these muscles strengthen the capsule and stabilize it. During abduction of the arm (by the deltoid and the supraspinatus) these two muscles pull the head of the humerus downwards, and thus prevent it from getting stuck under the coraco-acromial arch.

Important relations:

The subscapularis and the teres major form the posterior wall of the axilla, and are related to the contents of the axilla.

Musculotendinous cuff of shoulder

The tendons of the subscapularis, teres minor, supraspinatus and infraspinatus unite to form a cuff (covering) for the shoulder joint.

Quadrangular and Triangular spaces

These spaces are present just below the medial border of the scapula. Their boundaries are as follows.

The **quadrangular space** is bounded above by the teres minor and the subscapularis, below by the teres major, medially by the long head of the triceps, and laterally by the surgical neck of the humerus. The axillary nerve and the posterior circumflex humeral artery pass backwards through this space.

The upper and lower boundaries of the **triangular space** are the same as those of the quadrangular space. Its lateral boundary is formed by the long head of the triceps. The circumflex scapular branch of the subscapular artery passes through this space.

Compartments of The Arm

For purposes of description the arm can be divided into anterior and posterior compartments that are partially separated by the humerus and by the medial and lateral intermuscular septa. The muscles in each compartment are considered below.

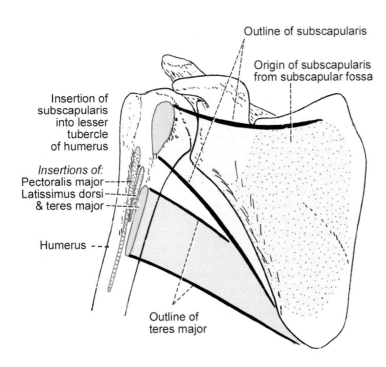

Fig. 24.7. Attachments of the subscapularis. The teres major is also shown.

MUSCLES OF THE ANTERIOR COMPARTMENT OF THE ARM

Biceps Brachii (Fig. 24.8)

Origin:

The biceps brachii arises from the scapula by two heads, long and short.

The long head arises from the supraglenoid tubercle.

The short head arises from the tip of the coracoid process (together with the coracobrachialis).

The tendon of the long head arches over the head of the humerus to enter the intertubercular sulcus. This part of the tendon lies within the cavity of the shoulder joint.

The two heads fuse to form a large belly which ends in a tendon.

Insertion:

The tendon crosses in front of the elbow joint and dips backwards to be inserted into the posterior part of the tuberosity of the radius.

Nerve Supply:

Musculocutaneous nerve (C5, C6).

Actions:

1. The muscle is a flexor of the forearm (at the elbow joint).

2. The biceps supinates the forearm at the superior and inferior radio-ulnar joints.

3. The short head is a flexor of the shoulder joint. The long head helps to maintain the head of the humerus in its normal position during movements at this joint.

Bicipital aponeurosis

The tendon of the biceps brachii gives off an extension called the bicipital aponeurosis. This aponeurosis passes medially and downwards (covering the brachial artery and the median nerve).

Coracobrachialis (Fig. 24.9)

Origin:

From tip of coracoid process of the scapula.

Insertion:

Into the medial border of the humerus near the middle of the shaft.

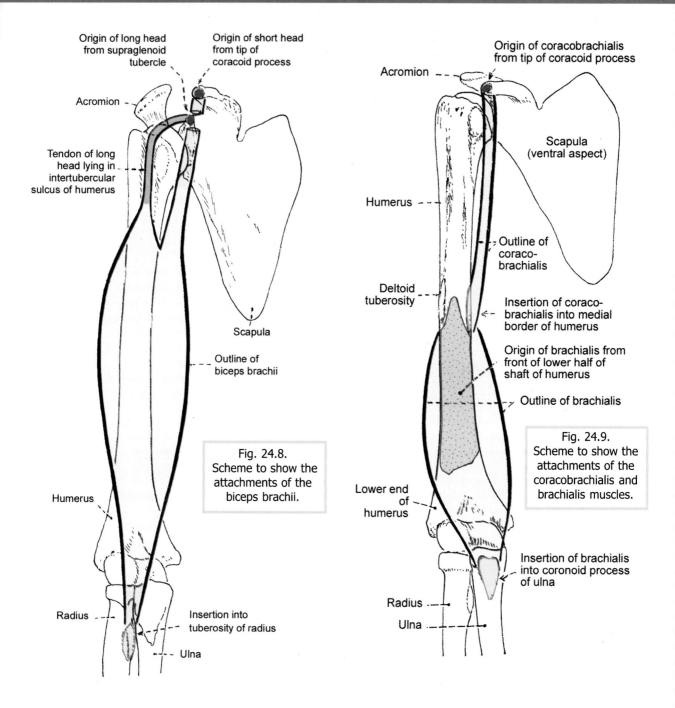

Fig. 24.8.
Scheme to show the attachments of the biceps brachii.

Fig. 24.9.
Scheme to show the attachments of the coracobrachialis and brachialis muscles.

Nerve Supply:
Musculocutaneous nerve (C5, 6, 7).

Action:
It is a flexor of the arm.

Brachialis (Fig. 24.9)

Origin:
The brachialis arises from the front of the lower half of the humerus (i.e., from the anteromedial and anterolateral surfaces).

Insertion:
Into the anterior surface of the coronoid process of the ulna, including the tuberosity of the ulna.

Nerve Supply:
The muscle receives its main supply from the musculocutaneous nerve (C5, 6). The lateral part of the muscle is supplied by the radial nerve (C7).

Action:
Flexor of the elbow joint.

CUBITAL FOSSA

The region where the front of the arm becomes continuous with the front of the forearm is marked by a triangular depression called the cubital fossa. (Cubit = elbow). For descriptive purposes the fossa can be said to have a roof, a floor, and superior, medial and lateral boundaries.

The superior boundary of the fossa is formed by an imaginary line connecting the medial and lateral epicondyles of the humerus.

The lateral boundary of the fossa is formed by the medial border of the brachioradialis.

The medial boundary of the fossa is formed by the lateral margin of the pronator teres.

The apex of the fossa lies inferiorly and is formed by crossing of the brachioradialis across the front of the pronator teres.

The floor of the fossa is formed by the lower end of the brachialis, above, and by the supinator muscle, below.

The roof of the fossa is formed by overlying fascia. The cephalic vein, the basilic vein, and the median cubital vein lie in this fascia. The medial and lateral cutaneous nerves of the forearm also lie in the roof.

The contents of the fossa are:

1. The tendon of the biceps brachii (along with the bicipital aponeurosis).

2. The lower end of the brachial artery (medial to the tendon), dividing into radial and ulnar arteries.

3. The median nerve (medial to the artery).

4. The radial nerve (in lateral part of fossa).

MUSCLE IN THE POSTERIOR COMPARTMENT OF ARM

Triceps (Fig. 24.10)

Origin:

As indicated by its name the muscle has three heads of origin.

1. The long head arises from the infraglenoid tubercle of the scapula.

2. The lateral head arises from a ridge on the posterior aspect of the humerus. The ridge corresponds to the upper part of the lateral border of the bone. The upper end of the ridge reaches the greater tubercle; the lower end lies near the deltoid tuberosity.

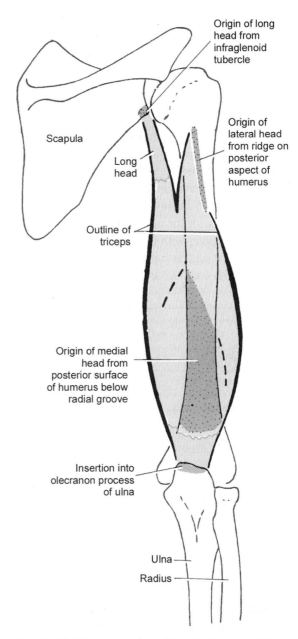

Fig. 24.10. Scheme to show the attachments of the triceps muscle.

3. The medial head arises from the posterior surface of the humerus below the radial groove; and also from the medial and lateral intermuscular septa.

Insertion:

The muscle is inserted into the posterior part of the superior surface of the olecranon process of the ulna.

Nerve supply:

Radial nerve .

Actions:

The triceps extends the forearm at the elbow joint.

MUSCLES OF THE FOREARM AND HAND

The forearm contains a large number of muscles. Most of them end in long tendons that enter the hand to gain insertion there. It is for this reason that we will consider the forearm and hand together. For convenience of description the structures in the forearm can be divided into those seen on the front and those seen on the back. At the wrist the front of the forearm becomes continuous with the palmar (anterior) aspect of the hand, while the back of the forearm becomes continuous with the dorsum of the hand.

MUSCLES OF FRONT OF FOREARM

Pronator Teres (Fig. 24.11)

Origin:

The pronator teres has two heads of origin. The **humeral head** (which is superficial) arises from (1) the lowest part of the medial supracondylar ridge, and (2) from the medial epicondyle (common flexor origin) of the humerus. The **ulnar head** (or deep head) arises from the medial side of the coronoid process of the ulna.

Insertion:

Into the lateral surface of the shaft of the radius at about the middle of the bone.

Nerve Supply:

Median nerve (C6, 7).

Actions:

As indicated by its name it pronates the forearm. It is also a weak flexor of the elbow.

Notes:

1. The lateral border of the pronator teres forms the medial boundary of the cubital fossa.

2. The median nerve passes between the humeral and ulnar heads.

3. The ulnar artery passes deep to the ulnar head. In other words, the ulnar head separates the ulnar artery from the median nerve.

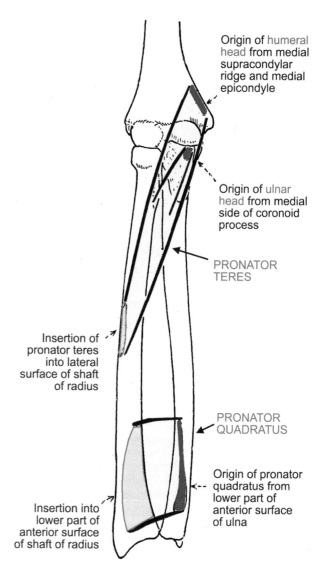

Fig. 24.11. Attachments of pronator teres and pronator quadratus.

Flexor Carpi Radialis (Fig. 24.12)

Origin:

From medial epicondyle of humerus (common flexor origin).

The muscle ends in a tendon which passes anterior to the wrist in its lateral part. Here the tendon passes through a tunnel, bounded laterally by a groove in the trapezium, and medially by two slips of the flexor retinaculum.

Insertion:

Bases of the second and third metacarpal bones.

Nerve Supply:

Median nerve (C6, 7).

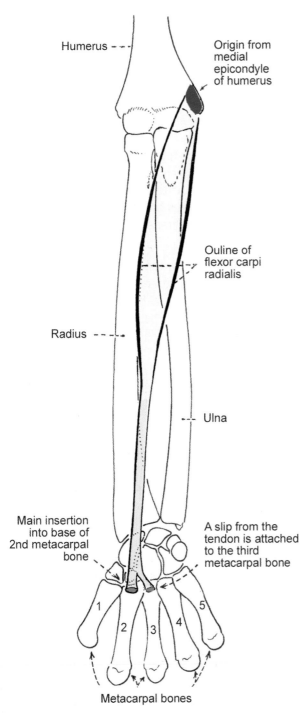

Fig. 24.12. Attachments of the Flexor carpi radialis.

Labels on figure:
- Humerus
- Origin from medial epicondyle of humerus
- Ouline of flexor carpi radialis
- Radius
- Ulna
- Main insertion into base of 2nd metacarpal bone
- A slip from the tendon is attached to the third metacarpal bone
- Metacarpal bones

Actions:
Flexion and abduction of the wrist.

Important Relation:
The radial artery lies just lateral to the tendon of this muscle (between it and the brachioradialis).

Flexor Carpi Ulnaris

Origin:
This muscle has two heads of origin. The **humeral head** arises from the medial epicondyle. The **ulnar head** arises from (a) the medial side of the olecranon process; and (b) from the upper two-thirds of the posterior border of the ulna (through an aponeurosis which also gives origin to the extensor carpi ulnaris and to the flexor digitorum profundus).

Some fibres of the muscle arise from a tendinous arch passing from the medial epicondyle of the humerus to the olecranon process of the ulna.

The muscle ends in a tendon which crosses the medial part of the wrist.

Insertion:
Into pisiform bone.

Nerve Supply:
Ulnar nerve (C7, 8).

Actions:
Flexion and adduction of the hand (at the wrist joint).

Note:
1. The ulnar nerve enters the forearm by passing deep to the tendinous arch connecting the humeral and ulnar heads of origin.

2. At the wrist the ulnar artery and nerve lie lateral to the tendon of this muscle.

Flexor Digitorum Superficialis (Fig. 24.13)

Origin:
The muscle has two heads of origin.

The **humero-ulnar head** arises from

a) the medial epicondyle of the humerus (common flexor origin).

b) the anterior part of the ulnar collateral ligament of the elbow joint, and

c) the medial margin of the olecranon process of the ulna.

The **radial head** arises from the anterior border of the radius (from the radial tuberosity above, up to the insertion of the pronator teres below (i.e., from the oblique line).

Insertion:
The muscle ends in a tendon which splits into four smaller tendons, one for each digit except the thumb.

Opposite the proximal phalanx the tendon for each digit splits to form two slips, medial and lateral that are attached to the sides of the middle phalanx.

Nerve Supply:
Median nerve (C7, 8, T1).

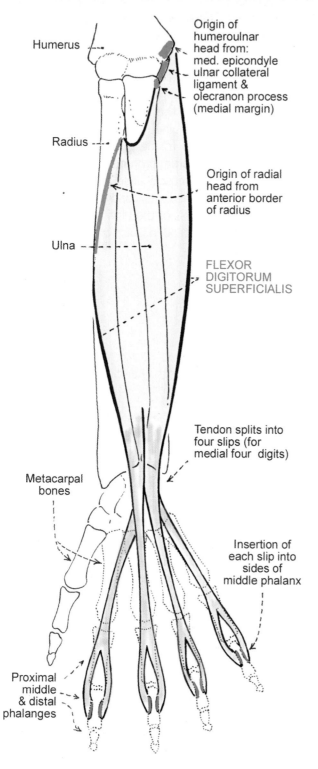

Fig. 24.13. Attachments of the flexor digitorum superficialis.

Actions:

Flexion of the middle and proximal phalanges of the digits concerned.

Flexor Digitorum Profundus (Fig. 24.14)

Origin:

The muscle arises from an extensive area extending on to the following parts of the ulna:

a) the medial surface of the coronoid process;

b) the upper three fourths of the anterior surface; and

c) the upper three fourths of the medial surface; and

d) the upper three fourths of the posterior border, by an aponeurosis which also gives origin to the flexor carpi ulnaris and the exterior carpi ulnaris .

The muscle also takes origin from the medial half of the interosseous membrane.

Insertion:

The muscle ends in a tendon which splits into four parts, one for each digit except the thumb. Each tendon passes through the interval between slips of the flexor digitorum superficialis to be inserted into the base of the distal phalanx.

Nerve Supply:

The muscle has a double supply: the medial part by the ulnar nerve and the lateral part by the median (through its anterior interosseous branch) (C8, T1).

Actions:

Flexion of the distal phalanges.

Some Additional facts about Flexor Digitorum Superficialis & Profundus

(1) Fibrous flexor sheaths:

During their course over the ventral aspect of the digits, the tendons of the flexor digitorum superficialis and profundus (for that digit) lie in a common canal bounded posteriorly, by the phalanges and anteriorly (and on the sides) by a fibrous membrane. This membrane is called the fibrous flexor sheath. It holds the tendons in place .

(2) Synovial sheaths:

At the wrist the four tendons of the flexor digitorum superficialis lie superficial to the four tendons of the profundus. All the eight tendons pass through the **carpal tunnel** which is bounded, in front by the flexor retinaculum; and behind by the carpal bones. Here the tendons are surrounded by a common synovial sheath (also called the **ulnar bursa**). Proximally, the sheath extends into the forearm for about 2.5 cm proximal to the flexor retinaculum. Distally it extends to the middle of the palm.

Over the digits the tendons are surrounded by a common digital synovial sheath, which lines the inside

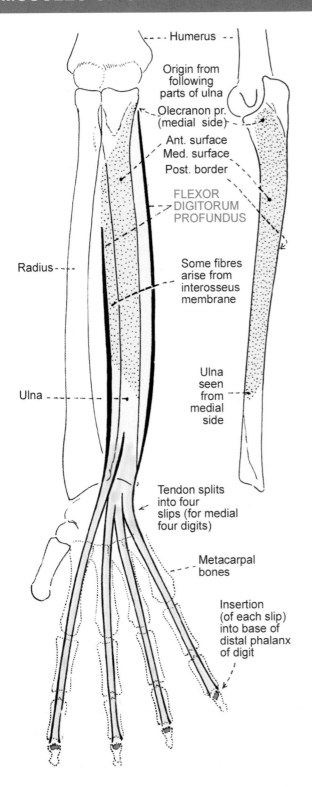

Humerus

Origin from following parts of ulna

Olecranon pr. (medial side)

Ant. surface
Med. surface
Post. border

FLEXOR DIGITORUM PROFUNDUS

Radius

Some fibres arise from interosseus membrane

Ulna

Ulna seen from medial side

Tendon splits into four slips (for medial four digits)

Metacarpal bones

Insertion (of each slip) into base of distal phalanx of digit

Fig. 24.14. A. Attachments of the flexor digitorum profundus. B. Medial view of ulna to show area of origin of the muscle.

Flexor Pollicis Longus

Origin:
The muscle arises from:
a) the anterior surface of the radius (below the oblique line, and excluding the lower one fourth of the bone; and
b) the lateral part of the interosseous membrane (anterior aspect).

The muscle ends in a tendon which runs across the front of the wrist (lateral part). Here it lies in the carpal tunnel. The tendon then passes into the thumb. Here it is surrounded by a synovial sheath, and a fibrous flexor sheath, just like tendons of the digital flexors.

Insertion:
Base of the distal phalanx of the thumb on its ventral aspect.

Nerve Supply:
Median nerve through its anterior interosseous branch (C8, T1).

Action:
The muscle flexes the phalanges of the thumb.

Radial bursa:
The synovial sheath surrounding the tendon is called the radial bursa. Proximally the bursa extends into the forearm for about 2.5 cm above the flexor retinaculum. It surrounds the tendon as it passes through the carpal tunnel and extends up to the insertion of the tendon.

Pronator Quadratus (Fig. 24.11)

Origin:
Oblique ridge on lower part of the anterior surface of the ulna.

Insertion:
Anterior surface of the shaft of the radius (lower one fourth).

Nerve Supply:
Median nerve through its anterior interosseous branch (C8, T1).

Actions:
It is the chief pronator of the forearm.

of the fibrous flexor sheath. Each digital sheath extends from the level of the metacarpo-phalangeal joint (proximally) to the insertion of the profundus tendon (distally). The digital sheath of the little finger is continuous proximally with the ulnar bursa. For description of the radial bursa see below.

Fascia on front of the wrist & hand

Flexor Retinaculum

This is a strong band of fascia stretching across the ventral aspect of the carpus. The space between the retinaculum and the carpal bones is called the *carpal tunnel*. It transmits the tendons of the flexor digitorum superficialis and profundus, the tendon of the flexor pollicis longus and the median nerve.

Palmar aponeurosis

This is a triangular structure consisting of thickened deep fascia that covers the central part of the palm. The apex of the triangle is directed proximally. It is continuous with the tendon of the palmaris longus. Distally, the aponeurosis is broad. It divides into four processes, one for each finger.

MUSCLES OF THE HAND

Lumbrical Muscles

These are four small muscles that take origin from the tendons of the flexor digitorum profundus. They are numbered from lateral to medial side. Some details of their origin are shown in Fig. 24.15.

Insertion:

The tendons of each muscle passes backwards on the radial side of a metacarpo-phalangeal joint, to be inserted into the lateral basal angle of the extensor expansion.

Nerve Supply:

The first and second lumbricals receive branches from the median nerve (C8, T1); and the third and fourth from the deep branch of the ulnar (C8, T1).

Actions:

The lumbrical muscles flex the metacarpo-phalangeal joints, and extend the interphalangeal joints of the digit into which they are inserted.

THE THENAR & HYPOTHENAR MUSCLES

The thenar muscles are present in relation to the thumb and form the thenar eminence. They produce movements of the thumb.

The thenar muscles are:
1. Abductor pollicis brevis.
2. Flexor pollicis brevis.
3. Opponens pollicis.
4. Adductor pollicis.

The hypothenar muscles are present in relation to the little finger and form the hypothenar eminence. They produce movements of the little finger. The hypothenar muscles are:
1. Abductor digiti minimi.
2. Flexor digiti minimi.
3. Opponens digiti minimi.

Note the following important points about them:
a) The action of each muscle is indicated by its name.
b) Remember that movements of the thumb take place at right angles to those of other digits.
c) The opponens muscles are responsible for bringing the thumb and little finger in contact with each other. The opponens pollicis also brings the thumb into opposition with other digits.
d) Each abductor muscle, and each flexor muscle, arises in the region of the carpus and is inserted into the proximal phalanx of the digit concerned.
e) Each opponens muscle arises in the region of the carpus and is inserted into the shaft of the corresponding metacarpal bone.
f) All hypothenar muscles are supplied by the deep branch of the ulnar nerve. The thenar muscles are supplied partly by the median nerve and partly by the deep branch of the ulnar nerve.

For details about each muscle see Figs. 24.16 to 24.19.

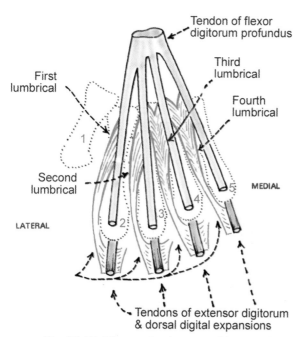

Fig. 24.15. Diagram to show attachments of lumbrical muscles.

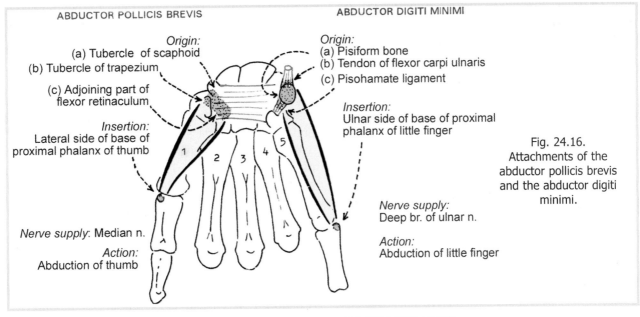

ABDUCTOR POLLICIS BREVIS

ABDUCTOR DIGITI MINIMI

Origin:
(a) Tubercle of scaphoid
(b) Tubercle of trapezium

(c) Adjoining part of
flexor retinaculum

Insertion:
Lateral side of base of
proximal phalanx of thumb

Origin:
(a) Pisiform bone
(b) Tendon of flexor carpi ulnaris
(c) Pisohamate ligament

Insertion:
Ulnar side of base of proximal
phalanx of little finger

Nerve supply: Median n.

Action:
Abduction of thumb

Nerve supply:
Deep br. of ulnar n.

Action:
Abduction of little finger

Fig. 24.16.
Attachments of the
abductor pollicis brevis
and the abductor digiti
minimi.

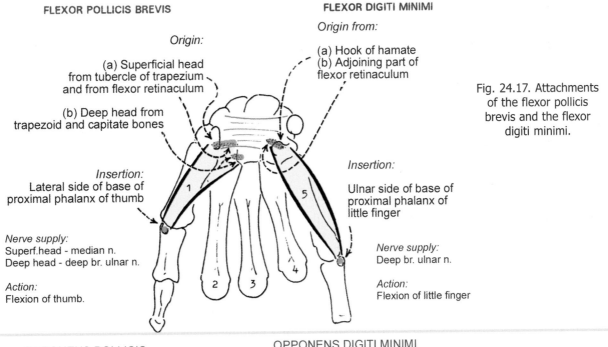

FLEXOR POLLICIS BREVIS

FLEXOR DIGITI MINIMI

Origin:

(a) Superficial head
from tubercle of trapezium
and from flexor retinaculum

(b) Deep head from
trapezoid and capitate bones

Insertion:
Lateral side of base of
proximal phalanx of thumb

Origin from:

(a) Hook of hamate
(b) Adjoining part of
flexor retinaculum

Insertion:

Ulnar side of base of
proximal phalanx of
little finger

Nerve supply:
Superf.head - median n.
Deep head - deep br. ulnar n.

Action:
Flexion of thumb.

Nerve supply:
Deep br. ulnar n.

Action:
Flexion of little finger

Fig. 24.17. Attachments
of the flexor pollicis
brevis and the flexor
digiti minimi.

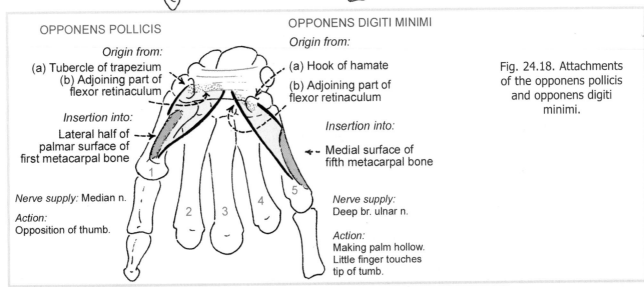

OPPONENS POLLICIS

OPPONENS DIGITI MINIMI

Origin from:
(a) Tubercle of trapezium
(b) Adjoining part of
flexor retinaculum

Insertion into:
Lateral half of
palmar surface of
first metacarpal bone

Origin from:
(a) Hook of hamate

(b) Adjoining part of
flexor retinaculum

Insertion into:
Medial surface of
fifth metacarpal bone

Nerve supply: Median n.

Action:
Opposition of thumb.

Nerve supply:
Deep br. ulnar n.

Action:
Making palm hollow.
Little finger touches
tip of tumb.

Fig. 24.18. Attachments
of the opponens pollicis
and opponens digiti
minimi.

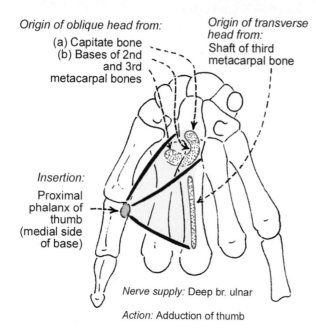

Origin of oblique head from:
   (a) Capitate bone
   (b) Bases of 2nd
      and 3rd
      metacarpal bones

Origin of transverse head from:
Shaft of third metacarpal bone

Insertion:
Proximal phalanx of thumb (medial side of base)

Nerve supply: Deep br. ulnar

Action: Adduction of thumb

Fig. 24.19. Attachments of adductor pollicis.

Palmar Interossei

These are four small muscles placed between the shafts of the metacarpal bones. They are numbered from lateral to medial side. There is one muscle each for the 1st, 2nd, 4th and 5th digits, there being none for the 3rd digit (Fig. 24.20).

Each muscle arises from one metacarpal bone and is inserted into the dorsal digital expansion of the same digit (see below).

All palmar interossei adduct the digit to which they are attached, towards the middle finger. In addition they flex the digit at the metacarpo-phalangeal joint and extend the digit at the interphalangeal joints.

All palmar interossei are supplied by the deep branch of the ulnar nerve (C8, T1). For details of attachment of each muscle see Fig. 24.20.

Dorsal Interossei

Like the palmar interossei the dorsal interossei are four small muscles placed between the metacarpal bones, and numbered from the lateral to the medial side (Fig. 24.21). Each muscle arises from the contiguous sides of two metacarpal bones. It is inserted (a) into a dorsal digital expansion, and (b) into one side of the base of a proximal phalanx.

All dorsal interossei are abductors of the digits i.e., they move the digits, away from the line of the middle finger. In addition (like the palmar interossei) they flex the metacarpo-phalangeal joint and extend the interphalangeal joint.

All dorsal interossei are supplied by the deep branch of the ulnar nerve (C8, T1).

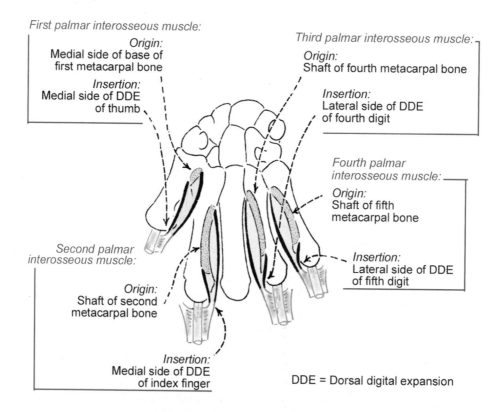

First palmar interosseous muscle:
   Origin:
   Medial side of base of first metacarpal bone
   Insertion:
   Medial side of DDE of thumb

Third palmar interosseous muscle:
   Origin:
   Shaft of fourth metacarpal bone
   Insertion:
   Lateral side of DDE of fourth digit

Fourth palmar interosseous muscle:
   Origin:
   Shaft of fifth metacarpal bone
   Insertion:
   Lateral side of DDE of fifth digit

Second palmar interosseous muscle:
   Origin:
   Shaft of second metacarpal bone
   Insertion:
   Medial side of DDE of index finger

DDE = Dorsal digital expansion

Fig. 24.20. Attachments of palmar interossei.

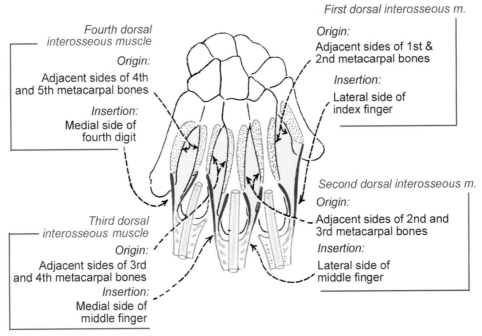

Fourth dorsal interosseous muscle

Origin:
Adjacent sides of 4th and 5th metacarpal bones

Insertion:
Medial side of fourth digit

First dorsal interosseous m.

Origin:
Adjacent sides of 1st & 2nd metacarpal bones

Insertion:
Lateral side of index finger

Second dorsal interosseous m.

Origin:
Adjacent sides of 2nd and 3rd metacarpal bones

Insertion:
Lateral side of middle finger

Third dorsal interosseous muscle

Origin:
Adjacent sides of 3rd and 4th metacarpal bones

Insertion:
Medial side of middle finger

Fig. 24.21. Attachments of dorsal interossei. Each insertion is partly into the dorsal digital expansion, and partly into the base of the proximal phalanx of the digit concerned.

MUSCLES OF THE BACK OF THE FOREARM

Brachioradialis

Origin:
The muscle arises from:
a) upper two thirds of lateral supracondylar ridge of humerus, and
b) lateral intermuscular septum.

Insertion:
Lateral side of the radius just above the styloid process.

Nerve Supply:
Radial nerve (C5, 6, 7).

Notes:
1. The fleshy part of the brachioradialis forms the lateral boundary of the cubital fossa. Here the radial nerve is deep to it (between it and the brachialis).
2. Near its insertion its tendon is crossed by tendons of the abductor pollicis longus and the extensor pollicis brevis (Fig. 6.23).
3. At the wrist the radial artery is medial to the tendon (between it and the tendon of the flexor carpi radialis).

Actions:
1. The muscle is a flexor of the forearm.
2. It supinates the fully pronated forearm; and pronates the fully supinated forearm.

Extensor Carpi Radialis Longus

Origin:
a) Lower one third of lateral supracondylar ridge of humerus;
b) Some fibres arise from the common extensor origin (i.e., lateral epicondyle).

Insertion:
Lateral side of the base of the second metacarpal bone.

Nerve Supply: Radial nerve (C6, C7).

Actions:
Extension and abduction of wrist.

Extensor Carpi Radialis Brevis

Origin:
a) Lateral epicondyle of the humerus (i.e., common extensor origin), and from
b) Radial collateral ligament of the elbow joint.

Insertion:
Dorsal aspect of the base of the second and third metacarpal bones.

Nerve Supply:
Deep branch of radial nerve (C7, C8).

Actions:
Extension and abduction of wrist.

Extensor Digitorum (Fig. 24.22)

Origin:

Lateral epicondyle of the humerus (common extensor origin).

The muscle ends in a tendon which passes deep to the extensor retinaculum. The tendon splits into four parts: one for each digit other than the thumb.

Insertion:

Each tendon is inserted into the base of the middle phalanx, and the base of the distal phalanx of the digit. (See Fig. 24.23 for details of insertion).

Nerve Supply:

Deep branch of radial nerve (C7, 8).

Actions:

The muscle produces extension at the:

a) interphalangeal joints,

b) metacarpophalangeal joints, and

c) wrist joint.

Notes:

1. As the tendons of the muscle pass under cover of the extensor retinaculum they are surrounded by a common synovial sheath.

2. The tendon for the index finger is joined by the tendon of the extensor indicis.

3. The tendon for the little finger is joined by the tendon of the extensor digiti minimi.

4. Over the proximal phalanx the tendon (of that digit) becomes embedded in a triangular membrane called the dorsal digital expansion.

Dorsal digital expansion and insertion of the extensor digitorum

The dorsal digital expansion is an aponeurosis present on the dorsal aspect of the proximal phalanx, and the metacarpo-phalangeal joint. The expansion is triangular (Fig. 24.23). It has an apex directed distally, and a broad base that lies dorsal to the metacarpo-phalangeal joint. The tendon of the extensor digitorum joins the central part of the the expansion. The expansion also gives attachment to the lumbrical and interosseous muscles of the digit. In addition to these muscles the expansion for the index finger receives the tendon of the extensor indicis and that of the little finger receives the tendon of the extensor digiti minimi.

Extensor Digit Minimi

Origin:

Lateral epicondyle of the humerus (common extensor origin).

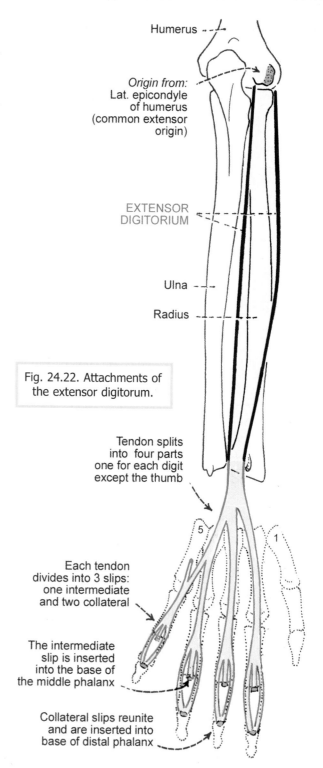

Humerus

Origin from:
Lat. epicondyle
of humerus
(common extensor
origin)

EXTENSOR
DIGITORIUM

Ulna

Radius

Fig. 24.22. Attachments of the extensor digitorum.

Tendon splits
into four parts
one for each digit
except the thumb

Each tendon
divides into 3 slips:
one intermediate
and two collateral

The intermediate
slip is inserted
into the base of
the middle phalanx

Collateral slips reunite
and are inserted into
base of distal phalanx

The tendon runs across the back of the wrist deep to the extensor retinaculum where it occupies a separate compartment just behind the radioulnar joint. Here the tendon is surrounded by a synovial sheath).

Insertion:

The tendon joins the tendon from the extensor digitorum for the little finger.

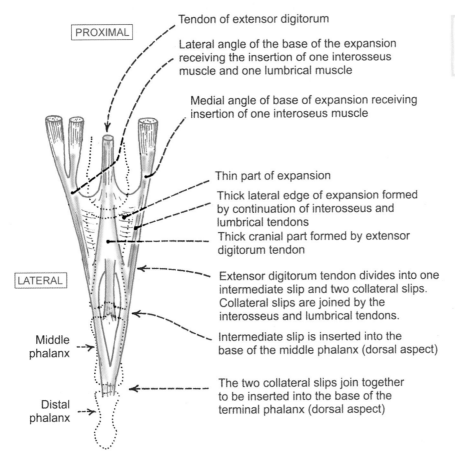

PROXIMAL

Tendon of extensor digitorum

Lateral angle of the base of the expansion receiving the insertion of one interosseus muscle and one lumbrical muscle

Medial angle of base of expansion receiving insertion of one interoseus muscle

Thin part of expansion

Thick lateral edge of expansion formed by continuation of interosseus and lumbrical tendons

Thick cranial part formed by extensor digitorum tendon

LATERAL

Extensor digitorum tendon divides into one intermediate slip and two collateral slips. Collateral slips are joined by the interosseus and lumbrical tendons.

Intermediate slip is inserted into the base of the middle phalanx (dorsal aspect)

Middle phalanx

The two collateral slips join together to be inserted into the base of the terminal phalanx (dorsal aspect)

Distal phalanx

Fig. 24.23. Dorsal digital expansion and insertion of the extensor digitorum.

Nerve supply: Deep branch of radial nerve.

Action: Extension of little finger.

Extensor Carpi Ulnaris

Origin:
a) Lateral epicondyle of the humerus (common extensor origin); and from
b) Posterior border of the ulna (by an aponeurosis common to it and to the flexor carpi ulnaris and the flexor digitorum profundus).

The muscle ends in a tendon which descends across the back of the wrist, lying deep to the extensor retinaculum. Here the tendon is surrounded by a synovial sheath.

Insertion:
Medial side of the base of the fifth metacarpal bone.

Nerve Supply:
Deep branch of radial nerve (C7, C8).

Actions:
1. Extension of the wrist.
2. Adduction of the hand.

Anconeus

This is a small triangular muscle on the back of the elbow. The muscle is a weak extensor of the elbow. It is supplied by the radial nerve.

Supinator (Fig. 24.24)

Origin:
The muscle has one continuous origin from the following structures:
1. Lateral epicondyle of the humerus.
2. Radial collateral ligament of the elbow.
3. Annular ligament.
4. Supinator crest of the ulna.

Insertion:
Upper one third of the lateral surface of the radius.

Nerve Supply:
Deep branch of the radial nerve.

Action:
Supination of the forearm.

Note:
The muscle has two layers, superficial and deep. The deep branch of radial nerve runs downwards between these layers.

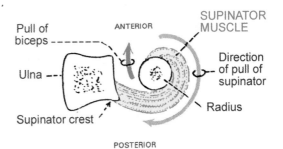

Pull of biceps

ANTERIOR

SUPINATOR MUSCLE

Ulna

Direction of pull of supinator

Radius

Supinator crest

POSTERIOR

Fig. 24.24. Schematic section across upper part of radius and ulna to show the arrangement of fibres of the supinator muscle.

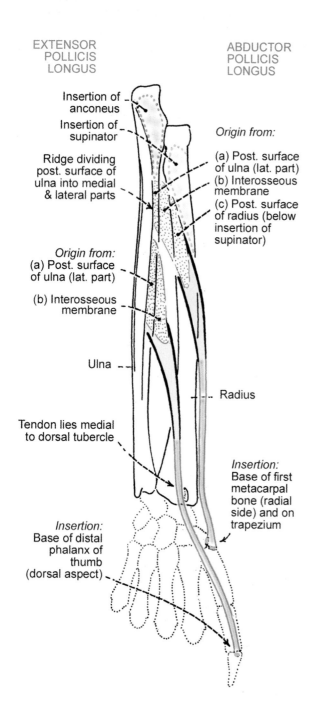

EXTENSOR
POLLICIS
LONGUS

ABDUCTOR
POLLICIS
LONGUS

Insertion of
anconeus

Insertion of
supinator

Origin from:

Ridge dividing
post. surface of
ulna into medial
& lateral parts

(a) Post. surface
of ulna (lat. part)
(b) Interosseous
membrane
(c) Post. surface
of radius (below
insertion of
supinator)

Origin from:
(a) Post. surface
of ulna (lat. part)

(b) Interosseous
membrane

Ulna

Radius

Tendon lies medial
to dorsal tubercle

Insertion:
Base of first
metacarpal
bone (radial
side) and on
trapezium

Insertion:
Base of distal
phalanx of
thumb
(dorsal aspect)

Fig. 24.25. Attachments of the extensor pollicis longus,
and of the abductor pollicis longus.

Extensor Pollicis Longus

Origin:
 a) Lateral part of posterior surface of the ulna (below the origin of the abductor pollicis longus), and from
 b) the adjoining part of the interosseous membrane.

Insertion:
 Base of the distal phalanx of the thumb on its dorsal aspect.

Actions:
 It extends the distal phalanx, the proximal phalanx and the metacarpal of the thumb.

Nerve Supply:
 Deep branch of radial nerve (C7, 8).

Abductor Pollicis Longus (Fig. 24.25)

Origin:
 a) The lateral part of the posterior surface of the ulna.
 b) Interosseous membrane.
 c) The posterior surface of the radius.

Insertion:
 Radial side of the base of the first metacarpal bone; and on the trapezium.

Nerve Supply:
 Deep branch of radial nerve (C7, 8).

Actions:
 Abduction and extension of the thumb.

Extensor Indicis

Origin :
 Posterior surface of the ulna below the origin of the extensor pollicis longus, and from interosseous membrane.

Insertion:
 The tendon ends by joining the extensor digitorum tendon for the index finger.

Nerve Supply:
 Deep branch of radial nerve (C7, 8).

Actions:
 The muscle extends the index finger.

Extensor Pollicis Brevis

Origin:

Posterior surface of the radius below the origin of the abductor pollicis longus, and from interosseous membrane.

Insertion:

Dorsal surface of the base of the proximal phalanx of the thumb.

Nerve Supply:

Deep branch of radial nerve (C7, 8).

Action:

The muscle extends the thumb.

Extensor Retinaculum

The extensor retinaculum is a thickened band of deep fascia that runs across the back (and sides) of the wrist. It is about 2.5 cm in width. It holds the extensor tendons in place and facilitates their action by acting as a pulley.

Laterally, the retinaculum is attached to the anterior border of the radius. Medially, it is attached to the triquetral and pisiform bones.

The space between the deep surface of the retinaculum and the underlying bones is divided into six compartments. Note the tendons passing through each compartment.

Synovial Sheaths

The tendons passing under the extensor retinaculum are surrounded by synovial sheaths. Normally, there are six sheaths; one for the tendons passing through each compartment under the extensor retinaculum.

25

Nerves of the Upper Extremity

Most of the nerves supplying structures in the upper limb are branches of the brachial plexus. Exceptions are: (a) the spinal accessory nerve, a cranial nerve, supplying the trapezius; (b) supraclavicular nerves, that arise from the cervical plexus; (c) some muscular branches from the cervical plexus, and (d) cutaneous branches derived from intercostal nerves to the lower part of the pectoral region.

CUTANEOUS NERVES OF THE PECTORAL REGION

The skin of the upper part of the pectoral region is supplied by nerves derived from spinal segments C3 and C4 (up to the level of the sternal angle). The area just below the level of the sternal angle is supplied by segment T2. The intervening nerves (C5 to T1) get 'pulled away' into the limb leaving the area for segment C4 in direct continuity with that for segment T2.

The cutaneous nerves of the pectoral region are as follows:

1. The supraclavicular nerves (derived from segments C3 and C4) arise in the neck from the cervical plexus. They enter the pectoral region by crossing in front of the clavicle. The main trunk divides into three branches called the medial, intermediate and lateral supraclavicular nerves. These branches descend over the posterior triangle of the neck. They pierce the deep fascia a little above the clavicle and then run downwards across this bone to reach the pectoral region.

The medial supraclavicular nerve supplies the skin of the upper and medial part of the thorax. A branch from the nerve supplies the sternoclavicular joint. The intermediate supraclavicular nerve supplies the skin over the upper part of the pectoralis major. The area of supply of the medial and intermediate supraclavicular nerves extends up to the level of the second rib. The lateral supraclavicular nerve supplies the skin over the shoulder.

2. Skin below the level of the sternal angle is supplied by anterior cutaneous branches of the 2nd to 6th intercostal nerves; and more laterally by lateral cutaneous branches of the 3rd to 6th intercostal nerves.

THE BRACHIAL PLEXUS AND ITS BRANCHES

Basic Plan of Brachial Plexus

The brachial plexus is shown in Fig. 25.1. The plexus consists of roots, trunks (and their divisions) and cords. The main branches arise as continuations of the cords: branches also arise from other parts of the plexus.

The roots of the plexus are the ventral rami of spinal nerves C5, C6, C7, C8 and T1. The roots from C5 and C6 join to form the upper trunk. The root from C7 continues as the middle trunk. The roots from C8 and T1 join to form the lower trunk. Each trunk divides into an anterior and a posterior division. The anterior divisions of the upper and middle trunks join to form the lateral cord. The anterior division of the lower trunk continues as the medial cord. The posterior divisions of all the three trunks join to form the posterior cord.

The main branches of the brachial plexus are the median, the ulnar and the radial nerves. The median nerve is formed by union of lateral and medial roots arising from the lateral and medial cords, respectively. The ulnar nerve arises from the medial cord; and the radial nerve from the posterior cord.

The brachial plexus lies partly in the neck and partly in the axilla. In the neck the plexus lies in the posterior triangle. It passes behind the medial part of the clavicle to enter the axilla through the cervico-axillary canal. In the axilla the cords and their main branches are closely related to the axillary artery.

Branches of Brachial Plexus

Branches arising from roots:

(1) Each root of the plexus gives branches to some muscles lying in the neck (scalene muscles and longus colli).

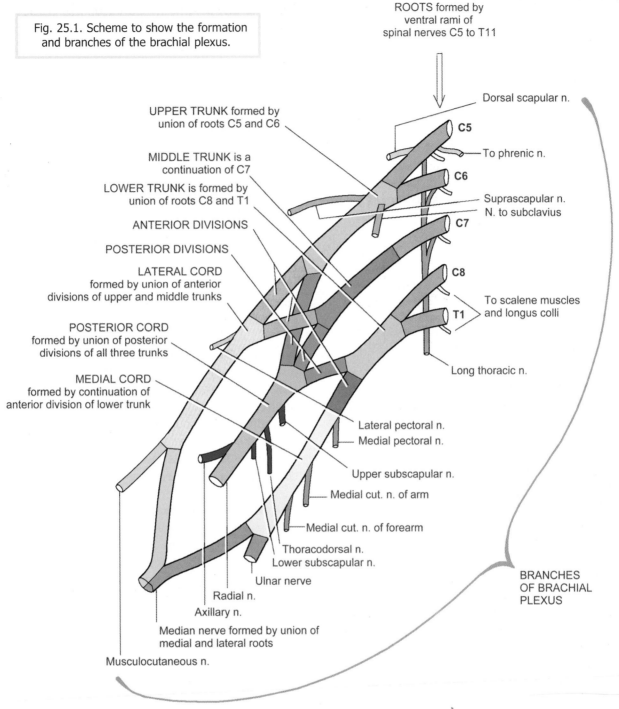

Fig. 25.1. Scheme to show the formation and branches of the brachial plexus.

ROOTS formed by ventral rami of spinal nerves C5 to T11

UPPER TRUNK formed by union of roots C5 and C6

MIDDLE TRUNK is a continuation of C7

LOWER TRUNK is formed by union of roots C8 and T1

ANTERIOR DIVISIONS

POSTERIOR DIVISIONS

LATERAL CORD formed by union of anterior divisions of upper and middle trunks

POSTERIOR CORD formed by union of posterior divisions of all three trunks

MEDIAL CORD formed by continuation of anterior division of lower trunk

Dorsal scapular n.

C5

To phrenic n.

C6

Suprascapular n.
N. to subclavius

C7

C8

To scalene muscles and longus colli

T1

Long thoracic n.

Lateral pectoral n.

Medial pectoral n.

Upper subscapular n.

Medial cut. n. of arm

Medial cut. n. of forearm

Thoracodorsal n.
Lower subscapular n.

Ulnar nerve

Radial n.

Axillary n.

Median nerve formed by union of medial and lateral roots

Musculocutaneous n.

BRANCHES OF BRACHIAL PLEXUS

(2) Root C5 gives a contribution to the phrenic nerve. The phrenic nerve descends into the thorax to supply the diaphragm.

(3) The dorsal scapular nerve arises from root C5.

(4) The long thoracic nerve is the nerve to the serratus anterior. It arises from roots C5, C6 and C7.

Branches arising from trunks:

The only branches arising from the trunks of the brachial plexus are the nerve to the subclavius and the suprascapular nerve. Both of these nerves arise from the upper trunk.

The nerve to the subclavius passes behind the clavicle to reach the subclavius.

The suprascapular nerve runs laterally and backwards over the shoulder.

Branches from cords:

The lateral pectoral nerve arises from the lateral cord. It is the main nerve supplying the pectoralis major. It also gives some fibres to the pectoralis minor.

The medial pectoral nerve arises from the medial cord. It is the main nerve of supply for the pectoralis minor. It also sends a few fibres to the pectoralis major.

The upper subscapular nerve arises from the posterior cord and supplies the subscapularis muscle.

The lower subscapular nerve arises from the posterior cord. It supplies the teres major and subscapularis.

The thoracodorsal nerve is the nerve to the latissimus dorsi. The nerve arises from the posterior cord between the upper and lower subscapular nerves.

The axillary nerve supplies the deltoid and teres minor.

The musculocutaneous nerve is a branch of the lateral cord.

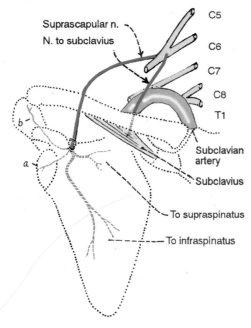

Fig. 25.2. Scheme to show the course of the suprascapular nerve, and the nerve to the subclavius.

The medial cutaneous nerve of the arm is a branch of the medial cord.

The medial cutaneous nerve of the forearm is a branch of the medial cord.

The ulnar nerve is the main continuation of the medial cord.

The radial nerve is the main continuation of the posterior cord. In the axilla it lies posterior to the third part of the axillary artery.

The median nerve is a continuation of the lateral cord and lies lateral to the third part of the axillary artery. It also receives a root from the medial cord.

Many of these nerves are considered in detail below.

Nerves supplying muscles of the upper limb seen on the back

Spinal part of accessory nerve

The accessory nerve is the eleventh cranial nerve. It has a cranial part, and a spinal part. The spinal part of the nerve reaches the trapezius in the lower part of the neck and descends into the back deep to this muscle, supplying it.

Dorsal scapular nerve

The dorsal scapular nerve arises from root C5 of the brachial plexus. It passes backwards and downwards through the lower part of the neck to reach the anterior aspect of the levator scapulae. It then descends into the back to reach the anterior (i.e., deep) aspect of the rhomboideus muscles. The dorsal scapular nerve supplies the rhomboideus major and minor and may give a branch to the levator scapulae.

NERVES OF SCAPULAR REGION

The nerves of the scapular region are the upper and lower subscapular nerves , the suprascapular nerve and the axillary nerve.

The upper subscapular nerve arises from the posterior cord and supplies the subscapularis muscle.

The lower subscapular nerve arises from the posterior cord and supplies th teres major and subscapularis.

The Suprascapular Nerve

The suprascapular nerve runs laterally and backwards over the shoulder (Fig. 25.2), deep to the trapezius. Reaching the upper border of the scapula it passes backwards through the suprascapular notch to enter the supraspinous fossa. After supplying the

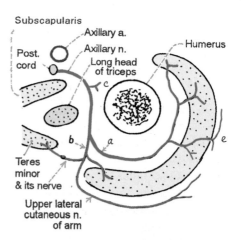

Fig. 25.3. Scheme to show the course and distribution of the axillary nerve. a – anterior branch. b – posterior branch. c – branch to shoulder joint. e – cutaneous twig from anterior branch.

supraspinatus the nerve enters the infraspinous fossa where it ends by supplying the infraspinatus. The nerve also gives branches to the shoulder joint and to the acromioclavicular joint.

The Axillary Nerve

The axillary nerve (Fig. 25.3) supplies the deltoid and the teres minor. It is a branch of the posterior cord of the brachial plexus. At its origin it lies behind the axillary artery. It descends over the subscapularis, and reaching its lower border it passes backwards through the quadrangular space. The nerve ends by dividing into an anterior and a posterior branch. The anterior branch passes round the surgical neck of the humerus and ends by supplying the deltoid. Some ramifications reach the skin. The posterior branch supplies the posterior part of the deltoid and also the teres minor. Its terminal part becomes the upper lateral cutaneous nerve of the arm: this nerve supplies the skin over the lower part of the deltoid muscle.

CUTANEOUS NERVES OF THE ARM & FOREARM

These are listed below. Their areas of distribution are indicated by their names, and are shown in Figs. 25.4 and 25.5.

1. Lateral supraclavicular nerve supplies skin over the upper part of the deltoid muscle.

2. Upper lateral cutaneous nerve of arm (branch of axillary nerve) supplies skin over the lower part of the deltoid muscle.

3. Lower lateral cutaneous nerve of arm (branch of radial nerve) supplies the lateral side of the arm.

4. Posterior cutaneous nerve of arm (branch of radial nerve) supplies an area on the back of the arm.

5. Intercostobrachial nerve (lateral cutaneous branch of second intercostal nerve) supplies skin of axilla and upper part of medial side of arm.

6. Medial cutaneous nerve of arm (branch of medial cord of brachial plexus) supplies skin over medial side of lower part of arm.

7. Medial cutaneous nerve of forearm (branch of medial cord of brachial plexus) supplies skin over medial side of forearm; and on the front of the arm.

8. Lateral cutaneous nerve of the forearm (continuation of musculocutaneous nerve) supplies skin on lateral side of the forearm, and the thenar eminence.

9. Posterior cutaneous nerve of forearm (branch of radial nerve) supplies skin on the back of the forearm, and the lower part of the back of the arm.

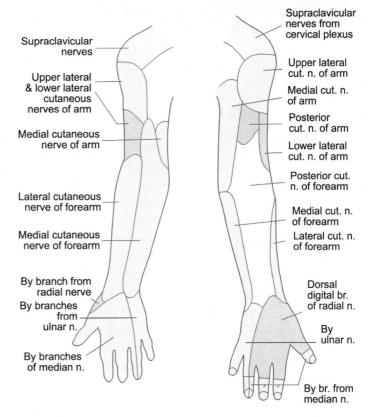

Fig. 25.4. Cutaneous nerve supply of front of upper extremity.

Fig. 25.5. Cutaneous nerve supply of the back of the upper extremity.

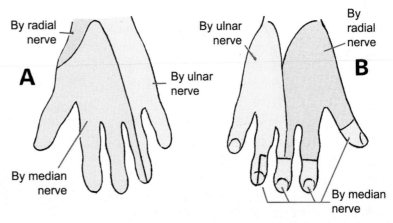

Fig. 25.6. Cutaneous nerve supply of the hand. . Palmar aspect. B. Dorsal aspect.

CUTANEOUS NERVES OF THE HAND

The skin on the palmar aspect of the hand is supplied mainly by branches of the ulnar and median nerves (Fig. 25.6). The ulnar nerve supplies the medial one and half digits and the corresponding part of the palm. The rest of the palmar aspect is supplied by branches of the median nerve. Small parts of the hand near the wrist are supplied by cutaneous nerves of the forearm.

The nerve supply of the skin on the dorsum of the hand is shown in Fig. 25.6B. Note that the dorsal aspects of the terminal phalanges of each digit are supplied by nerves that wind round from the palmar aspect. Over the medial one and half fingers the supply is by the ulnar nerve, and over the other digits it is by the median nerve. The rest of the dorsum of the hand is supplied in its lateral half (or so) by the radial nerve, and in its

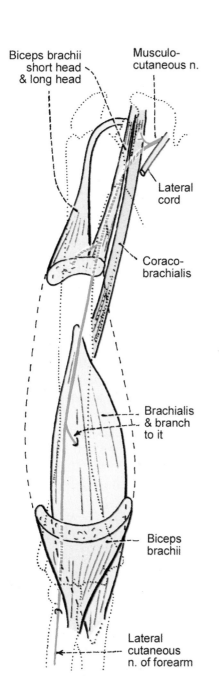

Fig. 25.7. Scheme to show the course and distribution of the musculocutaneous nerve. For areas of skin supplied by the lateral cutaneous nerve of the forearmm see Fig. 25.4.

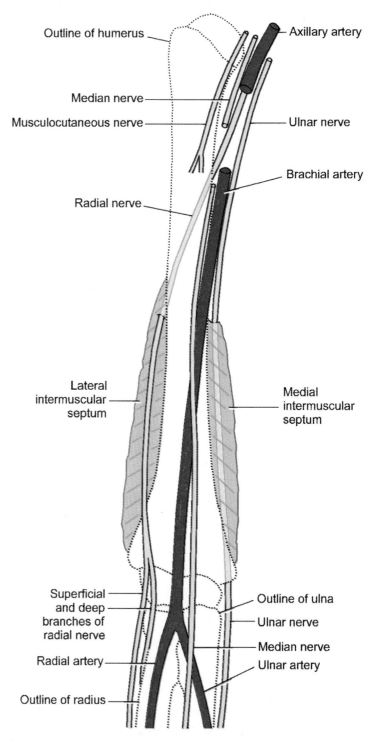

Fig. 25.8. Scheme to show the main nerves of the arm.

medial half (or so) by the ulnar nerve. Details of the branching pattern of these nerves will be considered when the hand is described.

NERVES OF THE ARM, FOREARM AND HAND

Musculocutaneous nerve

The musculocutaneous nerve is a branch of the lateral cord (Fig. 25.7). The nerve runs downwards and laterally through the front of the arm. It then crosses in front of the elbow to enter the forearm. Here the nerve becomes superficial and is called the lateral cutaneous nerve of the forearm.

The musculocutaneous nerve supplies the coracobrachialis, the biceps brachii (both heads) and the brachialis. As the lateral cutaneous nerve of the forearm it supplies the skin of the lateral half of the front of the forearm. Its lowest part supplies the skin of the thenar eminence. The cutaneous nerve supply of the forearm and hand has been described on page 36. The main nerves of the forearm are the median, ulnar and radial nerves. These are described below.

THE MEDIAN NERVE

The median nerve (Fig. 25.9) is formed by union of lateral and medial roots that arise from the corresponding cords of the brachial plexus. Its upper end lies in the axilla, lateral to the axillary artery. It continues into the arm lateral to the brachial artery. Near the middle of the arm it crosses superficial to the artery to reach its medial side, and descends in this position to the cubital fossa. The nerve leaves the cubital fossa by passing between the superficial and deep heads of the pronator teres.

The median nerve runs down the forearm in the plane between the flexor digitorum superficialis and the flexor digitorum profundus. At the wrist the nerve lies between the tendons of the flexor digitorum superficialis (medially) and the flexor carpi radialis (laterally). The nerve enters the hand by passing deep to the flexor retinaculum.

The nerve is distributed as follows.

A. Muscular branches:

1. The pronator teres is supplied by a branch that arises in the lower part of the arm.

2. Direct branches arising in the upper part of the forearm supply the flexor carpi radialis, the palmaris longus and the flexor digitorum superficialis.

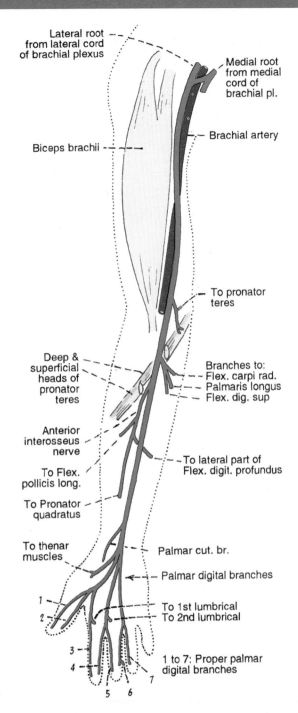

Fig. 25.9. Scheme to show the course and branches of the median nerve.

3. The anterior interosseus nerve arises from the median nerve as the latter passes between the two heads of the pronator teres. It runs down the forearm in front of the interosseus membrane. The muscles supplied through it are the flexor pollicis longus, the lateral part of the flexor digitorum profundus and the pronator quadratus.

4. A muscular branch arising in the palm supplies three thenar muscles namely the flexor pollicis brevis, the abductor pollicis brevis and the opponens pollicis.

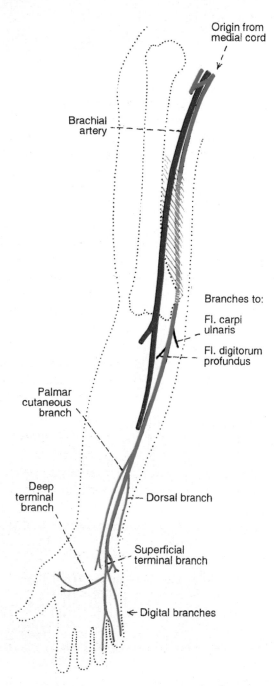

Fig. 25.10. Scheme to show the course and branches of the ulnar nerve.

5. The first and second lumbrical muscles of the hand are supplied by branches from the digital nerves (see below).

B. Cutaneous branches:

1. The palmar cutaneous branch (superficial palmar branch) arises in the lower part of the forearm. It supplies the skin over the thenar eminence and over the middle of the palm.

2. The median nerve ends by dividing into a variable number of palmar digital branches that subdivide so that ultimately seven proper palmar digital nerves are formed: two each (one medial and one lateral) for the thumb, the index and the middle fingers, and one for the lateral half of the ring finger. Through these branches the median nerve supplies the palmar surface of the lateral three and a half digits (Fig. 25.6). It also supplies the dorsal surfaces of the terminal parts of the same digits including the nail beds, the skin over the terminal phalanx of the thumb, and over the middle and terminal phalanges of the index and middle fingers and the lateral half of the ring finger.

C. Articular branches:

1. Articular branches arising directly from the median nerve near the elbow supply the elbow joint and the superior radioulnar joint.

2. The distal radioulnar joint and the wrist joint are supplied through the anterior interosseus nerve.

3. The metacarpophalangeal and interphalangeal joints are supplied through the digital branches.

THE ULNAR NERVE

The ulnar nerve is a branch of the medial cord of the brachial plexus (Fig. 25.10). It extends from the axilla to the hand. At its origin it lies medial to the axillary artery (between it and the axillary vein). It runs down into the front of the arm where it lies medial to the brachial artery. At the middle of the arm the nerve passes into the posterior compartment by piercing the medial intermuscular septum. It descends and passes behind the medial epicondyle of the humerus. The nerve enters the forearm by passing deep to the tendinous arch joining the humeral and ulnar heads of the flexor carpi ulnaris.

The ulnar nerve enters the forearm by passing deep to the tendinous arch joining the humeral and ulnar heads of the flexor carpi ulnaris. The nerve runs down the medial side of the front of the forearm lying superficial to the flexor digitorum profundus. In the lower two thirds of the forearm the nerve is accompanied by the ulnar artery which lies lateral to it. In the upper part of the forearm the nerve is deep to the flexor carpi ulnaris and to the flexor digitorum superficialis.

The nerve becomes superficial in the lower one third of the forearm: here it lies between the tendons of the flexor carpi ulnaris (medially) and that of the flexor digitorum superficialis (laterally). The nerve enters the hand by passing between the superficial and deep layers of the flexor retinaculum, lying just lateral to the pisiform bone.

The ulnar nerve is distributed to skin, muscle and joints through the following branches.

A. Cutaneous branches:

1. The palmar cutaneous branch supplies the skin of the medial one third of the palm.

2. The dorsal branch reaches the back of the wrist and hand. It supplies the skin of the medial part of the dorsum of the hand and gives two or three dorsal digital branches. The most medial digital branch supplies the medial side of the little finger. The next supplies the adjoining sides of the little and ring fingers. A third branch is present occasionally: when present it supplies the adjacent sides of the ring and middle fingers. The area of skin supplied by the dorsal digital branches extends only up to the middle phalanx: the skin over the distal phalanx (and over part of the middle phalanx) is supplied by the ventral branches.

3. The superficial terminal branch of the ulnar nerve arises after the nerve enters the hand. It divides into two palmar digital branches: one for the medial side of the little finger; and the other for the contiguous sides of the little and ring fingers. These nerves supply the skin on the palmar surfaces of the digits. They also supply the nail bed and the skin over the dorsal surface of the distal phalanx and part of the middle phalanx of the digit concerned.

B. Muscular branches:

1. Two main branches arising directly from the ulnar nerve supply the flexor carpi ulnaris and the medial part of the flexor digitorum profundus.

2. The deep terminal branch of the ulnar nerve arises in the hand. It supplies several muscles as follows.

   a) The proximal part of the nerve supplies the hypothenar muscles, namely the abductor digiti minimi, the opponens digiti minimi and the flexor digiti minimi.

   After supplying the hypothenar muscles the nerve runs transversely across the palm deep to the flexor tendons, along the deep palmar arch. Here it supplies the following:

   b) All the palmar and dorsal interossei of the hand;

   c) the third and fourth lumbrical muscles;

   d) the adductor pollicis, and frequently the flexor pollicis brevis.

3. The palmaris brevis is supplied either by the palmar cutaneous branch, or by the superficial terminal branch.

C. Articular branches:

Branches arising from the ulnar nerve or from its branches supply the elbow joint, the wrist joint, and various joints in the medial part of the hand.

THE RADIAL NERVE

The radial nerve is the main continuation of the posterior cord of the brachial plexus. At its upper end (i.e., in the axilla) it lies behind the third part of the axillary artery. In the upper part of the arm it lies behind the upper part of the brachial artery. It leaves the front of the arm by passing backwards (between the long and medial heads of the triceps).

In the posterior compartment the nerve passes downwards and laterally lying in the radial groove. Near the elbow, the nerve pierces the lateral intermuscular septum and enters the cubital fossa. Here it passes forwards in the interval between the brachialis (medially) and the brachioradialis (laterally). Finally it divides into superficial and deep branches. The superficial branch descends into the front of the forearm. The deep branch enters the substance of the supinator muscle (and while within the muscle) winds round the radius to reach the back of the forearm (Fig. 25.11).

Branches of radial nerve in the arm:

1. Near its upper end, the nerve gives branches to the medial and long heads of the triceps.

2. In the radial groove, the nerve gives branches to the medial and lateral heads of the triceps; and to the anconeus.

3. After piercing the lateral intermuscular septum, the nerve gives branches to the brachialis, the brachioradialis, and the extensor carpi radialis longus.

The superficial terminal branch runs downwards in front of the lateral part of the forearm. In the lower third of the forearm the nerve passes backwards round the lateral side of the radius to reach the dorsum of the hand where it ends by dividing into four or five digital branches.

The deep terminal branch is also called the posterior interosseus nerve. It enters the substance of the supinator muscle. Within the substance of the muscle it runs downwards winding round the lateral side of the radius. It appears in the back of the forearm through the lower part of the supinator muscle and gives several branches that supply the muscles of this region.

A. Muscular branches

We have already seen that the brachioradialis and the extensor carpi radialis longus receive branches arising from the main stem of the radial nerve in the lower part of the arm.

Muscles supplied by the deep terminal branch as follows.

1. Extensor carpi radialis brevis.
2. Supinator.
3. Extensor digitorum
4. Extensor digiti minimi.
5. Extensor carpi ulnaris
6. Extensor pollicis longus.
7. Extensor indicis.
8. Abductor pollicis longus.
9. Extensor pollicis brevis.

Note that all extensor muscles of the arm and forearm are supplied by the radial nerve directly or through its deep terminal branch.

B. Cutaneous branches to forearm and hand

These are as follows:

1. The posterior cutaneous nerve of the forearm arises from the radial nerve while the latter lies in the radial groove. It supplies an extensive area of skin on the back of the arm and on the back of the forearm.

2. Four to five dorsal digital branches arise from the superficial terminal branch of the radial nerve. The first (most lateral) supplies the skin of the lateral side of the thumb; the second the medial side of the thumb. The third branch supplies the lateral side of the index finger. The fourth branch supplies the contiguous sides of the index and middle fingers; while the fifth (when present) supplies the contiguous sides of the middle and ring fingers. The dorsal digital branches do not extend to the distal ends of the digits. The skin over the distal phalanges, and the whole or part of the middle phalanges is supplied by palmar digital branches of the median nerve.

C. Articular branches:

1) Direct branches from the radial nerve help to supply the elbow joint.

2) Joints in the region of the wrist are supplied by branches from the lower end of the deep terminal branch.

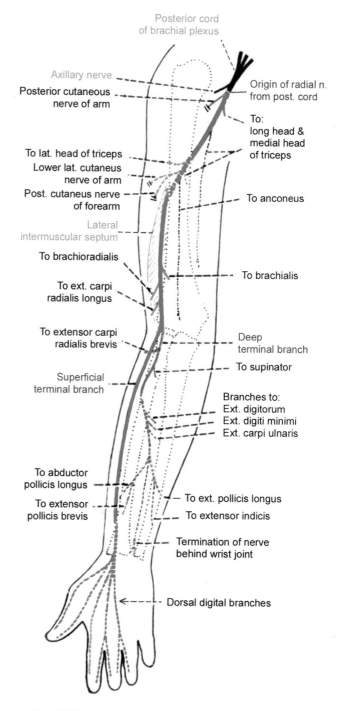

Fig. 25.11. Scheme to show the course and branches of the radial nerve.

26

Blood Supply of the Upper Extremity

ARTERIES OF THE UPPER EXTREMITY

THE AXILLARY ARTERY

The axillary artery is a continuation of the subclavian artery. It begins at the outer border of the first rib and ends at the lower border of the teres major (by becoming the brachial artery). The artery is crossed by the pectoralis minor which divides it into first, second and third parts.

A. *Relationship to muscles*

(a) The first part of the artery rests (posteriorly) on the muscles of the first intercostal space and the upper part of the serratus anterior.

(b) The second part and the upper portion of the third part of the artery lie on the subscapularis muscle. The lower portion of the third part lies on the teres major muscle and the tendon of the latissimus dorsi.

(c) The entire artery except its lowermost part is overlapped by the pectoralis major. The second part is also covered by the pectoralis minor. The first part is also covered by the clavipectoral fascia (which extends from the pectoralis minor to the clavicle).

(d) The coracobrachialis is lateral to the second and third parts of the artery.

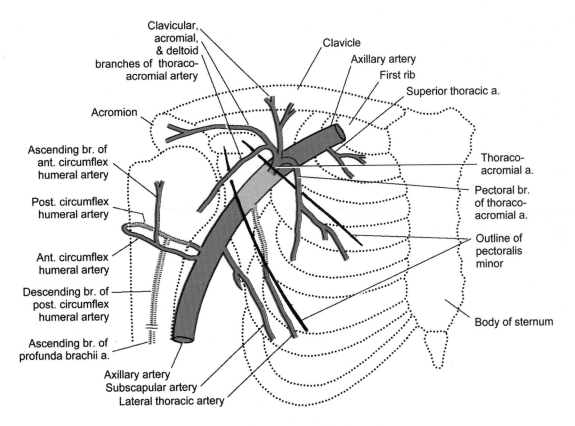

Fig. 26.1. Axillary artery and its branches.

B. Relationship to veins:

The axillary artery is accompanied by the axillary vein: the vein lies anteromedial to the artery.

C. Relationship to brachial plexus

The first and second parts of the artery are related to the cords of the plexus; and the third part of the artery to their branches.

Branches Of The Axillary Artery

The first part of the artery gives rise to one branch: the superior thoracic (Fig. 26.1). The second part of the artery gives two branches: the thoracoacromial and the lateral thoracic. The third part gives off three branches: the subscapular and the anterior and posterior circumflex humeral.

The ***superior thoracic artery*** arises from the first part of the axillary. It supplies the pectoral muscles and part of the thoracic wall.

The ***thoracoacromial artery*** arises from the second part of the axillary. It divides into four branches, pectoral, acromial, clavicular and deltoid.

The ***lateral thoracic artery*** runs downwards near the lateral margin of the pectoralis minor. In the female it gives off branches to the breast.

The ***subscapular artery*** runs downwards along the lateral border of the scapula. The artery gives off a large circumflex scapular branch. This branch winds

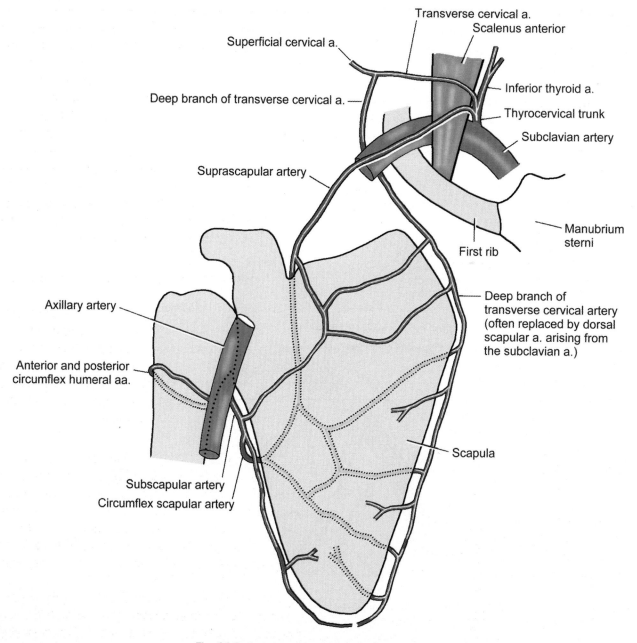

Fig. 26.2. Anastomoses around the scapula.

round the lateral border of the scapula passing backwards through the triangular space. It takes part in forming the anastomoses round the scapula (Fig. 26.2).

The *anterior circumflex humeral artery* (Fig. 26.1) runs laterally in front of the surgical neck of the humerus: it anastomoses with the posterior circumflex humeral artery (see below) to form an arterial circle round the neck.

The *posterior circumflex humeral artery* (Fig. 26.1) runs backwards (accompanied by the axillary nerve) through the quadrangular space. It then passes laterally behind the surgical neck of the humerus to anastomose with the anterior circumflex humeral artery.

ARTERIES OF SCAPULAR REGION

In the back and scapular region we see some arteries that begin in the neck as (direct or indirect) branches of the subclavian artery. Like the axillary artery, the subclavian artery is divided into first, second and third parts (by a muscle called the scalenus anterior). A short artery called the *thyrocervical trunk* arises from the junction of the first and third parts of the subclavian artery (Fig. 26.2). The thyrocervical trunk divides into three arteries, inferior thyroid, suprascapular and the transverse cervical. The suprascapular and transverse cervical arteries are encountered in the scapular region.

The Transverse Cervical Artery (Fig. 26.2)

This artery divides into superficial and deep branches. The *superficial branch* runs laterally across the posterior triangle of the neck to reach the trapezius. It then ascends deep to the trapezius, supplying it and neighbouring structures. The *deep branch* of the transverse cervical passes laterally and backwards in the lower part of the posterior triangle of the neck to reach the upper angle of the scapula. It then runs along the medial border of this bone up to the inferior angle (deep to the levator scapulae and rhomboideus muscles). It supplies these muscles and the trapezius. It gives branches that anastomose with the suprascapular and subscapular arteries (See below).

The Suprascapular artery (Fig. 26.2)

This artery arises in the neck from the thyrocervical trunk. It passes downwards to reach the superior border of the scapula: here it passes above the transverse scapular ligament and enters the supraspinous fossa (on dorsal surface of scapula above the spine). After giving some branches to the supraspinatus it passes into the infraspinous fossa by passing through the spinoglenoid notch. In the infraspinous fossa it divides into a number of branches that supply the infraspinatus. Branches are also given to some other muscles, to the shoulder joint, the acromioclavicular joint and skin.

Anastomosis around the scapula (Fig. 26.2)

1) On the back of the body of the scapula the suprascapular artery anastomoses with the deep branch of the transverse cervical artery and with the circumflex scapular branch of the subscapular artery.

2) On the ventral surface of the body of the scapula branches of the suprascapular artery anastomose with the subscapular artery and with the deep branch of the transverse cervical artery.

3) Over the acromion branches of the suprascapular artery anastomose with the thoracoacromial and posterior circumflex humeral arteries.

The anastomoses described above connect the first part of the subclavian artery to the third part of the axillary artery.

THE BRACHIAL ARTERY

The brachial artery begins at the lower border of the teres major as the continuation of the axillary artery. Its upper part lies on the medial aspect of the arm. As it descends it gradually passes forwards, so that its lower end lies in front of the elbow (cubital fossa). Here it terminates (at the level of the neck of the radius) by dividing into the radial and ulnar arteries. The relations of the artery are considered below.

Relationship to nerves:

a) The radial nerve lies behind the uppermost part of the brachial artery.

b) The median nerve descends along the lateral side of the upper half of the artery. It then crosses in front of the artery and comes to lie along its medial side.

c) The ulnar nerve lies medial to the upper half of the artery. Lower down it parts company from the artery as it pierces the medial intermuscular septum to enter the posterior compartment of the arm.

Relationship to veins:

The brachial artery is accompanied by venae comitantes. The basilic vein comes to lie medial to the artery a little above the elbow, but is separated from it by deep fascia. The vein pierces the deep fascia near the middle of the arm, and thereafter lies close to the artery. At the upper end of the brachial artery the venae comitantes join the basilic vein to form the axillary vein.

Branches Of The Brachial Artery (Fig. 26.3)

The *profunda brachii artery* arises a little below the upper end of the brachial artery. Accompanying

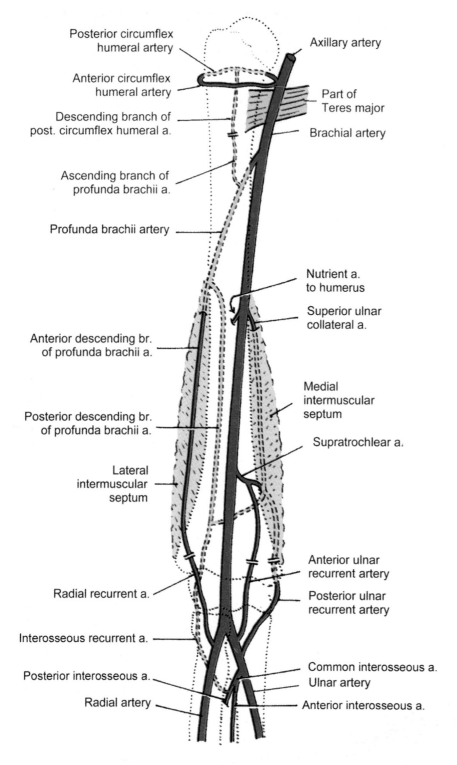

Fig. 26.3. Scheme to show arteries of the arm.

(**b**) The *ascending branch* anastomoses with the descending branch of the posterior circumflex humeral artery.

(**c**) The *posterior descending (or middle collateral) branch* anastomoses with the recurrent branch of the posterior interosseous artery.

(**d**) The *anterior descending (or radial collateral) artery* pierces the lateral intermuscular septum and enters the anterior compartment of the arm. It runs along the radial nerve in the lower lateral part of the arm and ends by anastomosing with the recurrent branch of the radial artery.

The **superior ulnar collateral** artery arises from the brachial artery near the middle of the arm. Accompanying the ulnar nerve this artery pierces the medial intermuscular septum to enter the posterior compartment of the arm. It runs downwards to reach the back of the medial epicondyle. The artery ends by anastomosing with the posterior recurrent branch of the ulnar artery and with the supratrochlear artery.

The **supratrochlear artery** arises from the brachial artery a little above the elbow. It pierces the medial intermuscular septum and enters the posterior compartment of the arm. Branches of the artery anastomose with the anterior recurrent branch of the ulnar

the radial nerve it enters the posterior compartment of the arm. Here it passes laterally and downwards behind the humerus, where it lies in the radial groove. It gives off the following branches.

(**a**) A *nutrient artery* is given off to the humerus.

artery (in front of the elbow); and with the posterior descending branch of the profunda brachii artery, and the interosseous recurrent artery (behind the elbow).

In Fig. 26.3 note the arteries helping to form the arterial anastomoses around the elbow joint.

ARTERIES OF THE FOREARM

The main arteries of the forearm are the radial and ulnar branches of the brachial artery. They are described below.

The Radial Artery

The radial artery begins in front of the elbow at the level of the neck of the radius (Fig. 26.2). It first passes downwards and laterally reaching the lateral border of the forearm about its middle. It then descends along the lateral margin of the forearm to the wrist. Thereafter, it winds round the lateral side of the carpus to reach the back of the hand (Fig. 26.4). It passes forwards through the space between the first and second metacarpal bones to reach the palm. Finally it runs transversely across the palm as the deep palmar arch, and ends by anastomosing with the deep palmar branch of the ulnar artery.

Branches of radial artery:

1. The **radial recurrent artery** arises near the upper end of the radial artery (Fig. 26.3). It ascends to anastomose with the radial collateral (anterior descending) branch of the profunda brachii artery.

All other branches of the radial artery arise near the wrist and hand (Fig. 26.4).

2. The **palmar carpal branch** passes medially in front of the carpus to anastomose with a corresponding branch from the ulnar artery to form the palmar carpal arch.

3. The **dorsal carpal branch** passes medially behind the carpus to anastomose with a corresponding branch from the ulnar artery to form the dorsal carpal arch.

4. The **superficial palmar branch** often joins the ulnar artery to complete the superficial palmar arch.

5. The **first dorsal metacarpal** artery arises on the dorsum of the hand. It divides into two branches, one for the medial side of the thumb and the other for the lateral side of the index finger.

6. The **princeps pollicis** artery arises just as the radial artery enters the palm after passing forwards between the first and second metacarpal bones. It supplies the lateral side of the thumb.

7. The **radialis indicis** artery arises near the princeps pollicis and runs along the lateral side of the index finger.

The Ulnar Artery

The ulnar artery begins in front of the elbow, at the level of the neck of the radius (Fig. 26.3). It passes downwards and medially to reach the medial margin of the forearm (at about its middle) and then runs vertically along this margin (Fig. 26.5). It runs across the wrist superficial to the flexor retinaculum. Entering the palm it runs laterally across it as the superficial palmar arch (Fig. 26.6). This arch is completed laterally by anastomosis with a branch of the radial artery which is usually the superficial palmar, but may be the princeps pollicis or the radialis indicis.

Branches of Ulnar artery (Fig. 26.5):

1. The **anterior ulnar recurrent** artery arises near the upper end of the ulnar artery. It passes upwards in front of the elbow to anastomose with the supratrochlear artery (Also see Fig. 26.3).

2. The **posterior ulnar recurrent** artery also arises near the upper end of the ulnar artery. It passes upwards behind the medial epicondyle and anastomoses with the superior ulnar collateral artery (Also see Fig. 26.3).

3. The **common interosseous** artery divides into anterior and posterior interosseous branches.

The **anterior interosseous** artery descends in front of the interosseous membrane. Near the upper border of the pronator quadratus it pierces the membrane and runs downwards behind it to the back of the wrist. The anterior interosseous artery also gives off a branch which accompanies the median nerve.

The posterior interosseous artery passes backwards above the upper margin of the interosseous membrane and then descends between muscles of the back of the forearm supplying them.

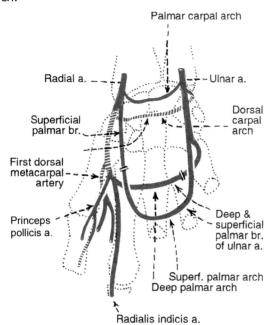

Palmar carpal arch

Radial a.

Ulnar a.

Superficial palmar br.

Dorsal carpal arch

First dorsal metacarpal artery

Princeps pollicis a.

Deep & superficial palmar br. of ulnar a.

Superf. palmar arch
Deep palmar arch

Radialis indicis a.

Fig. 26.4. Schematic diagram to show branches of the radial artery in the hand. Some branches of the ulnar artery are also shown. The various arches are formed by corresponding branches of the radial and ulnar arteries.

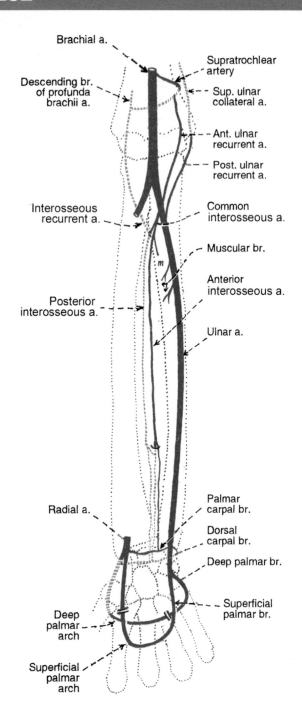

Fig. 26.5. Scheme to show branches of the ulnar artery.

Near its origin the posterior interosseous artery gives off an interosseous recurrent artery that runs upwards behind the elbow to anastomose with the posterior descending branch of the profunda brachii artery and with the supratrochlear artery (Also see Fig. 26.3).

4. The *palmar and dorsal carpal branches* of the ulnar artery arise at the wrist. They anastomose with the palmar and dorsal carpal branches of the radial artery to form the palmar and dorsal carpal arches.

5. The *deep palmar branch* of the ulnar artery arises just distal to the pisiform bone. It ends by anastomosing with the radial artery to complete the deep palmar arch.

6. After giving off its deep branch the ulnar artery continues into the palm as the *superficial palmar branch*. This branch runs transversely across the palm forming the superficial palmar arch: this arch lies distal to the deep palmar arch. The arch is completed laterally by a branch of the radial artery: usually the superficial palmar, but sometimes the radialis indicis or the princeps pollicis.

ARTERIES OF THE HAND

The palm and digits receive a series of branches from the various arterial arches formed in the region. They are:

1. Four *dorsal metacarpal arteries*. Each dorsal metacarpal artery ends by dividing into two dorsal digital arteries.

2. Four *palmar metacarpal arteries* end by joining the common palmar digital arteries (see below) of the corresponding intermetacarpal space.

3. The *common palmar digital arteries* arise from the superficial palmar arch. Each artery divides into two palmar digital branches.

Arteries on the dorsal and ventral aspect of the hand are united by a series of perforating arteries.

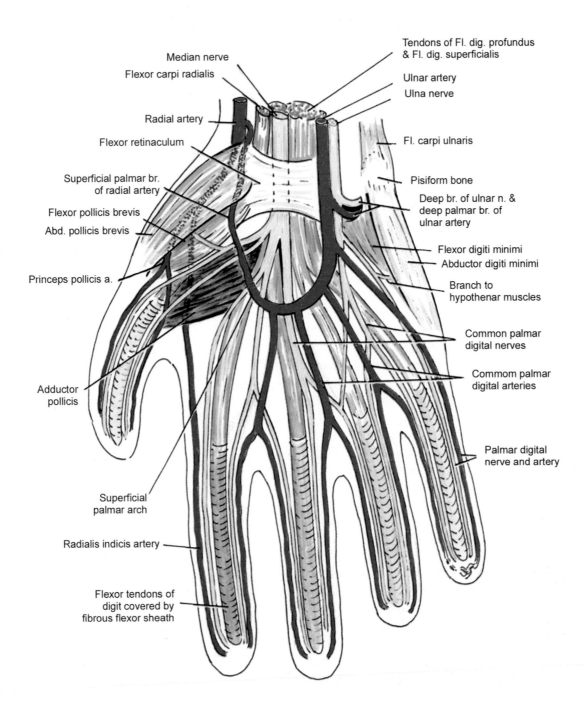

Fig. 26.6. Arteries and nerves of the palm.

VEINS OF THE UPPER LIMB

The venous drainage of the limbs is carried out through two separate sets of veins. Most of the blood is returned through superficial veins that lie in the superficial fascia and have no relationship to arteries of the limb. The other set, the deep veins, run along the arteries.

A. Superficial Veins

The dorsal digital veins from the fingers end in dorsal metacarpal veins which in turn join each other to form a dorsal venous network over the dorsum of the hand. The palmar digital veins drain into a superficial plexus in the palm. The veins of the hand are further drained by two main superficial veins. These are the cephalic and basilic veins.

The cephalic vein begins from the lateral side of the hand. It first ascends along the radial side of the forearm, but higher up it lies on the anterior surface. Crossing the lateral part of the elbow it runs upwards into the arm. Here it lies along the lateral side of the biceps brachii. In the upper part of the arm it comes to lie in the groove between the anterior margin of the deltoid muscle and the pectoralis major. A little below the clavicle it pierces the clavipectoral fascia and ends in the axillary vein. The cephalic vein is connected to the basilic vein by the median cubital vein (See below).

The basilic vein begins from the ulnar side of the venous network on the dorsum of the hand. It ascends along the ulnar side of the forearm, first on its posterior aspect and then winding round the ulnar border to reach the anterior aspect. Crossing in front of the medial part of the elbow it runs upwards along the medial side of the biceps brachii muscle. At about the middle of the arm it pierces the deep fascia and comes to lie medial to the brachial artery. It ascends in this position up to the lower border of the teres major where it becomes the axillary vein.

The median cubital vein lies in front of the elbow joint. It passes upwards and medially from the cephalic vein to the basilic vein.

Some other superficial veins seen in the limb are shown in Fig. 26.7.

B. Deep Veins

The deep veins accompany the arteries of the limb. Such veins are called venae comitantes. They are found

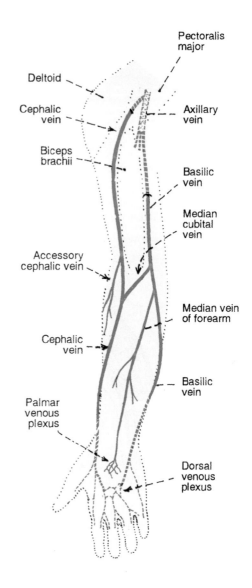

Fig. 26.7. Superficial veins of the upper limb.

in relation to the radial and ulnar arteries, and to the brachial artery. The veins accompanying the brachial artery are joined (near the lower border of the teres major) by the basilic vein to form the axillary vein.

THE AXILLARY VEIN

The axillary vein accompanies the axillary artery through the axilla. It is formed at the lower border of the teres major by joining together of the venae comitantes of the brachial artery and the basilic vein. It ends at the outer border of the first rib by becoming continuous with the subclavian vein . The vein lies medial to the axillary artery.

PART FIVE

THE
LOWER
EXTREMITY

27

Bones of the Lower Extremity

A brief introduction to the bones of the lower extremity has been given in Chapter 2. The bones are described one by one in this chapter.

THE HIP BONE

Introductory remarks (Figs. 27.1, 27.2)

Along with the sacrum and coccyx, the right and left hip bones form the bony pelvis. Each hip bone consists of three parts. These are the ilium, the pubis, and the ischium. These three parts meet at the **acetabulum** which is a large deep cavity placed on the lateral aspect of the bone. The acetabulum takes part in forming the hip joint along with the head of the femur. Below and medial to the acetabulum the hip bone shows a large oval or triangular aperture called the **obturator foramen**. The **ilium** consists, in greater part, of a large plate of bone which lies above and behind the acetabulum, and forms the side wall of the greater pelvis. Its upper border is in form of a broad ridge that is convex upwards: this ridge is called the **iliac crest**.

The posterior part of the ilium bears a large rough articular area on its medial side for articulation with the sacrum. The **pubis** lies in relation to the upper and medial part of the obturator foramen. It forms the most anterior part of the hip bone. The two pubic bones meet in the middle line, in front, to form the pubic symphysis. The lowest part of the hip bone is formed by the **ischium** which lies below and behind the acetabulum and the obturator foramen. Using the information given above, a given hip bone can be correctly orientated and its side determined.

The Ilium

In addition to the features already mentioned note the following.

The anterior end of the iliac crest projects forwards as the **anterior superior iliac spine**. The posterior end of the crest forms a projection called the **posterior superior iliac spine**. The iliac crest may be subdivided into a **ventral segment**, consisting of the anterior two thirds of the crest, and a **dorsal segment** consisting of the posterior one third. The ventral segment shows a broad intermediate area which is bounded by inner and outer lips. The outer lip of the iliac crest is most prominent about 5cm behind the anterior superior iliac spine. This prominence is called the **tubercle of the iliac crest**. The dorsal segment of the iliac crest has medial and lateral surfaces separated by a ridge.

The anterior border of the ilium extends from the anterior superior iliac spine to the acetabulum. Its lowest part presents a prominence called the **anterior inferior iliac spine**.

The posterior border of the ilium extends from the posterior superior iliac spine to the back of the acetabulum. A few centimetres below the posterior superior iliac spine the posterior border presents another prominence called the **posterior inferior iliac spine**. The lower part of the posterior border forms the upper boundary of a deep notch called the **greater sciatic notch**.

The lateral aspect of the ilium constitutes its **gluteal surface**. This surface is marked by three ridges called the anterior, posterior and inferior gluteal lines.

The **posterior gluteal line** is vertical. It extends from the iliac crest, above, to the posterior inferior iliac spine below. The **anterior gluteal line** is convex upwards and backwards. Its anterior end meets the iliac crest in front of the tubercle; while its posterior end reaches the greater sciatic notch. The **inferior gluteal line** is horizontal. Its anterior end lies just above the anterior inferior iliac spine; and its posterior end reaches the greater sciatic notch. The gluteal surface of the ilium bears a prominent groove just above the acetabulum. The lower part of the gluteal surface extends behind the acetabulum where it becomes continuous with the ischium. The lowest part of the ilium forms the upper two fifths of the acetabulum.

The medial surface of the ilium is divisible into the following parts. The **iliac fossa** is smooth and concave

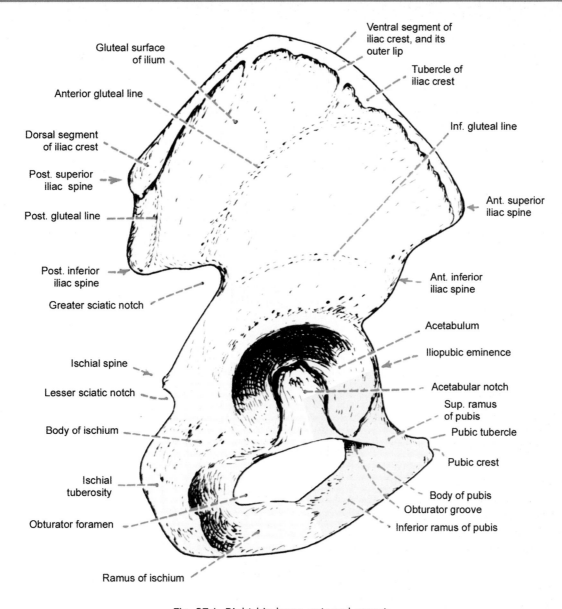

Fig. 27.1. Right hip bone, external aspect.

and forms the wall of the greater pelvis: it occupies the anterior part of the medial surface. The **sacropelvic surface** lies behind the iliac fossa. It can be subdivided into three parts. The upper part is rough and constitutes the **iliac tuberosity**. The middle part articulates with the lateral side of the sacrum. This part is called the **auricular surface** because of a resemblance to the pinna. The **pelvic part** of the medial surface lies below and in front of the auricular surface. It is smooth and takes part in forming the wall of the lesser pelvis. This surface is often marked (specially in the female) by a rough groove called the **preauricular sulcus**. The iliac fossa and the sacropelvic surface are separated by the medial border of the ilium. Its lower part is rounded and forms the **arcuate line**. The lower end of the arcuate line reaches the junction of the ilium and pubis.

This junction shows an enlargement called the **iliopubic eminence**.

The Ischium

The ischium consists of a main part called the **body**, and a projection called the **ramus**. The upper end of the body forms the inferior and posterior part of the acetabulum. The lower part of the body has three surfaces: dorsal, femoral and pelvic. The lower part of the dorsal surface has a large rough impression called the **ischial tuberosity**. This tuberosity is divided into upper and lower parts by a transverse ridge. Each of these parts is again divided into medial and lateral parts. Superiorly the dorsal surface becomes continuous with the gluteal surface of the ilium. The posterior border of the dorsal surface of the ischium forms part of the lower

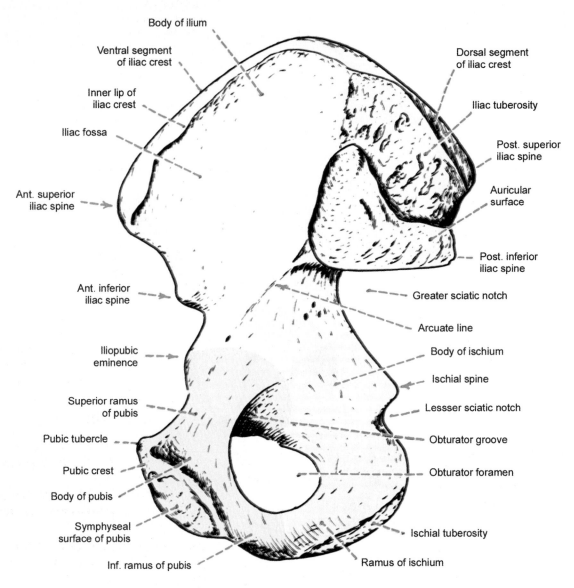

Fig. 27.2. Right hip bone, internal aspect.

margin of the greater sciatic notch. Just below this notch the border projects backwards and medially as the ischial spine. Between the ischial spine and the upper border of the ischial tuberosity we see a shallow *lesser sciatic notch*.

The *ramus of the ischium* is attached to the medial side of the lower end of the body. The ramus has an anterior (external) surface and a posterior (internal) surface.

The Pubis

The pubis consists of a body, a superior ramus and an inferior ramus. The *body* (Fig. 27.3) forms the anterior and most medial part of the hip bone. It has an anterior surface and a posterior surface. The upper border of the body of the pubis is called the pubic crest.

The crest ends laterally in a projection called the pubic tubercle.

The *superior ramus* of the pubis runs upwards backwards and laterally from the body. Its lateral extremity takes part in forming the pubic part of the acetabulum. It meets the ilium at the iliopubic eminence. The superior ramus is triangular in cross section. It has three borders and three surfaces.

The anterior border is called the *obturator crest*. The posterior border is sharp and forms the *pecten pubis* or *pectineal line*. The inferior border is also sharp and forms the upper margin of the obturator foramen. The surface between the obturator crest and the pecten pubis is the *pectineal surface*. The pelvic surface lies between the pecten pubis and the inferior

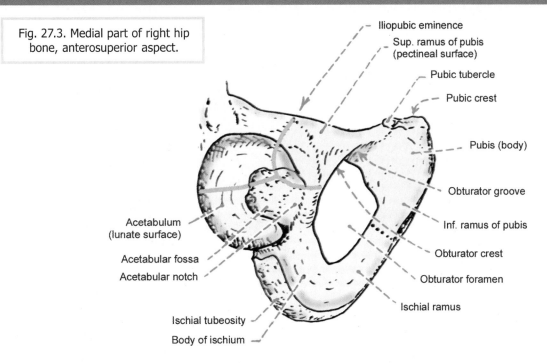

Fig. 27.3. Medial part of right hip bone, anterosuperior aspect.

Labels (clockwise from top):
- Iliopubic eminence
- Sup. ramus of pubis (pectineal surface)
- Pubic tubercle
- Pubic crest
- Pubis (body)
- Obturator groove
- Inf. ramus of pubis
- Obturator crest
- Obturator foramen
- Ischial ramus
- Body of ischium
- Ischial tuberosity
- Acetabular notch
- Acetabular fossa
- Acetabulum (lunate surface)

border. The surface between the obturator crest and the inferior border is called the *obturator surface*. A groove runs forwards and downwards across it and is called the *obturator groove*.

The *inferior ramus* of the pubis passes downwards and laterally to meet the ramus of the ischium. These two rami form the medial boundary of the obturator foramen. In the intact pelvis the conjoined rami of the pubis and ischium of the two sides form the boundaries of the *pubic arch* which lies below the pubic symphysis.

The Acetabulum

The acetabulum forms the hip joint with the head of the femur. It is directed laterally and somewhat downwards and forwards. The margin of the acetabulum is deficient in the anteroinferior part: the gap in the margin is called the *acetabular notch*. The floor of the acetabulum is partly articular and partly non-articular. The articular area for the head of the femur is shaped like a horse-shoe and is called the *lunate surface*. The non-articular part of the floor of the acetabulum is called the *acetabular fossa*. The contributions to the acetabulum by the ilium, the ischium and the pubis are shown in Fig. 27.3 in which the lines of junction of the three parts are indicated by grey lines.

The Obturator Foramen

The obturator foramen is bounded above by the superior ramus of the pubis; medially by the body of the pubis, by its inferior ramus and by the ramus of the ischium; and laterally by the body of the ischium. In

the intact body the foramen is filled by a fibrous sheet called the *obturator membrane*. The membrane is deficient in the uppermost part of the foramen.

Some Important Attachments on the Hip Bone

A. The muscles attached to the iliac crest are as follows (Figs. 27.4, 27.5).

1. The internal oblique muscle of the abdomen arises from the intermediate area of the ventral segment of the iliac crest.

2. The external oblique muscle of the abdomen is inserted into the anterior two thirds of the outer lip of the ventral segment of the iliac crest.

3. The lowest fibres of the latissimus dorsi take origin from the outer lip of the iliac crest just behind its highest point.

4. The tensor fasciae latae arises from the anterior part of the outer lip of the iliac crest.

5. The transversus abdominis arises from the anterior two thirds of the inner lip of the ventral segment of the iliac crest.

6. The quadratus lumborum arises from the posterior one third of the inner lip of the ventral segment of the iliac crest.

7. The gluteus maximus arises from the lateral surface of the dorsal segment of the iliac crest and from the gluteal surface of the ilium behind the posterior gluteal line.

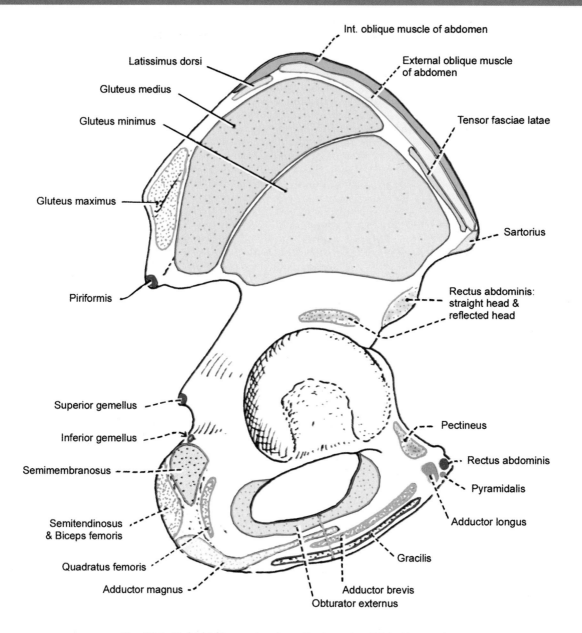

Fig. 27.4. Right hip bone showing attachments. External aspect.

B. The muscles attached to the external aspect of the hip bone (excluding the iliac crest) are as follows (Fig. 27.4).

1. The gluteus maximus arises from the lateral surface of the dorsal segment of the iliac crest and from the gluteal surface of the ilium behind the posterior gluteal line.

2. The gluteus medius arises from the gluteal surface of the ilium between the anterior and posterior gluteal lines.

3. The gluteus minimus arises from the gluteal surface of the ilium between the anterior and inferior gluteal lines.

4. The sartorius arises from the anterior superior iliac spine.

5. The straight head of the rectus femoris arises from the anterior inferior iliac spine; and its reflected head from the groove above the acetabulum.

7. The pectineus arises from the upper part of the pectineal surface of the superior ramus of the pubis.

8. The rectus abdominis (lateral head) arises from the pubic crest.

9. The adductor longus arise from the anterior surface of the body of the pubis.

10. The gracilis arises from the anterior surface of the body, and the inferior ramus, of the pubis; and from the ramus of the ischium.

11. The adductor brevis arises from the anterior surface of the body of the pubis and its inferior ramus.

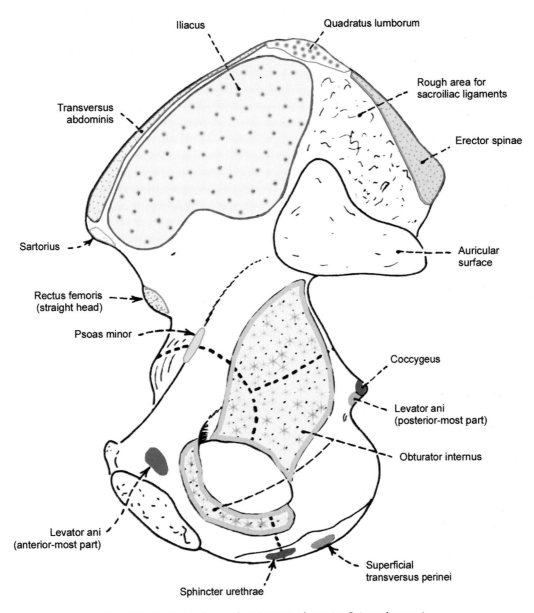

Fig. 27.5. Right hip bone showing attachments. Internal aspect.

12. The obturator externus arises from the superior and inferior rami of the pubis, and from the ramus of the ischium, immediately around the obturator foramen.

13. The adductor magnus arises from the lower lateral part of the ischial tuberosity, and from the ramus of the ischium.

14. The semitendinosus and the biceps femoris (long head) arise from the upper medial part of the ischial tuberosity.

15. The semimembranosus arises from the upper lateral part of the ischial tuberosity.

16. The quadratus femoris arises from the femoral surface of the ischium just lateral to the ischial tuberosity.

C. The muscles arising from the internal aspect of the hip bone are as follows (Fig. 27.5).

1. The iliacus arises from the upper two thirds of the iliac fossa.

2. The obturator internus arises from the pelvic surfaces of the superior and inferior rami of the pubis, and the ramus of the ischium, immediately adjoining the obturator foramen; and from the pelvic surfaces of the ischium and of the ilium.

3. The psoas minor is inserted into the pecten pubis and into the iliopectineal eminence.

Greater and Lesser Sciatic Foramina

The greater and lesser sciatic notches are converted into foramina by the sacrotuberous and sacrospinous ligaments. The greater sciatic foramen transmits the following structures:

Piriformis; the superior and inferior gluteal nerves and vessels; the internal pudendal vessels; the pudendal and sciatic nerves; the posterior cutaneous nerve of the thigh; and the nerves to the obturator internus and to the quadratus femoris.

Having emerged from the greater sciatic foramen the pudendal nerve, the nerve to the obturator internus, and the internal pudendal vessels pass behind the ischial spine to enter the lesser sciatic foramen. The tendon of the obturator internus emerges from the pelvis through this foramen.

PELVIS AS A WHOLE

We have seen that the bony pelvis is made up of the two hip bones, the sacrum and the coccyx (Fig. 27.6). It may be subdivided into the *greater (or false) pelvis* and the *lesser (or true) pelvis*. The walls of the greater pelvis are formed by the broad upper parts of the two iliac bones (iliac fossae), and posteriorly by

the base of the sacrum. The communication between the greater and lesser pelvis is called the *superior pelvic aperture* or *pelvic inlet*. The margins of the aperture constitute the *pelvic brim*. The pelvic brim is formed behind by the sacral promontory, and the ridge separating the superior and anterior surfaces of the sacrum; on either side by the arcuate line of the ilium (also see Fig. 27.2); and anteriorly by the pecten pubis and by the pubic crest. The arcuate line, the pecten pubis and the pubic crest are collectively referred to as the *linea terminalis*.

The *cavity of the lesser pelvis* is bounded in front by the body and rami of the pubis; on either side by the pelvic surfaces of the ilium and ischium; and behind by the anterior surfaces of the sacrum and coccyx.

The *inferior pelvic aperture* is highly irregular. It is bounded anteriorly by the pubic arch; laterally, in that order, by the ischial tuberosity, the lesser sciatic notch, the ischial spine and the greater sciatic notch. Posteriorly, it is formed by the lateral margin of the sacrum and coccyx. When the ligaments are intact the lateral margins are formed by the sacrotuberous ligaments (that stretch from the side of the sacrum and coccyx to the ischial tuberosity. The inferior aperture then appears to be rhomboidal.

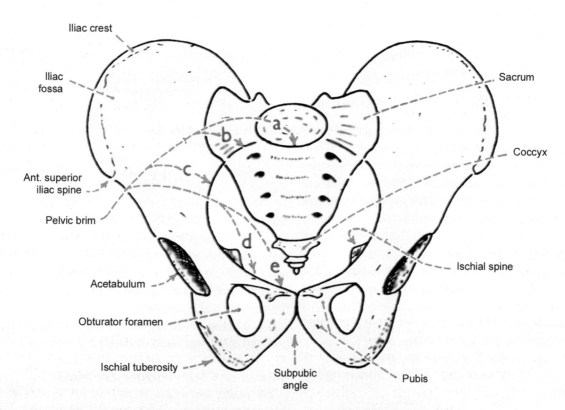

Fig. 27.6. Pelvis seen from the front.

THE FEMUR

The femur (Figs. 27.7, 27.8) is a long bone having a shaft, an upper end and a lower end. The upper end is easily distinguished from the lower end by the presence of a rounded head which is joined to the shaft by an elongated neck. The head is directed medially to articulate with the acetabulum of the hip bone. The anterior and posterior aspects of the bone can be distinguished by examining the shaft: it is convex forwards and the anterior aspect is smooth, while the posterior aspect is marked by a prominent vertical ridge called the linea aspera. The information given above is sufficient to distinguish between a femur of the right or left side.

The Upper End

Apart from the head and the neck the upper end of the femur has two projections called the greater and lesser trochanters.

The **head** is directed medially, upwards and somewhat forwards. It is slightly more than half a sphere. Near the centre of the head there is a pit or **fovea**.

The **neck** connects the head to the shaft. It joins the shaft at an angle of about 125 degrees. The greater and lesser trochanters are situated near the junction of the neck with the shaft.

The **greater trochanter** forms a large quadrangular projection on the lateral aspect of the upper end of the femur. Its upper and posterior part projects upwards beyond the level of the neck and thus comes to have a medial surface. On this surface we see a depressed area called the **trochanteric fossa**. The anterior aspect of the greater trochanter shows a large rough area for muscle attachments. The lateral surface of the greater trochanter is also marked by a ridge that runs downwards and forwards across the lateral surface.

The **lesser trochanter** is a conical projection attached to the shaft where the lower border of the neck meets the shaft. The posterior parts of the greater and lesser trochanters are joined together by a prominent ridge called the **intertrochanteric crest**. A little above its middle this crest bears a rounded elevation called the **quadrate tubercle**. Anteriorly, the junction of the neck and the shaft is marked by a much less prominent **intertrochanteric line**. The upper end of this line reaches the anterior and upper

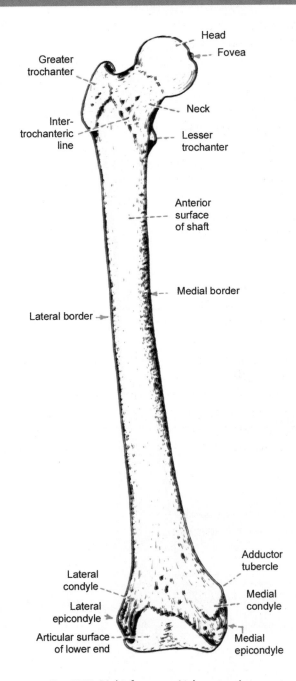

Fig. 27.7. Right femur, anterior aspect.

part of the greater trochanter; its lower end lies a little in front of the lesser trochanter. Here it becomes continuous with the **spiral line** which runs downwards and backwards across the medial aspect of the shaft to reach its posterior aspect.

The Shaft

The shaft of the femur has a forward convexity and is smooth anteriorly. Its posterior aspect is marked by a rough vertical ridge called the **linea aspera**. The shaft is triangular having three borders (lateral, medial and posterior) and three surfaces (anterior, lateral and

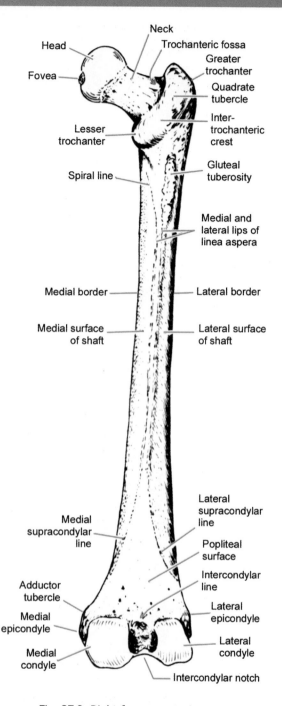

Fig. 27.8. Right femur, posterior aspect.

(posterior) over the upper one third of the shaft. The two lips of the linea aspera also diverge from each other over the lower one third of the shaft to become continuous with ridges called the medial and lateral supracondylar lines. Here again, the shaft has an additional surface directed posteriorly: this surface is triangular and is called the *popliteal surface*.

The Lower End

The lower end of the femur consists of two large condyles, medial and lateral. The two condyles are joined together anteriorly and, on this aspect, they lie in the same plane as the lower part of the shaft. Posteriorly, the two condyles project much beyond the plane of the shaft, and here they are separated by a deep *intercondylar notch* or fossa.

When viewed from the side the lower margin of each condyle is seen to form an arch that is convex downwards. When seen from below it is seen that the long axis of the lateral condyle is straight and is directed backwards and somewhat laterally. In contrast the medial condyle is slightly curved having a medial convexity.

The anterior aspect of the two condyles is marked by an articular area for the patella. The area is concave from side to side to accommodate the convex posterior surface of the patella. It is divided into medial and lateral parts. The lateral part is much larger.

Inferiorly, the condyles articulate with the tibia to form the knee joint. For this purpose each condyle bears a large convex articular surface which is continuous anteriorly with the patellar surface. The articular surface covers the inferior and posterior aspects of each condyle.

When seen from the lateral aspect the lateral condyle of the femur is seen to be more or less flat. A little behind the middle it is marked by a prominence called the *lateral epicondyle*. Behind and below the epicondyle there is a prominent groove that is divided into an anterior deeper part and a shallower posterior part.

When seen from the medial aspect the medial condyle is seen to be convex. The most prominent point on it is called the *medial epicondyle*. The uppermost part of the medial condyle is marked by a prominence called the *adductor tubercle* (Fig. 27.8).

Important Attachments on the Femur

A. The muscles inserted into the femur are as follows (Figs. 27.9, 27.10) .

1. The gluteus minimus is inserted on the anterior aspect of the greater trochanter.

medial). The lateral and medial borders are rounded. The posterior border corresponds to the linea aspera. The linea aspera has distinct medial and lateral lips. When traced upwards to the upper one third of the shaft the lips diverge. The medial lip becomes continuous with the spiral line. The lateral lip of the linea aspera becomes continuous with a broad rough area called the *gluteal tuberosity*. The upper end of the gluteal tuberosity reaches the greater trochanter. The area between the gluteal tuberosity (laterally) and the spiral line (medially) constitutes a fourth surface

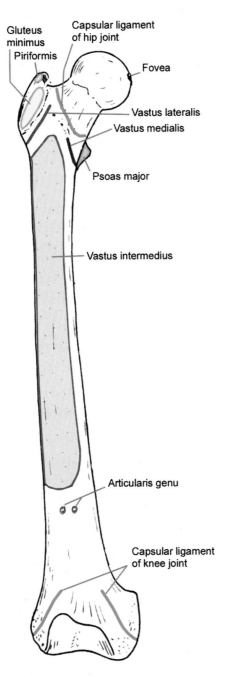

Fig. 27.9. Right femur, showing attachments, seen from the front.

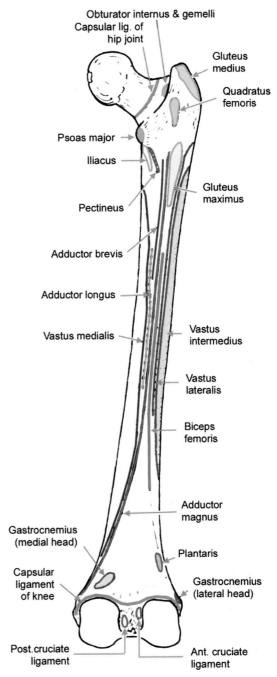

Fig. 27.10. Right femur, showing attachments, seen from behind.

2. The gluteus medius is inserted into the oblique strip running downwards and forwards across the lateral surface of the greater trochanter.

3. The piriformis is inserted into the upper border of the greater trochanter.

4. The obturator internus and gemelli are inserted into the anterior part of the medial surface of the greater trochanter.

5. The obturator externus is inserted into the trochanteric fossa on the medial surface of the greater trochanter.

6. The psoas major is inserted into the medial part of the anterior surface of the lesser trochanter.

7. The iliacus is inserted into the medial side of the base of the lesser trochanter, and into a small area below the latter.

8. The pectineus is inserted along a line descending from the root of the lesser trochanter to the upper end of the linea aspera. The insertion lies between the gluteal tuberosity and the spiral line.

9. The quadratus femoris is inserted on the quadrate tubercle, and into a small area below the latter.

10. The deep fibres of the gluteus maximus are inserted into the gluteal tuberosity.

11. The upper part of the adductor brevis is inserted between the insertions of the pectineus (medially) and the adductor magnus (laterally) (see below). The lower part of the muscle is inserted into the linea aspera.

12. The adductor longus is inserted into the middle one third of the linea aspera.

13. The adductor magnus is inserted into the medial margin of the gluteal tuberosity, the linea aspera, and the medial supracondylar line. The hamstring part of the muscle ends in a tendon which is attached to the adductor tubercle.

B. The muscles taking origin from the femur are as follows.

1. The vastus lateralis has a long linear origin. The line begins at the upper end of the intertrochanteric line, and passes along the anterior and lower borders of the greater trochanter, the lateral margin of the gluteal tuberosity, and the lateral lip of the linea aspera.

2. The vastus medialis also has a long linear origin from the lower part of the intertrochanteric line, the spiral line, the medial lip of the linea aspera, and the medial supracondylar line right up to the adductor tubercle.

3. The vastus intermedius arises from the upper three fourths of the anterior and lateral surfaces of the shaft. The medial surface of the shaft does not give origin to the muscle, but is covered by it.

4. The articularis genu arises from small areas on the anterior surface of the shaft below the origin of the vastus intermedius.

5. The short head of the biceps femoris arises from the linea aspera and from the upper part of the lateral supracondylar line.

6. The medial head of the gastrocnemius arises from the popliteal surface a little above the medial condyle. The lateral head of the muscle arises from the lateral surface of the lateral condyle.

7. The plantaris arises from the lower part of the lateral supracondylar line.

8. The popliteus arises (by a tendon) from the anterior part of the groove on the lateral aspect of the lateral condyle.

C. Other attachments on the femur.

1. The capsular ligament of the hip joint is attached to the neck of the femur most of which is intracapsular. Anteriorly, the capsule is attached to the intertrochanteric line, but posteriorly the capsule is attached about 1cm medial to the intertrochanteric crest.

2. The ligament of the head is attached to the fovea on the head of the femur.

3. The capsular ligament of the knee joint is attached to the femoral condyles and to the posterior margin of the intercondylar fossa.

THE PATELLA

The tendons of some muscles have, embedded in them, small bones that help them to glide over bony surfaces. Such bones are called **sesamoid bones**. The largest sesamoid bone in the body is to be seen in the tendon of the quadriceps femoris as it passes in front of the knee joint. It is called the patella.

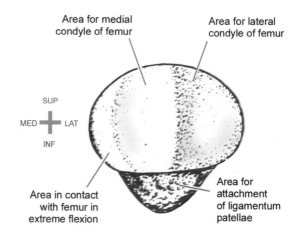

Fig. 27.11. Right patella, posterior aspect.

The patella is shaped somewhat like a disc (Fig. 27.11). It is roughly triangular in outline. It has anterior and posterior surfaces that are separated by three borders: superior, medial, and lateral. The superior border is also called the **base**. The inferior part of the bone shows a downward projection representing the **apex** of the triangle.

The **anterior surface** is rough and can be felt through the overlying skin. The upper part of the **posterior surface** is articular. This part articulates with the patellar surface on the anterior aspect of the condyles of the femur. It consists of a larger lateral part and a smaller medial part, the two parts being separated by a ridge. The lower part of the posterior surface is nonarticular. It is rough for attachment of the ligamentum patellae.

Some Attachments on the Patella

1. The superior border gives attachment to the rectus femoris and to the vastus intermedius.

2. The apex gives attachment to the ligamentum patellae.

THE TIBIA

The tibia is the medial bone of the leg. It has a shaft, an upper end and a lower end (Figs. 27.12, 27.13). The upper end can be distinguished from the lower end as it is much larger. The medial and lateral sides of the bone can be distinguished by examining the lower end: this end has a prominent downward projection, the medial malleolus, on its medial side. The anterior and posterior aspects of the bone can be distinguished by examining the shaft. The shaft is triangular in section and has a sharp anterior border. The side to which a tibia belongs can be determined from the information given above.

The Upper End

The upper end of the tibia consists of two parts called the medial and lateral **condyles** that are separated by an **intercondylar area**. The anterior aspect of the upper end of the tibia is marked by another projection called the **tibial tuberosity**.

The upper surfaces of the medial and lateral condyles bear large, slightly concave, articular surfaces that take part in forming the knee joint (Fig. 27.16). The medial articular surface is oval, and is larger than the lateral surface which is rounded. The articular surfaces are separated by the intercondylar area which is non-articular. The intercondylar area is raised in its central part to form the **intercondylar eminence**. The medial and lateral parts of the eminence are more prominent than its central part and constitute the medial and lateral **intercondylar tubercles**. The medial and lateral condylar articular surfaces extend on to the sides of the intercondylar tubercles.

In addition to its upper surface the medial condyle has rough anterior, medial and posterior surfaces that are distinctly marked off from the shaft by a ridge (Fig. 27.13). The lateral condyle has similar anterior, lateral and posterior surfaces. The posterior surface of the medial condyle is marked by a groove. The posterolateral part of the lateral condyle bears an oval articular facet for the upper end of the fibula. The anterior surfaces of the medial and lateral condyles

merge to form a large rough triangular area. The apex of the triangle is placed inferiorly and is raised to form a large projection called the **tibial tuberosity**. The tuberosity has an upper smooth part and a lower rough part. The lateral margin of the triangle mentioned above has a prominent impression (which is also triangular).

The Shaft

The shaft of the tibia is triangular. It has anterior, medial and lateral (or interosseous) borders; and medial, lateral and posterior surfaces.

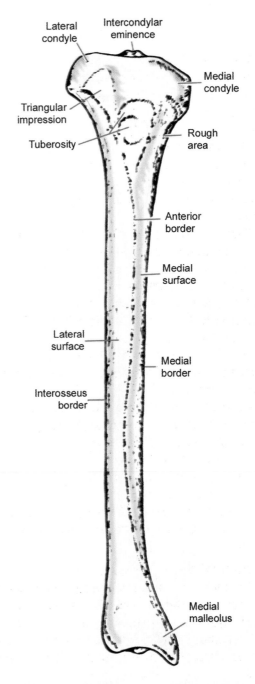

Fig. 27.12. Right tibia, anterior aspect.

The ***anterior border*** runs downwards from the tibial tuberosity. Its lower part turns medially and reaches the anterior margin of the medial malleolus.

The ***interosseous*** or ***lateral border*** begins a little below and in front of the articular facet for the fibula. It descends along the lateral aspect of the shaft. Its lower end forms the anterior margin of a rough triangular area seen on the lateral aspect of the lower end.

The upper end of the ***medial border*** lies below the most medial part of the medial condyle. Its lower end

becomes continuous with the posterior margin of the medial malleolus.

The ***medial surface*** lies between the anterior and medial borders. The upper end of the surface is rough just in front of the medial border. The rest of the surface is smooth and can be felt through the overlying skin.

The ***lateral surface*** lies between the anterior and interosseous borders. Because of the fact that the anterior border turns medially in its lower part, the lateral surface extends on to the anterior aspect of the lower part of the shaft.

The ***posterior surface*** lies between the medial and interosseous borders. Over the upper one third of the shaft this surface is marked by a prominent ridge that runs downwards and medially across it. This ridge is called the soleal line. The part of the posterior surface above the soleal line is triangular. The part below the line is subdivided into medial and lateral parts by a faint vertical ridge.

The Lower End

The lower end of the tibia is much less expanded than the upper end. Its medial part shows a downward projection called the ***medial malleolus***. The posterior aspect of the malleolus is marked by a prominent groove. The lateral aspect of the lower end shows a triangular ***fibular notch*** for articulation with the fibula. It consists of an upper part which is rough and a lower part which is smooth. The inferior surface of the lower end bears an articular area that articulates with the upper surface of the talus to form the ankle joint. The area is continuous with another articular area on the lateral aspect of the medial malleolus that articulates with the medial side of the talus.

Some Attachments on the Tibia

A. The muscles inserted into the tibia are as follows (Figs. 27.14, 27.15).

1. The pull of the quadriceps femoris is transmitted to the tibia through the ligamentum patellae which is attached to the smooth upper part of the tuberosity of the tibia.

2. The sartorius, the gracilis, and the semitendinosus are inserted on the upper part of the medial surface. The area for the sartorius is most anterior and that for the semitendinosus is most posterior.

3. The semimembranosus is inserted into the posterior and medial aspects of the medial condyle.

4. The popliteus is inserted into the posterior surface of the shaft, on the triangular area above the soleal line.

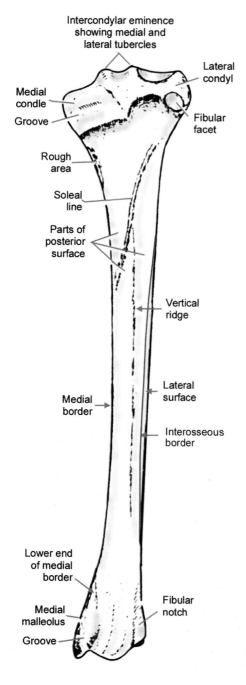

Intercondylar eminence showing medial and lateral tubercles

Lateral condyl

Medial condle

Groove

Fibular facet

Rough area

Soleal line

Parts of posterior surface

Vertical ridge

Lateral surface

Medial border

Interosseous border

Lower end of medial border

Medial malleolus

Groove

Fibular notch

Fig. 27.13. Right tibia. Posterior aspect.

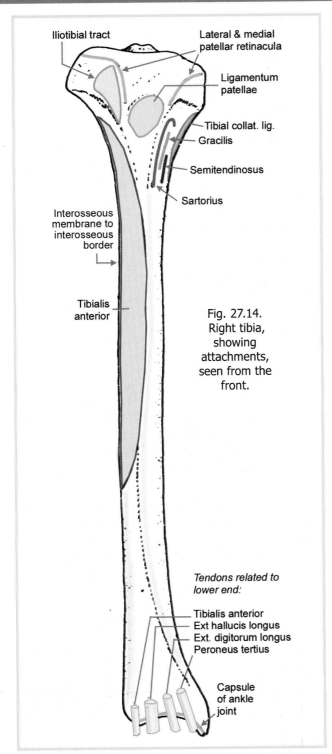

Iliotibial tract

Lateral & medial patellar retinacula

Ligamentum patellae

Tibial collat. lig.

Gracilis

Semitendinosus

Sartorius

Interosseous membrane to interosseous border

Tibialis anterior

Fig. 27.14. Right tibia, showing attachments, seen from the front.

Tendons related to lower end:

Tibialis anterior
Ext hallucis longus
Ext. digitorum longus
Peroneus tertius

Capsule of ankle joint

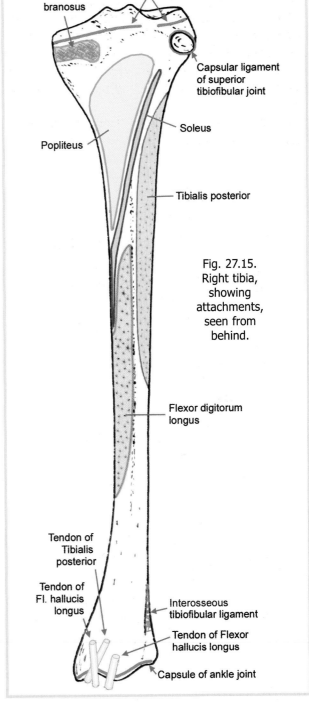

Semimem-branosus

Capsular ligament of knee joint (note gap)

Capsular ligament of superior tibiofibular joint

Popliteus

Soleus

Tibialis posterior

Fig. 27.15. Right tibia, showing attachments, seen from behind.

Flexor digitorum longus

Tendon of Tibialis posterior

Tendon of Fl. hallucis longus

Interosseous tibiofibular ligament

Tendon of Flexor hallucis longus

Capsule of ankle joint

B. The muscles taking origin from the tibia are as follows.

1. The tibialis anterior arises from the upper two thirds of the lateral surface of the shaft.

2. The soleus arises from the soleal line, and from the middle one third of the medial border of the shaft.

3. The tibialis posterior arises from the upper two thirds of the lateral part of the posterior surface of the shaft, below the soleal line.

4. The flexor digitorum longus arises from the medial part of the posterior surface of the shaft below soleal line.

C. Other attachments on the tibia

1. The capsular ligament of the knee joint is attached to the condyles of the tibia a little below the margins of the articular surfaces.

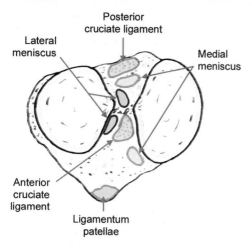

Fig. 27.16. Right tibia, showing attachments, seen from above.

2. The intercondylar area, on the superior aspect of the upper end of the tibia, gives attachment to the medial and lateral menisci and to the cruciate ligaments. For details see Fig. 27.16.

3. The margins of the fibular facet give attachment to the capsule of the superior tibiofibular joint.

4. The interosseous membrane is attached to the interosseous border.

5. The articular capsule of the ankle joint is attached to the margins of the articular surface on the lower end of the bone.

THE FIBULA

The fibula has a **Shaft**, an **upper end** and a **lower end** (Figs. 27.17, 27.18). The upper end is irregularly expanded in all directions. In contrast the lower end is flattened from side to side and forms the **lateral malleolus**. The medial side of the malleolus bears a triangular articular surface (for the talus). Just behind this articular surface the malleolus shows a deep **malleolar fossa**; and this fact enables the anterior and posterior aspects of the bone to be distinguished from one another. The side to which a fibula belongs can be determined with the help of the information given above.

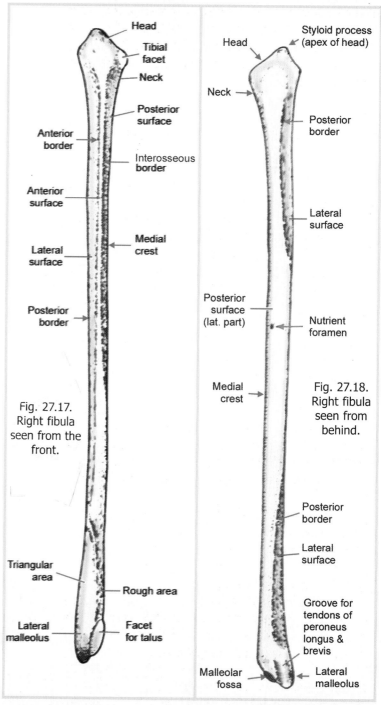

Fig. 27.17. Right fibula seen from the front.

Fig. 27.18. Right fibula seen from behind.

The Upper End

The upper end of the fibula is also called the **head**. Its posterior and lateral part shows an upward projection called the **styloid process**. In front of, and medial to, the styloid process the head shows a circular facet for articulation with the tibia (to form the superior tibiofibular joint). The part of the bone immediately below the head is called the **neck**.

The Lower End

The lower end of the fibula is called the **lateral malleolus**. It has a lateral surface that can be felt through the overlying skin.

The medial surface of the malleolus bears a triangular facet. This facet articulates with the lateral surface of the talus and forms part of the ankle joint. Behind the facet the medial surface of the malleolus shows a deep *malleolar fossa*.

The Shaft

The shaft has three borders: anterior, posterior and interosseous (or medial).

The *anterior border* is sharp (Fig. 27.17). It begins just below the anterior aspect of the head. Near its lower end it turns laterally to join the apex of the triangular area of the shaft already identified above the lateral malleolus. The lowest part of the anterior border forms the posterior margin of the triangle.

The upper end of the *posterior border* lies in line with the styloid process. Its lower end reaches the medial part of the posterior surface of the lateral malleolus.

The *interosseous border* lies very near the anterior border and may be indistinguishable from the latter in the upper part of the shaft. When traced downwards it passes medially and merges with the upper part of the rough area above the talar facet of the lateral malleolus.

The *lateral surface* of the fibula lies between the anterior and posterior borders. The lower part of the lateral surface faces backwards and becomes continuous with the posterior aspect of the lateral malleolus.

The *medial surface* lies between the anterior and interosseous borders. It is very narrow in the upper half of the shaft. Its lower broader part faces forwards and medially. This surface is, therefore, sometimes called the anterior surface.

The *posterior surface* lies between the interosseous and posterior borders. Over its upper three fourths it is divided into two distinct parts, medial and lateral, by a vertical ridge called the *medial crest*.

Attachments on the Fibula

A. The muscles attached to the fibula are as follows (Figs. 27.19, 27.20).

1. The biceps femoris is inserted into the head of the fibula.

2. The narrow medial surface gives origin to the following.

(**a**) The extensor digitorum longus arises from the upper three fourths of this surface.

(**b**) The peroneus tertius arises from an area on the medial surface below that for the extensor digitorum longus.

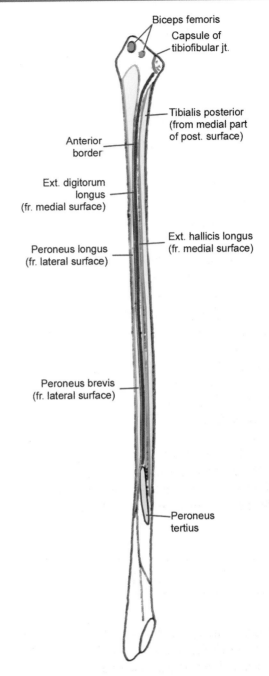

Fig. 27.19. Right fibula, showing attachments, seen from the front.

(**c**) The extensor hallucis longus arises from the middle two fourths of the medial surface, medial to the origin of the extensor digitorum longus.

3. The lateral surface gives origin to the following.

(**a**) The peroneus longus arises from the upper two thirds of the lateral surface. Part of the muscle also arises from the lateral aspect of the head of the fibula. The common peroneal nerve lies between the two areas of origin.

(**b**) The peroneus brevis arises from the lower two thirds of the lateral surface.

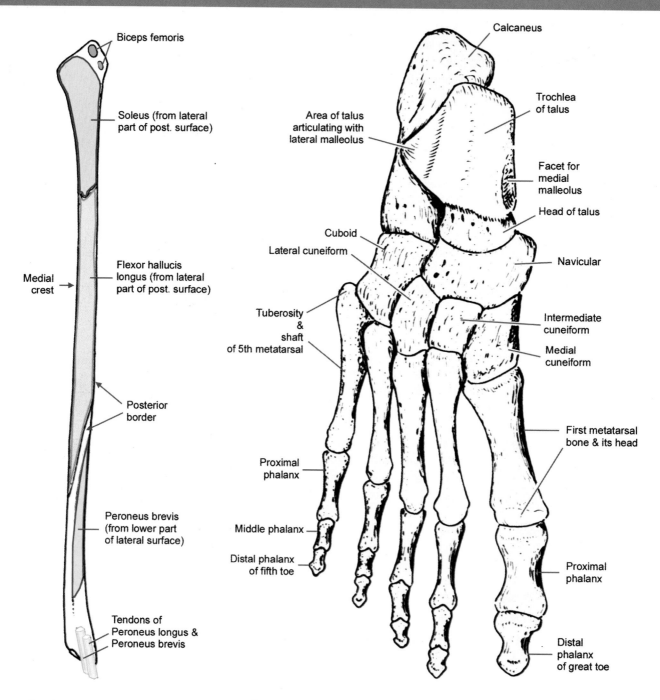

Fig. 27.20. Right fibula , showing attachments, seen from behind.

Fig. 27.21. Skeleton of the foot seen from above (dorsal aspect).

4. The following muscles are attached to the posterior surface.

(**a**) The tibialis posterior arises from the upper two thirds of the medial part of the posterior surface.

(**b**) The soleus arises from the posterior aspect of the head and from the upper one fourth of the lateral part of the posterior surface.

(**c**) The flexor hallucis longus arises from the lower two thirds of the lateral part of the posterior surface.

Some Relations Of The Fibula

1. The common peroneal nerve winds round the lateral aspect of the neck of the fibula.

2. The tendons of the peroneus longus and the peroneus brevis pass downwards just behind the lateral malleolus.

THE SKELETON OF THE FOOT

The skeleton of the foot is seen from above (dorsal aspect) in Fig. 27.21, and from below (plantar aspect) in Fig. 27.22. The posterior half (or so) of the foot is made up of seven *tarsal bones*. The largest tarsal bone is called the *calcaneus*: it is the bone that forms the heel. Placed above the calcaneus there is another large bone called the *talus*. The talus articulates with the lower ends of the tibia and fibula to form the *ankle joint*. Anterior (or distal) to the calcaneus and the talus there are two bones of intermediate size. These are the *navicular bone* placed medially, and the *cuboid bone* placed laterally. Distal to the navicular bone there are three smaller bones. These are the *medial cuneiform*, the *intermediate cuneiform*, and the *lateral cuneiform* bones.

Anterior to the tarsal bones we see five *metatarsal bones*. Distal to the metatarsal bones there are the *phalanges*: three (proximal, middle, distal) for each digit except the great toe which has only two phalanges, proximal and distal.

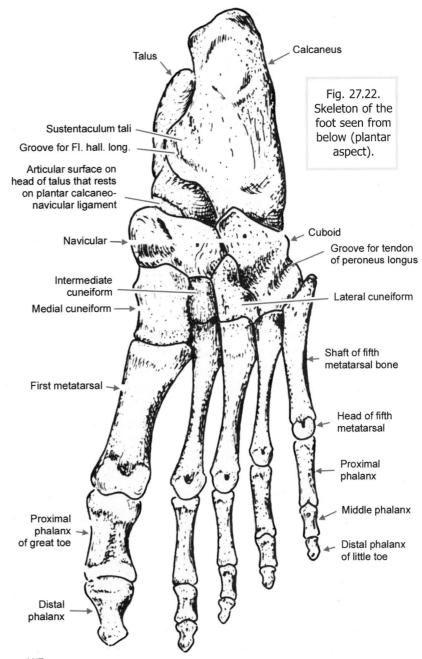

Talus — Calcaneus

Sustentaculum tali
Groove for Fl. hall. long.
Articular surface on head of talus that rests on plantar calcaneo-navicular ligament
Navicular
Intermediate cuneiform
Medial cuneiform
First metatarsal
Proximal phalanx of great toe
Distal phalanx

Cuboid
Groove for tendon of peroneus longus
Lateral cuneiform
Shaft of fifth metatarsal bone
Head of fifth metatarsal
Proximal phalanx
Middle phalanx
Distal phalanx of little toe

Fig. 27.22. Skeleton of the foot seen from below (plantar aspect).

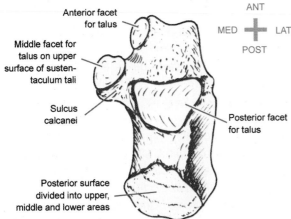

Anterior facet for talus
Middle facet for talus on upper surface of sustentaculum tali
Sulcus calcanei
Posterior surface divided into upper, middle and lower areas

ANT
MED — LAT
POST

Posterior facet for talus

Fig. 27.23. Right calcaneus seen from above.

The Calcaneus

The calcaneus can be correctly orientated, and its side determined using the following information (Fig. 27.23) .

(1) The bone is elongated anteroposteriorly. The anterior aspect is easily distinguished from the posterior as it is covered by a large articular facet, while the posterior aspect is non-articular.

(2) The superior aspect can be distinguished from the inferior as it bears three facets, while the inferior aspect is nonarticular.

(3) The medial aspect can be distinguished from the lateral aspect as it bears a prominent projection.

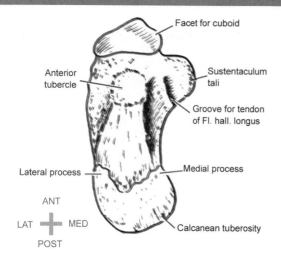

Fig. 27.24. Right calcaneus seen from below.

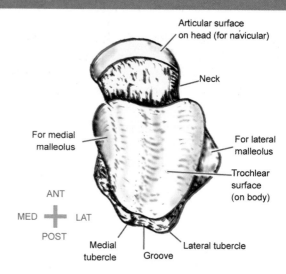

Fig. 27.25. Right talus, seen from above.

Having orientated the bone correctly the following facts can now be appreciated.

The calcaneus has anterior, posterior, superior, inferior, medial and lateral surfaces. The *anterior surface* is fully covered by a large articular facet for the cuboid bone. The *posterior surface* is non-articular. It is divisible into upper, middle and inferior parts. The *lateral surface* is more or less flat. Its anterior part shows a small elevation called the *peroneal trochlea* (or *tubercle*). The *medial surface* is easily distinguished as it bears a large projection called the *sustentaculum tali* that projects medially from its anterior and upper part. The *superior or dorsal surface* bears three facets: anterior, middle and posterior that articulate with corresponding facets on the talus.

The *plantar (or inferior) surface* of the calcaneus shows a prominence in its posterior part called the calcaneal tuberosity. The lateral and medial parts of the tuberosity extend further forwards than its central part and are called the *lateral and medial processes*, respectively, of the tuberosity. The anterior part of the plantar surface shows another elevation called the *anterior tubercle*.

The Talus

The talus can be orientated correctly, and its side determined using the following information (Fig. 27.25).

(**1**). The bone is elongated anteroposteriorly. The anterior end (or head) can be distinguished from the posterior end as it is rounded and has a large convex articular surface.

(**2**). The superior aspect of the bone bears a large pulley shaped surface that is convex upwards. The inferior aspect bears three facets.

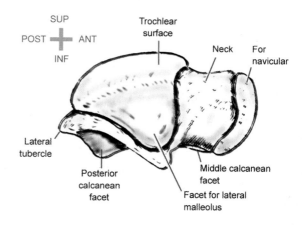

Fig. 27.26. Right talus, seen from the lateral side.

(**3**). The lateral surface bears a large triangular facet, while the medial side shows a 'comma' shaped facet.

The talus has a *head*, a *neck* and a *body*. The distal surface of the head has a large convex surface that articulates with the navicular bone. The upper surface of the body of the talus is covered by a large *trochlear articular surface* which articulates with the lower end of the tibia.

The *lateral surface* bears a large triangular facet for articulation with the lateral malleolus of the fibula, while the *medial surface* bears a 'comma' shaped facet that is broad anteriorly and tapers off posteriorly. This facet articulates with the medial malleolus of the tibia.

The lower and posterior part of the body of the talus projects backwards. This projection is called the *posterior process*. A groove divides this process into *medial and lateral tubercles.*

When the talus is viewed from below we see that the articular area on the head, for the navicular bone, extends on to the inferior aspect of the head.

Behind this there are three facets, anterior middle and posterior, that articulate with corresponding facets on the upper surface of the calcaneus. The middle and posterior facets are separated by a deep groove called the sulcus tali.

The Navicular Bone

The navicular bone articulates proximally with the head of the talus, distally with the three cuneiform bones, and laterally with the cuboid. The medial part of the bone has a projection called the *tuberosity*.

The Cuboid Bone

The cuboid bone articulates proximally with the calcaneus; distally with the fourth and fifth metatarsal bones; and medially with the navicular and lateral cuneiform bones. The lateral and plantar aspects of the bone show a groove that is limited posteriorly by a ridge. The lateral end of this ridge forms a projection called the *tuberosity*.

The Medial Cuneiform Bone

The medial cuneiform bone is the largest of the cuneiform bones.

It can be distinguished by the fact that it bears a large kidney-shaped facet on one side. It articulates proximally with the navicular bone; distally with the first metatarsal bone; and laterally with the intermediate cuneiform and second metatarsal bones.

The Intermediate Cuneiform Bone

The intermediate cuneiform bone is the smallest of the cuneiform bones. It is shaped like a typical wedge. It articulates proximally with the navicular bone, distally with the second metatarsal bone, medially with the medial cuneiform bone, and laterally with the lateral cuneiform bone.

The Lateral Cuneiform Bone

The lateral cuneiform bone articulates proximally with the navicular bone; distally with the third metatarsal bone; medially with the intermediate cuneiform and second metatarsal bones; and laterally with the cuboid and fourth metatarsal bones.

The Metatarsal Bones

The metatarsal bones are five in number (Fig. 27.21). They are numbered from medial to lateral side (in contrast to the metacarpal bones which are numbered from lateral to medial side). The metatarsal bones are similar in structure to the metacarpal bones. Each bone has a distal end or head; a proximal end or base and an intervening shaft. The head is rounded. The base is enlarged and has proximal, dorsal, plantar, medial and lateral surfaces. The shaft is slightly convex on its dorsal side and concave on the plantar side.

The Phalanges of the Foot

The phalanges of the foot are arranged on a pattern similar to that in the hand (Figs. 27.21, 27.22). There are three phalanges in each toe except the great toe: proximal, middle and distal. The great toe has only two phalanges, proximal and distal. The phalanges of the foot are similar in shape to those of the hand, but are much shorter and thinner than the latter.

The skeleton of the foot gives attachment to numerous muscles and ligaments. These will be considered in the sections on muscles and joints.

28

Joints of the Lower Extremity

THE HIP JOINT

This is a synovial joint of the ball and socket variety. The rounded head of the femur fits into the deep cavity provided by the acetabulum of the hip bone. The depth of the acetabulum is increased by the presence of a rim of fibrocartilage called the *acetabular labrum*.

The cavity of the *acetabulum* is partly articular and partly non-articular. The articular surface is shaped like a horse-shoe. The inferior part of the acetabulum is non-articular and is called the *acetabular fossa*. Here the rim of the acetabulum is also deficient the gap being called the *acetabular notch*. A part of the acetabular labrum bridges across the notch as the *transverse ligament of the acetabulum*.

The *head of the femur* is somewhat more than half a sphere. It faces upwards, medially and slightly forwards. Near its centre it is marked by a pit called the *fovea*.

The proximal and distal articular surfaces are joined together by a capsular ligament, and directly by a ligament passing from the head of the femur to the acetabulum. This ligament is called the *ligament of*

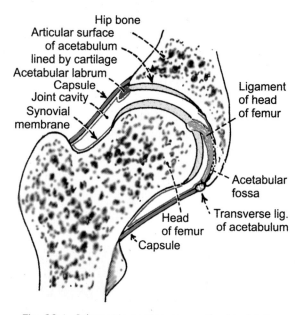

Fig. 28.1. Schematic section across the hip joint.

the head of the femur. It is attached, laterally, to the fovea on the head of the femur, and medially to the two ends of the acetabular notch, and between them to the transverse ligament.

The *capsular ligament* of the hip joint is strong. Medially it is attached to the hip bone around the

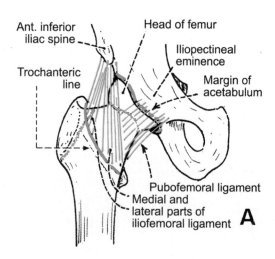

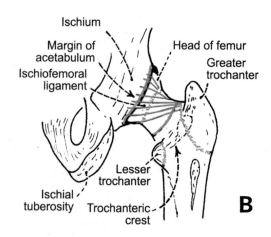

Fig. 28.2. Hip joint. A. Anterior aspect. B. Posterior aspect.

margins of the acetabulum. Laterally, it covers the greater part of the neck of the femur. Anteriorly it is attached to the trochanteric line; posteriorly to the neck of the femur a short distance medial to the trochanteric crest; above to the base of the greater trochanter; and inferiorly to the neck near the lesser trochanter (Fig. 28.2).

The capsule is strengthened by the presence of three ligaments: iliofemoral, pubofemoral and ischiofemoral. The *iliofemoral ligament* is the strongest. It is attached above to the anterior inferior iliac spine (Fig. 28.2A). Inferiorly, its fibres diverge to form two bands, medial and lateral. The medial band runs vertically to be attached to the lower part of the trochanteric line.

The lateral band is attached to the upper part of the same line. Because of its shape it is also called the Y-shaped ligament.

The *pubofemoral ligament* (Fig. 28.2A) is attached above and medially to the iliopectineal eminence and the superior ramus of the pubis. It passes downwards and laterally to blend with the medial band of the iliofemoral ligament and with the capsular ligament.

The *ischiofemoral ligament* (Fig. 28.2B) is attached medially to the ischium just beyond the acetabulum and laterally to the greater trochanter.

The *synovial membrane* of the hip joint is extensive. It lines the inside of the capsular ligament, the intracapsular part of the neck of the femur, both surfaces of the acetabular labrum, the acetabular fossa, and the ligament of the head of the femur (Fig. 28.1).

The hip joint is supplied by branches from the obturator, medial circumflex femoral, superior gluteal and inferior gluteal arteries; by the femoral, obturator and superior gluteal nerves, and by the nerve to the quadratus femoris.

The movements at the hip joint are flexion, extension, abduction, medial rotation and lateral rotation. The muscles responsible for them are shown in Fig. 28.3.

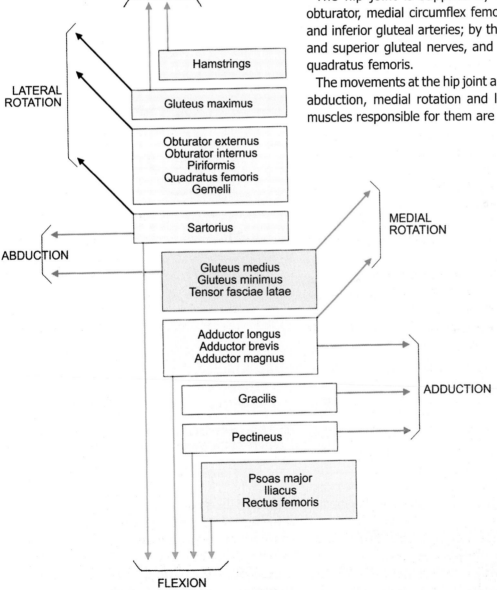

Fig. 28.3. Scheme to show the muscles responsible for movements at the hip joint.

THE KNEE JOINT

The knee joint is a synovial joint of the condylar variety. It is a compound joint having two distinct articular surfaces on the medial and lateral condyles of the femur, for articulation with corresponding surfaces on the medial and lateral condyles of the tibia. The anterior aspect of the lower end of the femur articulates with the posterior aspect of the patella. The knee joint is also complex because its cavity is partially divided into upper and lower parts by plates of cartilage called the medial and lateral menisci.

The ***proximal articular surface*** covers the anterior, inferior and posterior aspects of the medial and lateral condyles of the femur (Fig. 28.4). Anteriorly, the medial and lateral articular surfaces are continuous with each other, but posteriorly they are separated by the intercondylar notch. The part of the femoral articular surface situated on the anterior aspect of its lower end articulates with the patella. It is concave from side to side and is subdivided by a vertical groove into a larger lateral part and a smaller medial part. A small part of the inferior surface of the medial condyle, adjacent to the anterior part of the intercondylar notch comes in contact with the patella in extreme flexion of the joint. The tibial articular surface of each femoral condyle is convex anteroposteriorly, the curvature being much more marked in the posterior part. The condyles are also convex from side to side. The long axis of the lateral condylar articular surface (4) is straight and is placed anteroposteriorly. The axis of the medial condylar surface (5) shows an anteroposterior curve, the convexity of the curve being directed medially.

The ***distal articular surfaces*** of the knee joint are present on the upper surfaces of the medial and lateral condyles of the tibia (Fig. 28.5). These surfaces are slightly concave centrally, and flat at the periphery, where they are covered by the corresponding menisci. The articular surface of the medial condyle is oval. The articular surface of the lateral condyle is almost circular.

The posterior surface of the patella bears a large articular area for the femur. It is convex and is divided by a ridge into a larger lateral part and a smaller medial part.

The attachment of the ***capsule*** of the knee joint is complicated because of the presence of the patella anteriorly, and because of the fact that anteriorly the capsule blends indistinguishably with the lower tendinous part of the quadriceps femoris muscle. To

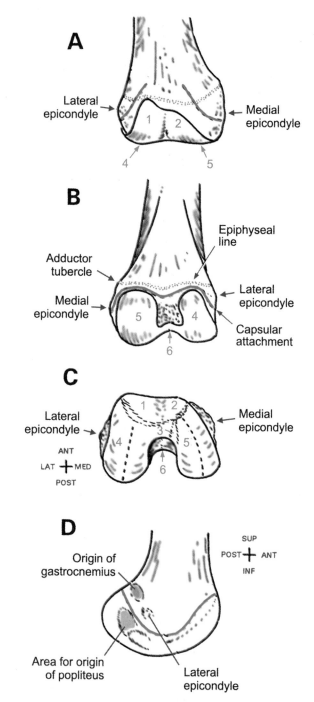

Fig. 28.4. Lower end of femur showing attachments of the capsule of the knee joint (green). Epiphyseal lines are shown in purple. A. Anterior aspect. B. Posterior aspect. C. Inferior aspect. D. Lateral aspect.

understand the attachments on the femur we may begin on the medial side. Here the capsule is attached to the medial and posterior aspects of the condyle just beyond the articular surface (Fig. 28.4A).

Traced laterally the line of attachment passes along the posterior margin of the intercondylar notch to the posterior surface of the lateral condyle (Fig. 28.4B),

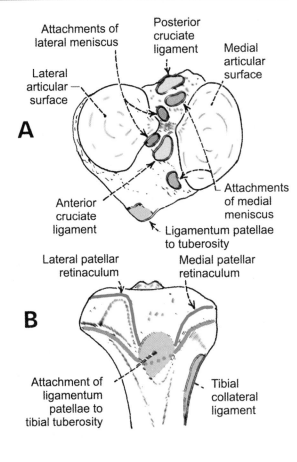

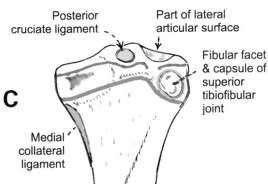

attached to the medial margin of the medial condyle of the tibia. Traced posteriorly the line of attachment passes (in that order) on to the posterior aspect of the medial condyle (Fig. 28.5), the posterior margin of the intercondylar area, the posterior and then the lateral margin of the lateral condyle. There is a gap in the capsular attachment behind the lateral condyle. The popliteus, which arises from within the knee joint, leaves it through this gap. Here the lower margin of the capsule is attached to a band of fibres called the **arcuate popliteal ligament**. This ligament passes from the head of the fibula to the posterior margin of the intercondylar area of the tibia (Fig. 28.16). Anteriorly, the expansions from the vastus medialis and the vastus lateralis gain attachment to the anterior aspect of the medial and lateral condyles of the tibia: here these expansions are called the **medial and lateral patellar retinacula** (Fig. 28.5).

The capsule is strengthened in several situations by ligaments and expansions as follows.

(**a**) Anteriorly, below the patella the capsule is replaced by the **ligamentum patellae**. This ligament is attached above to the non-articular lower part of the posterior surface of the patella and below to the upper smooth part of the tibial tuberosity.

(**b**) On the medial and lateral sides of the joint there are strong collateral ligaments. The **tibial collateral ligament** is attached above to the medial surface of the medial condyle of the femur just below the adductor tubercle (Fig. 28.6). Inferiorly, the deeper fibres of the ligament are attached to the medial condyle of the tibia: they are adherent to the medial meniscus and blend with the capsule. The more superficial fibres of the ligament gain attachment to the upper part of the

Fig. 28.5. Upper end of right tibia to show attachments of the capsule of the knee joint (green). A. Superior asspect. B. Anterior aspect. C. Posterior aspect.

and then to the lateral side of the condyle where it is attached above the origin of the popliteus muscle (Fig. 28.4D). Anteriorly, the capsule merges with expansions from two muscles: the vastus medialis (medially) and the vastus lateralis (laterally). These expansions are attached to the upper, lateral and medial borders of the patella; and below the patella to the medial and lateral sides of the ligamentum patellae.

The inferior attachment of the capsule may also be traced beginning from the medial side (Fig. 28.5). It is

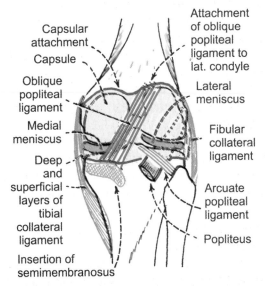

Fig. 28.6. Schematic diagram showing some structures on the posterior aspect of the knee joint.

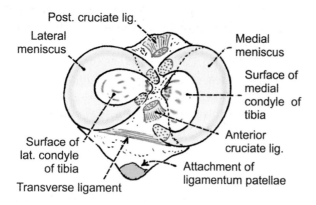

Fig. 28.7. Menisci of the knee joint seen from above after removing the femur.

medial surface of the shaft of the tibia (Figs. 28.6, 28.7). The **fibular collateral ligament** is attached above to the lateral epicondyle of the femur (Fig. 28.4) above the groove for the popliteus. Below it is attached to the head of the fibula. The ligament is separated from the lateral meniscus by the tendon of the popliteus and is, therefore, not adherent to the meniscus.

The posterior aspect of the capsule is strengthened by the **oblique popliteal ligament**. This ligament is an expansion from the tendon of the semimembranosus (Fig. 28.6). It passes upwards and laterally from the posterior aspect of the medial condyle of the tibia to be attached to the femur on the lateral part of the intercondylar line and to the lateral condyle.

Apart from the capsular ligament and its associated ligaments, the femur and tibia are united by two strong ligaments that lie within the joint. These are the anterior and posterior cruciate ligaments (so called because they cross each other). The **anterior cruciate ligament** is attached below to the anterior part of the intercondylar area of the tibia (Figs. 28.5, 28.7). Its upper end is attached to the medial aspect of the lateral condyle of the femur (i.e., on the lateral wall of the intercondylar notch). The **posterior cruciate ligament** is attached below to the posterior part of the intercondylar area of the tibia. Its upper end is attached above to the lateral surface of the medial condyle of the femur.

The **medial and lateral menisci** of the knee joint are intra-articular discs made of fibrocartilage. They have a thick peripheral border and a thin inner border. They intervene between the femoral and tibial condyles (Fig. 28.6). In accordance with the shape of the tibial condyles the lateral meniscus is smaller and its outline more nearly circular than that of the medial meniscus (Fig. 28.7). The anterior and posterior ends of the lateral meniscus are attached to the intercondylar area of the tibia just in front of and behind the intercondylar

eminence (Fig. 28.5A). The anterior end of the medial meniscus is attached to the most anterior part of the intercondylar area of the tibia in front of the anterior cruciate ligament. Its posterior end is attached to the posterior part of the intercondylar area in front of the attachment of the posterior cruciate ligament. The anterior margins of the two menisci are connected by a band of fibres called the transverse ligament (Fig. 28.7). The menisci provide for better adaptation of the articular surfaces of the joint. They participate in gliding movements (see below) and assist in lubrication of the joint.

The **synovial membrane** of the knee joint covers all structures within the joint excepting the articular surfaces and the surfaces of the menisci. It lines the inner side of the tendinous expansion of the quadriceps femoris (that replaces the capsule anteriorly) and some parts of the tibia and femur enclosed within the capsule.

The main **movements** at the knee joint are those of flexion and extension. The tibia and menisci glide forwards relative to the femoral condyles in extension; and backwards in flexion. Further, flexion is associated with lateral rotation of the femur (or medial rotation of the tibia if the foot is off the ground); and extension is associated with medial rotation. The medial rotation of the femur is most marked during the last stages of extension. This rotation **locks** the knee joint in the position of full extension. Locking is produced by continued action of the same muscles that produce extension, namely the quadriceps femoris. When the knee is locked the position of extension can be maintained without much muscular activity. The 'locked' knee can be flexed only after it is unlocked by a reversal of the rotation. Unlocking is brought about by the action of the popliteus muscle.

The muscles responsible for movements of the knee joint are as follows. Flexion is produced mainly by the hamstring muscles. It is assisted by the gastrocnemius, popliteus, sartorius, gracilis and plantaris muscles. Extension is produced by the quadriceps femoris and by the tensor fasciae latae. Muscles producing locking and unlocking of the joint have been mentioned in the preceding paragraph.

The knee joint is supplied by branches of the descending genicular, popliteal, anterior tibial and lateral circumflex arteries; and by branches from the obturator, femoral, tibial and common peroneal nerves.

The knee joint is surrounded by several muscles. The posterior aspect of the joint is related to the popliteal vessels and to the tibial nerve, and more laterally to the common peroneal nerve.

THE ANKLE JOINT

The ankle joint is a synovial joint of the hinge variety. The bones taking part are the lower end of the tibia, the lower end of the fibula, and the upper part of the talus.

Three distinct surfaces on the talus take part in the formation of the joint. The superior or trochlear surface (**a** in Fig. 28.8) is convex from front to back. It is slightly concave from side to side, so that it is like a pulley and hence the name trochlear surface. It comes in contact with a reciprocally shaped surface on the lower end of the tibia (**e** in Fig. 28.9). The medial side of the talus bears a comma-shaped articular surface (**c**). The medial surface articulates with the lateral surface of the medial malleolus of the tibia (**f** in Fig. 28.9). The lateral surface of the talus has a large triangular surface (**b**), the apex of the triangle being directed downwards. It articulates with the medial surface of the lateral malleolus of the fibula (**d** in Fig. 28.9).

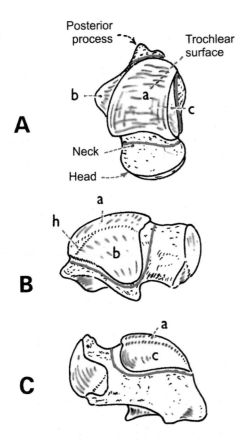

A

B

C

Fig. 28.8. Right talus showing attachments of capsular ligament of ankle joint. A. Superior aspect. B. Lateral aspect. C. Medial aspect.

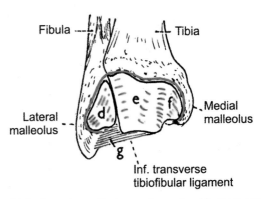

Fig. 28.9. Superior articular surface of ankle joint seen from the anteroinferior aspect.

The **capsular ligament** of the ankle joint is attached just beyond the margins of the articular surfaces. A small part of the neck of the talus is included within the joint cavity. The capsule is strengthened on the medial and lateral side by strong ligaments.

On the lateral side of the ankle there are three distinct bundles that constitute the **lateral ligament** of the joint (Fig. 28.10).

(**a**) The **anterior talofibular ligament** extends from the lateral malleolus to the anterior part of the talus.

(**b**) The **posterior talofibular ligament** passes from the lateral malleolus to the posterior process of the talus.

(**c**) The **calcaneofibular ligament** passes from the lateral malleolus. to the lateral surface of the calcaneus.

The **medial or deltoid ligament** is triangular (Fig. 28.11). Above it is attached to the medial malleolus. Its anterior fibres pass to the navicular bone and form the **tibionavicular ligament**. The middle fibres are attached, below, to the sustentaculum tali of the calcaneus and form the **tibiocalcanean ligament**. The posterior fibres are attached to the posterior part of the talus. They form the **posterior tibiotalar**

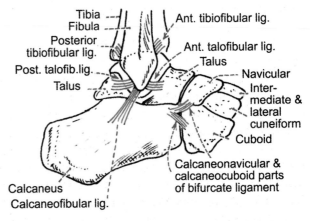

Fig. 28.10. Ligaments on the lateral aspect of the ankle joint.

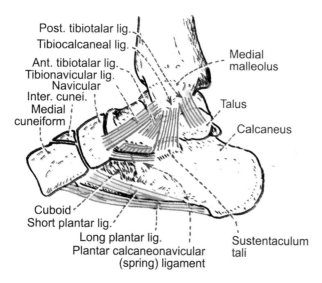

Fig. 28.11. Ligaments on the medial aspect of the ankle joint.

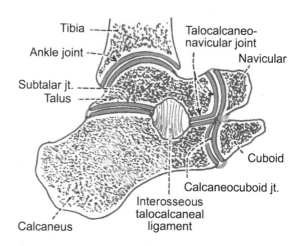

Fig. 28.12. Schematic vertical section along the long axis of the talus, to show the various joints formed by it.

ligament. Deeper fibres attached more anteriorly on the talus form the *anterior tibiotalar ligament*.

The ankle joint is supplied by branches from the anterior tibial and peroneal arteries and from the deep peroneal and tibial nerves.

The movements that take place at the ankle joint are those of plantar flexion and dorsiflexion. The muscles producing these movements are as follows. Dorsiflexion is produced by muscles of the anterior compartment of the leg viz., tibialis anterior, extensor digitorum longus, extensor hallucis longus and peroneus tertius. Plantar flexion is produced mainly by the gastrocnemius and soleus muscles. It is assisted by the plantaris, the tibialis posterior, the flexor hallucis longus and flexor digitorum longus. Note that plantar flexion provides the propulsive force for walking, running and jumping.

INTERTARSAL JOINTS

These will not be considered in detail. The three most important joints between the tarsal bones are:

(**1**) The *subtalar joint* (Fig. 28.12) between the posterior facet on the inferior surface of the talus and on the superior surface of the calcaneus .

(**2**) The *talocalcaneonavicular* joint in which the surface taking part are the head of the talus, which fits into a concavity on the posterior aspect of the navicular bone; and the anterior and middle facets on the inferior aspect of the talus and on the superior aspect of the calcaneus (Fig. 28.12).

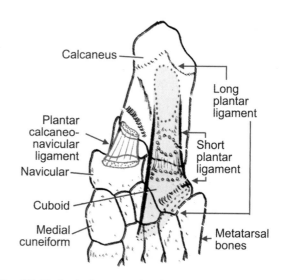

Fig. 28.13. Posterior part of right foot (plantar aspect) to show attachments of some ligaments.

(**3**) The *calcaneocuboid* joint in which reciprocally concavo-convex surfaces on the anterior surface of the calcaneus and the posterior aspect of the cuboid fit each other (Fig. 28.12).

The talocalcaneonavicular and the calcaneocuboid joints lie along the same transverse plane and are collectively referred to as the *transverse tarsal joint*.

Some important ligaments connecting the tarsal bones are as follows.

(**a**) The *long plantar ligament* (Fig. 28.13) is attached posteriorly to the plantar surface of the calcaneus, and anteriorly to the plantar surface of the cuboid bone distal to the groove for the peroneus longus (PL) It converts this groove into tunnel. Some fibres of the ligament are prolonged into the bases of the 2nd, 3rd and 4th metatarsal bones.

(**b**) The *short plantar ligament* (or *plantar calcaneocuboid ligament*) passes from the anterior tubercle of the calcaneus to the cuboid proximal to the groove for the peroneus longus.

(**c**) The ***plantar calcaneonavicular or spring ligament*** passes from the anterior margin of the sustentaculum tali of the calcaneus to the plantar surface of the navicular bone. This ligament is in contact above with the head of the talus and its upper surface forms part of the articular surface of the talocalcaneonavicular joint.

(**d**) The ***bifurcate ligament*** (Fig. 28.10) is Y-shaped. The stem of the Y is attached posteriorly to the anterior part of the upper surface of the calcaneus. Anteriorly it splits into two bands: one passing to the dorsal aspect of the cuboid bone and another to the dorsal aspect of the navicular bone.

(**e**) The ***interosseus talocalcaneal ligament*** lies deep between the talus and the calcaneus. It passes from the sulcus tali to the sulcus calcanei joining the talus and calcaneus in the interval between the subtalar and talocalcaneo-navicular joints (Fig.28.12).

Tibiofibular Joints

The tibia and fibula are joined to each other at the superior and inferior tibiofibular joints. The superior joint is a synovial joint of the plane variety. At the inferior tibiofibular joint the tibia and fibula are united by fibrous tissue(syndesmosis).

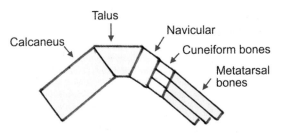

Fig. 28.14. Scheme to show constitution of the medial longitudinal arch of the foot

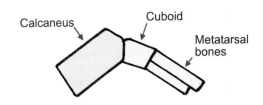

Fig. 28.15. Scheme to show constitution of the lateral longitudinal arch of the foot.

ARCHES OF THE FOOT

The bones of the foot are so arranged that they form a series of arches. There are two longitudinal arches, medial and lateral; and a number of transverse arches.

The ***medial longitudinal arch*** is formed (from posterior to anterior side) by the calcaneus; the talus; the navicular; the medial, intermediate and lateral cuneiform bones; and the medial three metatarsal bones. The arch rests posteriorly on the tubercles of the calcaneus, and anteriorly on the heads of the metatarsals. The summit of the arch is formed by the talus (Fig. 28.14).

The ***lateral longitudinal arch*** is formed by the calcaneus, the cuboid, and the lateral two metatarsal bones (Fig. 28.15). The calcaneus is thus common to both arches.

The ***transverse arches*** are best marked in the middle of the foot. As a result of the transverse arches the medial border of the foot remains off the ground in its middle part. Each foot has only half an arch the complete transverse arch being formed when the feet are placed together.

As a result of the presence of the arches body weight is transmitted to the ground only through the tuberosity of the calcaneus and the heads of the first and fifth metatarsal bones. The presence of the arches confers considerable resilience to the foot and makes it a more efficient lever for propulsion forwards of the body.

The ***factors that help to maintain the arches of the foot*** are:

(**a**) The configuration of the articular surfaces. The talus plays an important role in maintaining the medial longitudinal arch by acting as its key stone.

(**b**) Flattening of the arches is prevented by ligaments, specially those that run longitudinally on the plantar aspect of the foot. These include the long and short plantar ligaments and the plantar calcaneonavicular ligament.

(**c**) The plantar aponeurosis plays an important role by connecting the anterior and posterior ends of the longitudinal arches like a 'tie-beam'.

(**d**) The muscles and tendons running longitudinally on the plantar aspect of the foot have a similar action. The tendons of the tibialis posterior and the peroneus longus together form a sling that holds the longitudinal arches up.

Flattening of the arches is seen in some individuals. It is called ***flat foot***, or ***pes planus***. The reverse condition in which the arches are too marked is also known: it is termed ***pes cavus***.

29

Muscles of the Lower Extremity

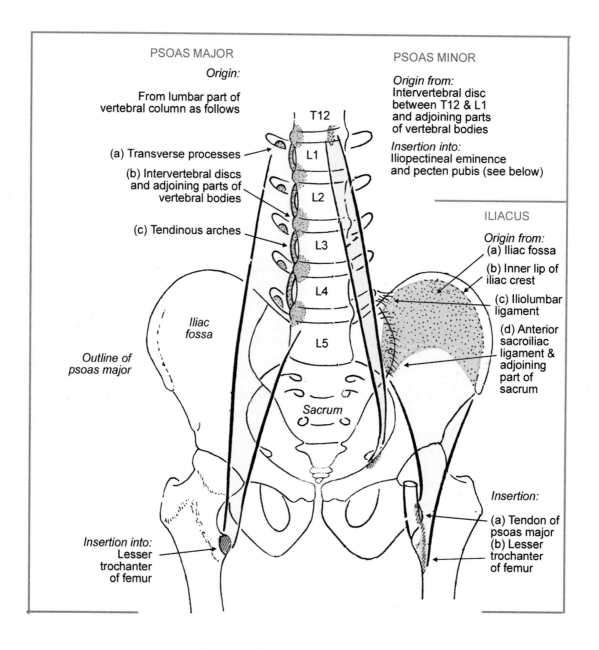

PSOAS MAJOR

Origin:

From lumbar part of vertebral column as follows

(a) Transverse processes

(b) Intervertebral discs and adjoining parts of vertebral bodies

(c) Tendinous arches

Outline of psoas major

Iliac fossa

Insertion into: Lesser trochanter of femur

PSOAS MINOR

Origin from: Intervertebral disc between T12 & L1 and adjoining parts of vertebral bodies

Insertion into: Iliopectineal eminence and pecten pubis (see below)

ILIACUS

Origin from:
(a) Iliac fossa
(b) Inner lip of iliac crest
(c) Iliolumbar ligament
(d) Anterior sacroiliac ligament & adjoining part of sacrum

Insertion:
(a) Tendon of psoas major
(b) Lesser trochanter of femur

T12, L1, L2, L3, L4, L5, Sacrum

Fig. 29.1 Scheme to show the attachments of the psoas major and iliacus. Note the small muscle the psoas minor.

MUSCLES OF THE FRONT OF THE THIGH

Psoas Major

The greater part of this muscle lies in the abdomen and pelvis. Its lower end enters the thigh (Fig. 29.1).

Origin:

(a) Through 5 slips attached to transverse processes and bodies of lumbar vertebrae; and to intervertebral discs.

(b) Through tendinous arches that run vertically along the sides of upper four lumbar vertebrae.

Insertion:

Into lesser trochanter of femur.

Nerve Supply:

By branches from ventral rami of spinal nerves L1, L2 and L3.

Actions:

1. Flexion of the thigh at the hip joint.

2. Flexion of the lumbar part of the vertebral column (as in sitting up from supine position).

Iliacus

Origin:

The iliacus arises from (Fig. 29.1):

1. Iliac fossa

2. Inner lip of the iliac crest.

3. Iliolumbar ligament.

4. Anterior sacro-iliac ligament.

5. Lateral part of upper surface of sacrum.

Insertion:

The iliacus is inserted into:

1. The tendon of psoas major.

2. Lesser trochanter of the femur.

Nerve Supply:

By the femoral nerve.

Actions:

1. Flexion of thigh.

2. Flexion of lumbar part of vertebral column.

Tensor Fasciae Latae (Fig. 29.2)

Origin:

1. Anterior part of the outer lip of the iliac crest, and

2. Outer aspect of the anterior superior iliac spine.

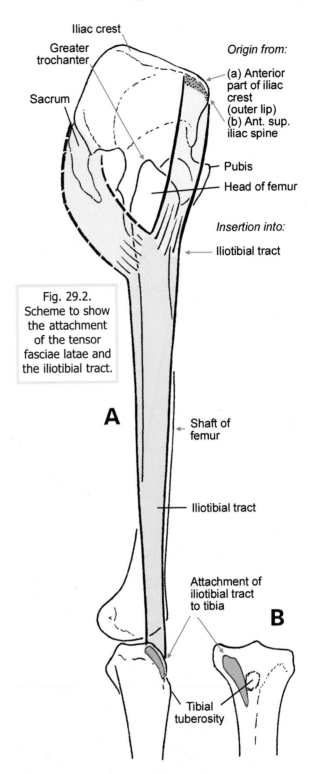

Fig. 29.2. Scheme to show the attachment of the tensor fasciae latae and the iliotibial tract.

Insertion:

Into the upper end of the iliotibial tract. The pull of the muscle is transmitted through this tract to the lateral condyle of the tibia. The attachment to the tibia is on a triangular area on the front of the lateral condyle.

Nerve Supply:

Branch from the superior gluteal nerve.

Actions:

1. It helps to maintain the erect posture (a) by stabilizing the pelvis on the head of the femur, and (b) by stabilizing the femur on the tibia.

2. It helps to extend the leg.

3. It helps in medial rotation of the thigh.

Sartorius

Origin:

The sartorius arises from the anterior superior iliac spine (Fig. 29.3).

Insertion:

It is inserted on the tibia along a vertical line on the upper part of the medial surface. The insertion is anterior to that of the gracilis and of the semitendinosus.

Note

1. The medial border of the upper part of the sartorius forms the lateral boundary of the femoral triangle (Fig. 29.11).

2. In the middle one third of the thigh the muscle forms the roof of the adductor canal (Fig. 29.12).

Nerve Supply: Femoral nerve.

Actions:

The sartorius helps in:

1. Flexion of the leg (at knee joint).

2. Flexion of thigh (at hip joint).

3. Abduction of thigh.

4. Lateral rotation of thigh.

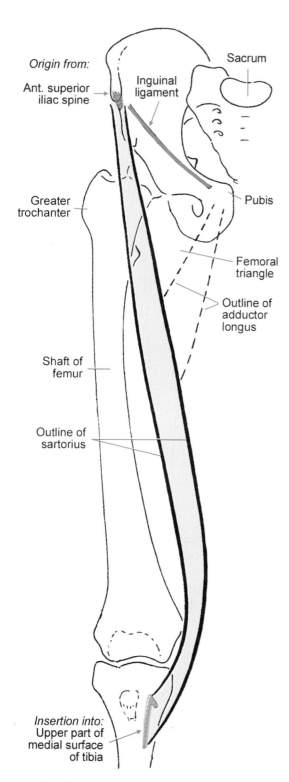

Fig. 29.3. Scheme to show the attachments of the sartorius.

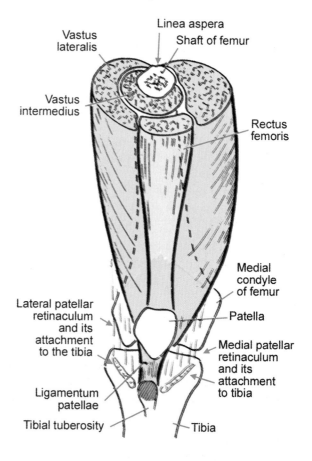

Fig. 29.4. Scheme to show the arrangement of the parts of the quadriceps femoris.

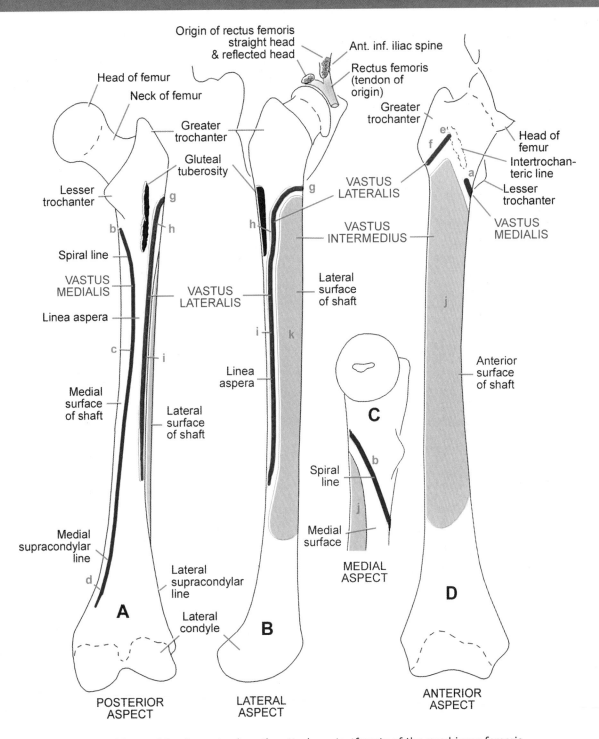

Fig. 29.5. Views of the femur to show the attachments of parts of the quadriceps femoris.

Quadriceps Femoris

This muscle consists of four parts (Figs. 29.4, 29.5). These are the *rectus femoris*, the *vastus lateralis*, the *vastus medialis,* and the *vastus intermedius.*

Origin:

The *rectus femoris* has a tendinous origin from the hip bone. It arises by two heads. The straight head arises from the anterior inferior iliac spine. The reflected head arises from the ilium just above the acetabulum.

The *vastus medialis* has a long linear origin from the following:

1. The lower part of intertrochanteric line.
2. The spiral line
3. The medial lip of the linea aspera.
4. The medial supracondylar line.

The *vastus intermedius* arises from a large area extending onto the following:

1. Anterior surface of shaft.

2. Lateral surface of shaft.

The *vastus lateralis* has a long linear origin from the following:

1. The upper end of the intertrochanteric line.
2. The anterior border of the greater trochanter.
3. The lower border of the greater trochanter.
4. The lateral margin of the gluteal tuberosity.
5. The lateral lip of the linea aspera.

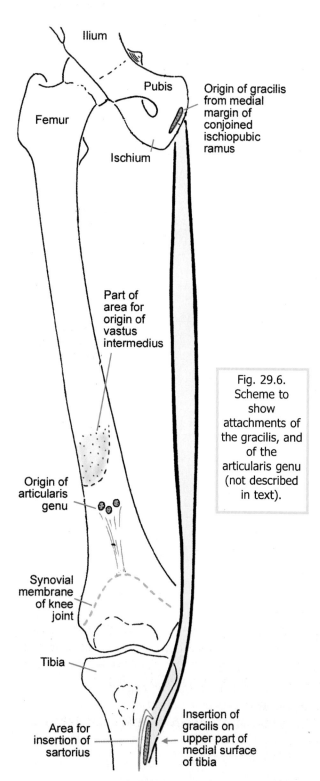

Fig. 29.6. Scheme to show attachments of the gracilis, and of the articularis genu (not described in text).

Insertion:

The *vastus lateralis* is inserted into (Fig. 29.4):
(1) the lateral border of the patella, and
(2) through the lateral patellar retinaculum into the lateral condyle of the tibia.

The *vastus medialis* is inserted into the medial border of the patella, and through the medial patellar retinaculum into the medial condyle of the tibia.

The *rectus femoris* is inserted into the upper border of the patella.

The *vastus intermedius* is also inserted into the upper border of the patella, but deep to the rectus femoris.

The pull of the quadriceps femoris is transmitted to the tibia through the ligamentum patellae.

Nerve Supply:
Femoral nerve.

Actions:

The muscle straightens the lower extremity at the knee (as in standing up from a sitting position). This involves extension of both the leg and the thigh (at the knee and hip joints).

The rectus femoris can produce flexion of the thigh (at the hip). With the thigh fixed (as in standing) it can rotate the pelvis forwards on the head of the femur.

The vastus medialis prevents lateral displacement of the patella during extension of the knee.

Note: The muscle is not active while standing upright because the knee is locked when the knee is fully extended.

MUSCLES OF MEDIAL SIDE OF THIGH

Gracilis (Fig. 29.6):

Origin:
Medial margin of pubic arch. The area of origin includes parts of
1. Body of the pubis.
2. Inferior ramus of pubis.
3. Ramus of ischium.

Insertion:
The gracilis is inserted into the upper part of the medial surface of the tibia (behind the insertion of the sartorius).

Nerve Supply:
Obturator nerve.

Actions:

The gracilis helps in:

1. Flexion of the leg (at the knee joint).

2. Medial rotation of thigh (at the hip joint)

3. Adduction of the thigh.

Pectineus (Fig. 29.7)

Origin:

The pectineus takes origin from the superior ramus of the pubis (pecten pubis and part of the pectineal surface).

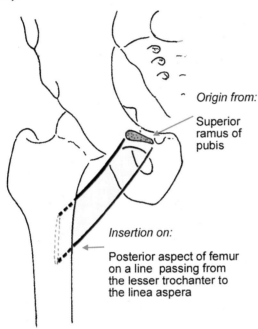

Origin from:

Superior
ramus of
pubis

Insertion on:

Posterior aspect of femur
on a line passing from
the lesser trochanter to
the linea aspera

Fig. 29.7. Scheme to show the attachments
of the pectineus.

Insertion:

The pectineus is inserted on the ***posterior*** aspect of the femur on a line passing from the lesser trochanter to the linea aspera.

Nerve Supply:

The muscle has a double nerve supply by branches from:

1. The femoral nerve.

2. The accessory obturator or the (main) obturator nerve.

Actions:

The muscle is an adductor and flexor of the thigh.

Adductor Longus (Fig. 29.8)

Origin:

Front of the body of the pubis.

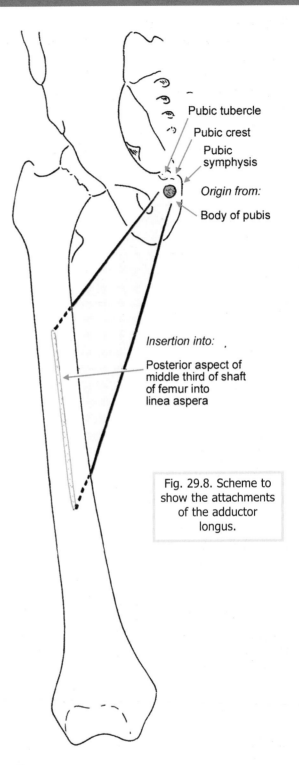

Pubic tubercle
Pubic crest
Pubic
symphysis

Origin from:

Body of pubis

Insertion into:

Posterior aspect of
middle third of shaft
of femur into
linea aspera

Fig. 29.8. Scheme to
show the attachments
of the adductor
longus.

Insertion:

Posterior aspect of the middle one third of the shaft of the femur. The insertion is into the linea aspera between that of the vastus medialis (medially), and of the adductor brevis magnus (laterally).

Nerve Supply:

This is through the anterior division of the obturator nerve.

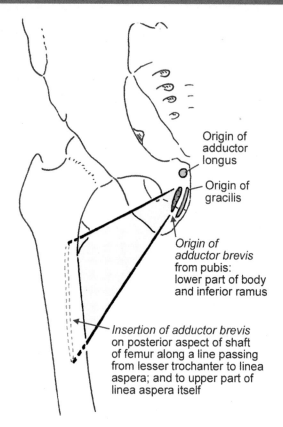

Origin of adductor longus

Origin of gracilis

Origin of adductor brevis from pubis: lower part of body and inferior ramus

Insertion of adductor brevis on posterior aspect of shaft of femur along a line passing from lesser trochanter to linea aspera; and to upper part of linea aspera itself

Fig. 29.9. Scheme to show the attachments of the adductor brevis.

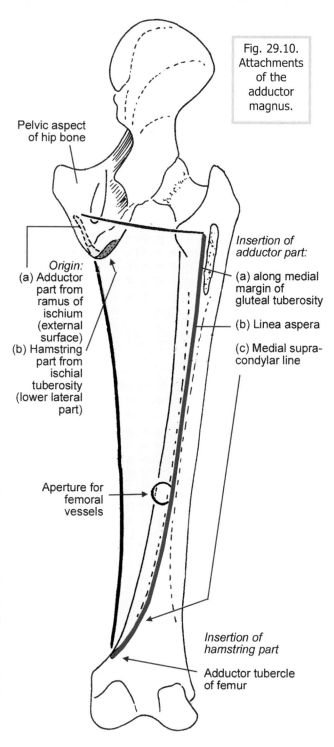

Fig. 29.10. Attachments of the adductor magnus.

Pelvic aspect of hip bone

Origin:
(a) Adductor part from ramus of ischium (external surface)
(b) Hamstring part from ischial tuberosity (lower lateral part)

Insertion of adductor part:
(a) along medial margin of gluteal tuberosity
(b) Linea aspera
(c) Medial supra-condylar line

Aperture for femoral vessels

Insertion of hamstring part

Adductor tubercle of femur

Actions:

The adductor longus helps in adduction and flexion of the thigh.

Adductor Brevis

Origin:

From the pubis: the area of origin includes the lower part of the body and the inferior ramus. The origin is lateral to that of the gracilis and below that of the adductor longus (Fig. 29.9).

Insertion:

Posterior aspect of the femur (i) along a line passing from the lesser trochanter to the linea aspera, and (ii) the upper part of the linea aspera itself.

Nerve Supply:

Obturator nerve.

Actions:

Adduction and flexion of the thigh.

Adductor Magnus

This muscle has an *adductor* part and a *hamstring* part (Fig. 19.10). Each part has its own origin, insertion and nerve supply. (The hamstring part belongs to the back of the thigh, but is considered here for completeness).

Origin:

(a) The **adductor part** arises from the ramus of ischium.

(b) The **hamstring part** arises from the inferior and lateral part of the ischial tuberosity.

Insertion:

(a) The ***adductor part*** is inserted along the medial margin of the gluteal tuberosity; into the linea aspera; and into the medial supracondylar line.

(b) The ***hamstring part*** is inserted (through a tendon) into the adductor tubercle (on medial condyle of the femur).

Actions:

Adduction of the thigh. The hamstring part of the muscle may produce extension of the thigh.

Note:

Near the insertion of the muscle there are a series of apertures for passage of blood vessels. The largest (and lowest) of these is for the femoral vessels. The others are for the profunda femoris and perforating arteries.

Nerve Supply:

The ***adductor part*** is supplied by the obturator nerve, and the ***hamstring part*** by the sciatic nerve (tibial part).

Femoral triangle

The region on the front of thigh medial to the upper part of the sartorius is called the femoral triangle. The region is of importance as it contains several vessels and nerves.

The ***boundaries*** of the triangle are as follows (Fig. 29.11). The ***upper boundary*** or ***base*** of the triangle is formed by the inguinal ligament. The triangle is bounded ***laterally***, by the <u>medial</u> margin of the sartorius; and medially, by the <u>medial</u> margin of the adductor longus. The apex of the triangle, directed inferiorly, lies where the medial and lateral borders meet.

The ***floor*** of the triangle is formed (from lateral to medial side) by the iliacus, the psoas major, the pectineus and the adductor longus. The ***roof*** of the triangle is formed by the fasciae over the region, and superficial structures within them. These include the saphenous opening, the cribriform fascia, the terminal part of the saphenous vein, and the superficial inguinal lymph nodes.

The main contents of the femoral triangle are as follows.

(1) Running down the middle of the femoral triangle we see the ***femoral artery***.

(2) Medial to the artery we see the ***femoral vein***.

(3) A short distance lateral to the artery we see the trunk of the ***femoral nerve***.

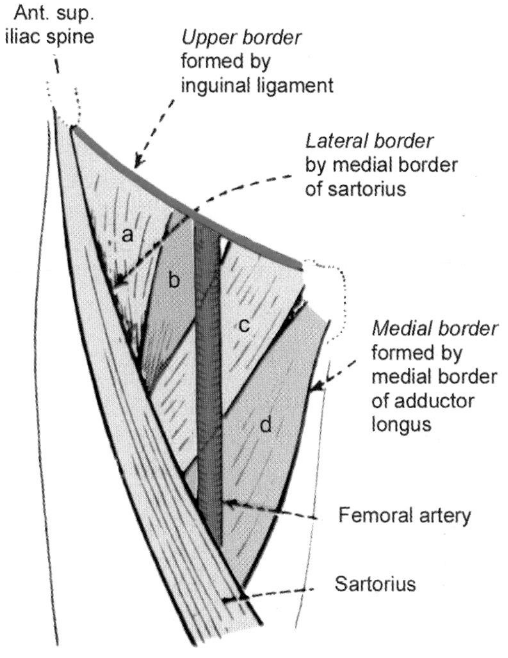

Adductor canal

The adductor canal is a space deep to the sartorius, over the middle one third of the thigh. For obvious reasons it is also called the ***subsartorial canal***. The boundaries of the canal can be visualized by examining a transverse section (Fig. 29.12). The canal is bounded ***anteriorly*** by the vastus medialis; ***posteriorly***, by the adductor longus (above) and the adductor magnus (below); and ***medially***, by a strong fibrous membrane lying deep to the sartorius.

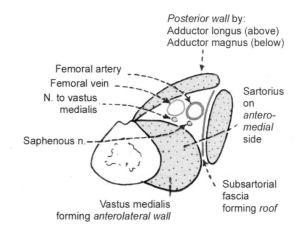

Fig. 29.12. Boundaries and contents of the adductor canal.

Fig. 29.11. Boundaries of the femoral triangle.

MUSCLES OF GLUTEAL REGION

Gluteus Maximus

Origin:

The gluteus maximus arises from one large area that extends onto the following (Fig. 29.13):

1. External surface of the ilium including the posterior gluteal line and the area behind it.

2. The sacrotuberous ligament.

3. The aponeurosis covering the erector spinae.

4. The lower lateral part of the posterior surface of the sacrum.

5. The lateral part of the posterior surface of the coccyx.

Insertion:

1. Most fibres of the muscle are inserted into the iliotibial tract.

2. Some deeper fibres are inserted into the gluteal tuberosity of the femur.

Nerve Supply:

Inferior gluteal nerve (L5, S1, S2).

Actions:

A. ***Acting from its origin*** the gluteus maximus produces ***extension*** of the thigh (as in standing up from a sitting position, climbing, or jumping). It also causes lateral rotation of the thigh.

B. ***Acting from its insertion*** (when the femur and tibia are fixed as in standing) the muscle can:

(a) straighten the trunk, after stooping, by rotating the pelvis backwards on the head of the femur; and

(b) maintain the upright position of the trunk by preventing the pelvis from rotating forwards on the head of the femur under the influence of gravity.

C. Through the ilio-tibial tract it steadies the femur on the tibia in standing.

Through a combination of all the actions described above it helps to maintain the upright position.

Gluteus Medius

Origin:

The gluteus medius arises from the outer surface of the ilium (Fig. 29.14). The area of origin is bounded above by the iliac crest (IC), behind by the posterior gluteal line (PGL), and in front by the anterior gluteal line (AGL).

Insertion:

It is inserted into the lateral surface of the greater trochanter of the femur. The insertion is on a ridge that runs downwards and forwards.

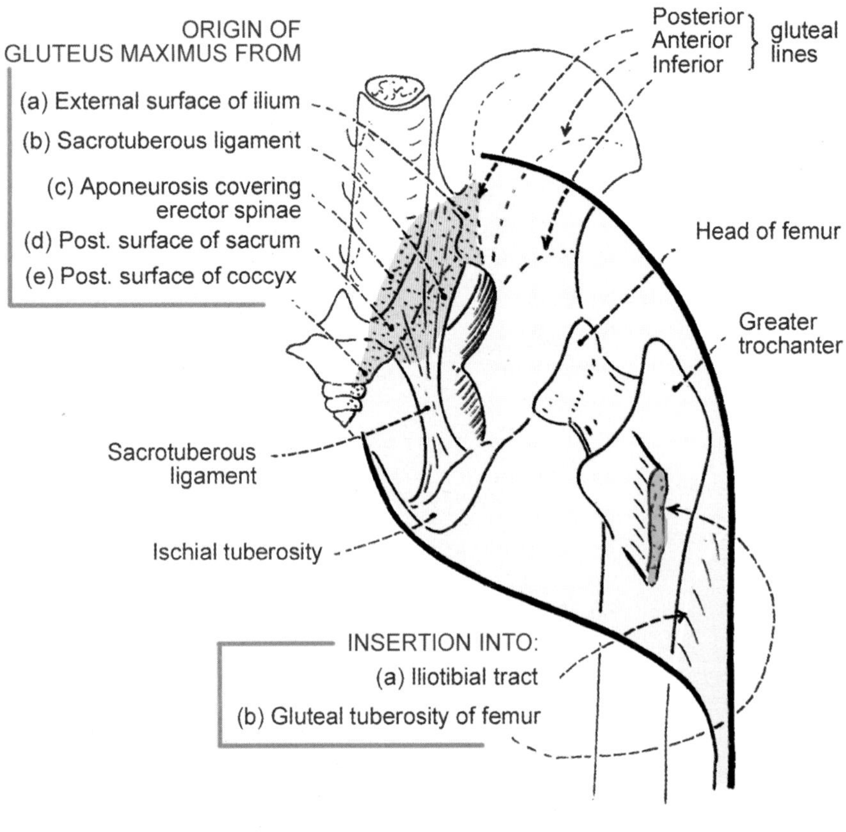

Nerve Supply of Gluteus Medius and Minimus

Both the gluteus medius and minimus are supplied by the superior gluteal nerve (L5, S1).

Actions of Gluteus Medius and Minimus:

Both the gluteus medius and minimus are abductors of the thigh. The minimus and the anterior fibres of the medius can act as flexors and medial rotators, whereas the posterior fibres of the medius can act as extensors and lateral rotators of the thigh.

With the femur fixed (as in standing) the medius and minimus pull the corresponding side of the pelvis downwards by rotating it over the head of the femur. As a result the opposite side of the pelvis is raised. In this way the muscles of one side prevent the opposite side of the pelvis from sinking downwards when the limb of that side is off

ORIGIN OF
GLUTEUS MAXIMUS FROM

(a) External surface of ilium
(b) Sacrotuberous ligament
(c) Aponeurosis covering erector spinae
(d) Post. surface of sacrum
(e) Post. surface of coccyx

Posterior
Anterior } gluteal
Inferior } lines

Head of femur

Greater trochanter

Sacrotuberous ligament

Ischial tuberosity

INSERTION INTO:
(a) Iliotibial tract
(b) Gluteal tuberosity of femur

Fig. 29.13. Scheme to show the attachments of the gluteus maximus.

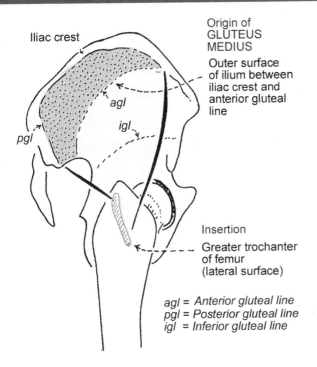

Fig. 29.14. Scheme to show attachments of the gluteus medius. The hip bone and femur are viewed from the lateral side.

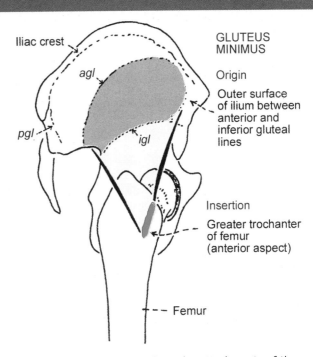

Fig. 29.15. Scheme to show the attachments of the gluteus minimus. The hip bone and femur are viewed from the lateral side.

the ground. In fact the pelvis on the unsupported side is somewhat higher than on the supported side. In paralysis of the medius and minimus the unsupported side becomes lower than the supported side. This is referred to as the **_Trendelenberg sign._**

Gluteus Minimus

Origin:
The gluteus minimus arises from the outer surface of the ilium between the anterior and inferior gluteal lines (IGL) (Fig. 29.15).

Insertion:
It is inserted on a ridge on the anterior aspect of the greater trochanter of the femur.

Nerve supply and action:
See under gluteus medius.

Piriformis

The muscle arises **_within_** the pelvis. It leaves the pelvis through the greater sciatic foramen to reach the gluteal region (Fig. 29.16).

Origin:
The piriformis arises from the lateral part of the **_anterior_** (or pelvic) aspect of the sacrum.

Insertion:
The muscle is inserted into the upper border of the greater trochanter of the femur.

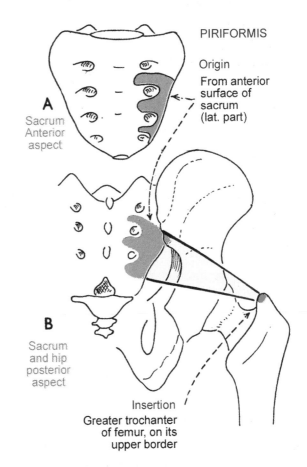

Fig. 29.16. A. Sacrum seen from the front to show the origin of the piriformis. B. Scheme to show the attachments of the piriformis. The pelvis and femur are viewed from behind.

Nerve supply:

The muscle is innervated by direct branches from L5, S1, S2.

Action:

The piriformis is a lateral rotator of the femur.

Obturator Internus

Origin:

This muscle arises from (Fig. 29.17):

(1) Inner (pelvic) surface of the hip bone. The areas of the hip bone include the body, the superior ramus, and the inferior ramus of the pubis; ramus and body of the ischium; and part of the pelvic surface of the ilium.

(2) The pelvic surface of the obturator membrane.

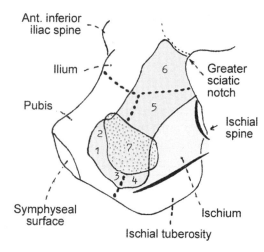

Fig. 29.17. Anterior part of hip bone seen from behind to show the origin of the obturator internus.

The fibres of the muscle converge towards a tendon which leaves the pelvis through the lesser sciatic foramen to enter the gluteal region. The tendon turns through 90 degrees and runs laterally behind the hip joint to reach its insertion.

Insertion:

The tendon is inserted into the anterior part of the medial surface of the greater trochanter of the femur. The insertion is above and in front of the trochanteric fossa.

Nerve supply:

The muscle is supplied by the nerve to obturator internus (L5, S1).

Actions:

The muscle is a lateral rotator of the femur.

Gemelli

These are two small muscles situated in the gluteal region, above and below the tendon of the obturator internus.

Origin:

The **superior gemellus** arises from the posterior aspect of the ischial spine.

The **inferior gemellus** takes origin from the uppermost part of the ischial tuberosity.

Insertion:

The gemelli are inserted into the tendon of the obturator internus (and exert their pull through it on the greater trochanter of the femur).

Nerve supply: The superior gemellus is supplied by the nerve to the obturator internus (L5, S1). The inferior gemellus is supplied by a branch from the nerve to the quadratus femoris (L5, S1).

Action: The gemelli help in lateral rotation of the femur.

Quadratus Femoris

Origin:

The quadratus femoris takes origin from the lateral border of the ischial tuberosity (Fig. 29.18).

Insertion:

It is inserted into the quadrate tubercle. This is a bony elevation present on the upper part of the trochanteric crest of the femur.

Nerve supply:

The nerve to the quadratus femoris is a branch from the sacral plexus (L4, L5, S1).

Action:

The quadratus femoris is a lateral rotator of the femur.

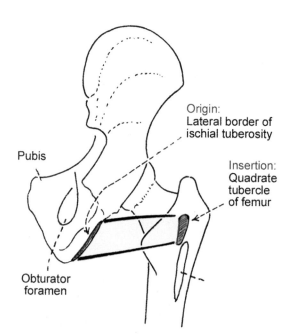

Fig. 29.18. Scheme to show attachments of the quadratus femoris.

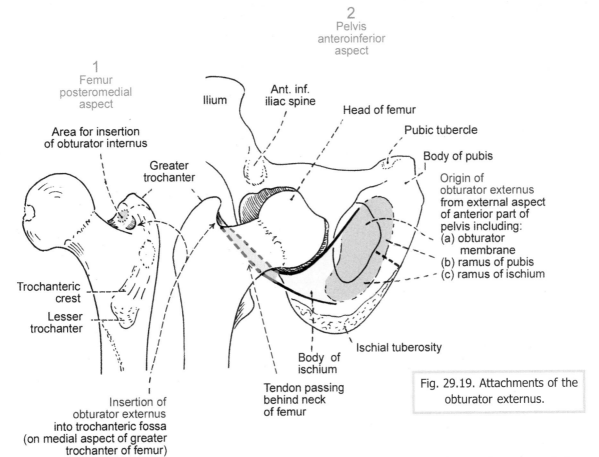

1
Femur
posteromedial
aspect

2
Pelvis
anteroinferior
aspect

Ilium

Ant. inf.
iliac spine

Head of femur

Pubic tubercle

Area for insertion
of obturator internus

Body of pubis

Greater
trochanter

Origin of
obturator externus
from external aspect
of anterior part of
pelvis including:
(a) obturator
     membrane
(b) ramus of pubis
(c) ramus of ischium

Trochanteric
crest

Lesser
trochanter

Ischial tuberosity

Body of
ischium

Tendon passing
behind neck
of femur

Insertion of
obturator externus
into trochanteric fossa
(on medial aspect of greater
trochanter of femur)

Fig. 29.19. Attachments of the
obturator externus.

Obturator Externus

Origin:

The obturator externus takes origin from the external surface of the anterior part of the pelvis. The area of origin covers parts of the following (Fig. 29.19):
(a) Ramus of ischium.
(b) Ramus of pubis.
(c) Obturator membrane (medial two thirds).
The muscle ends in a tendon that runs upwards and laterally behind the neck of the femur to reach the gluteal region.

Insertion:

The tendon is inserted into the trochanteric fossa (situated on the medial aspect of the greater trochanter) of the femur.

Nerve supply:

The muscle is supplied by a branch from the obturator nerve (L3, L4).

Actions:

It is a lateral rotator of the femur.

Note on actions of Small Muscles around the Hip Joint

Although the various small muscles related to the hip joint are described as medial or lateral rotators, their main action is to stabilize the joint.

MUSCLES OF BACK OF THIGH

Semitendinosus

The muscle is so called because its lower half is tendinous. It belongs to the hamstring group of muscles.

Origin:

The semitendinosus arises from the upper and medial part of the ischial tuberosity, in common with the biceps femoris (Fig.29.20).

Insertion:

Into upper part of medial surface of shaft of tibia. The area of insertion is behind that of the sartorius, and below and behind that for the gracilis.

Nerve supply:

Tibial part of sciatic nerve.

Actions (common to all hamstring muscles):

1. Acting from their origin (i.e., when the pelvis is fixed) the hamstring muscles flex the leg at the knee joint.

2. Acting from their insertion (i.e., when the knee is fixed, as in standing upright) they exert a downward pull on the ischial tuberosity. This is useful (a) in preventing the pelvis from rolling forwards on the head of the femur, and (b) in straightening the trunk after bending forwards.

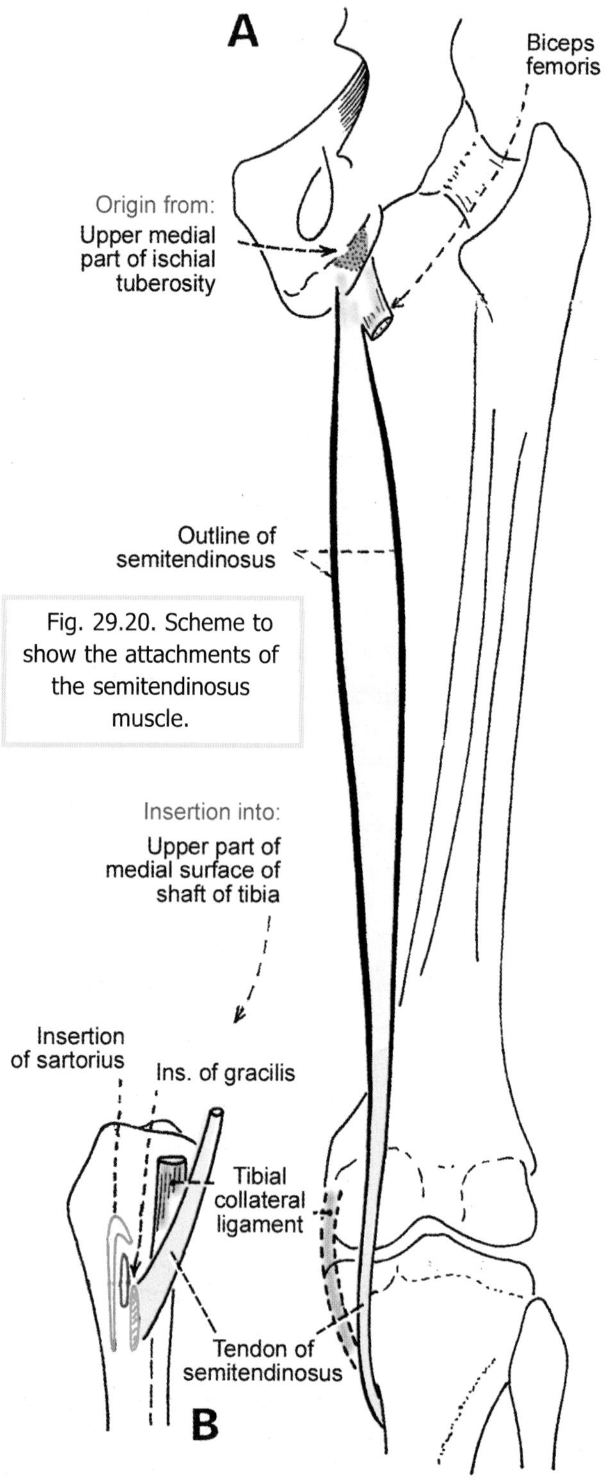

Semimembranosus

This is a muscle of the hamstring group (Fig. 29.21). The muscle is so called because its upper part is membranous.

Origin:
From upper lateral part of ischial tuberosity.

Insertion:
The muscle end in a tendon which is inserted into the medial condyle of the tibia.

Nerve supply:
Branch from tibial part of sciatic nerve.

Actions:
See under semitendinosus.

Biceps Femoris

Origin:
The muscle has two heads (Fig. 29.22).

(a) The **long head** arises from the upper medial part of the ischial tuberosity.

(b) The **short head** arises from the linea aspera of the femur (between the insertion of the adductor magnus, medially; and the origin of the vastus lateralis laterally.

Insertion:
The two heads end in a common tendon which is inserted into the head of the fibula.

Nerve supply:
By branches from the sciatic nerve (L5, S1, S2). The long head is supplied by the tibial part of the nerve and the short head by the peroneal part.

Actions:
See under semitendinosus.

Fig. 29.20. Scheme to show the attachments of the semitendinosus muscle.

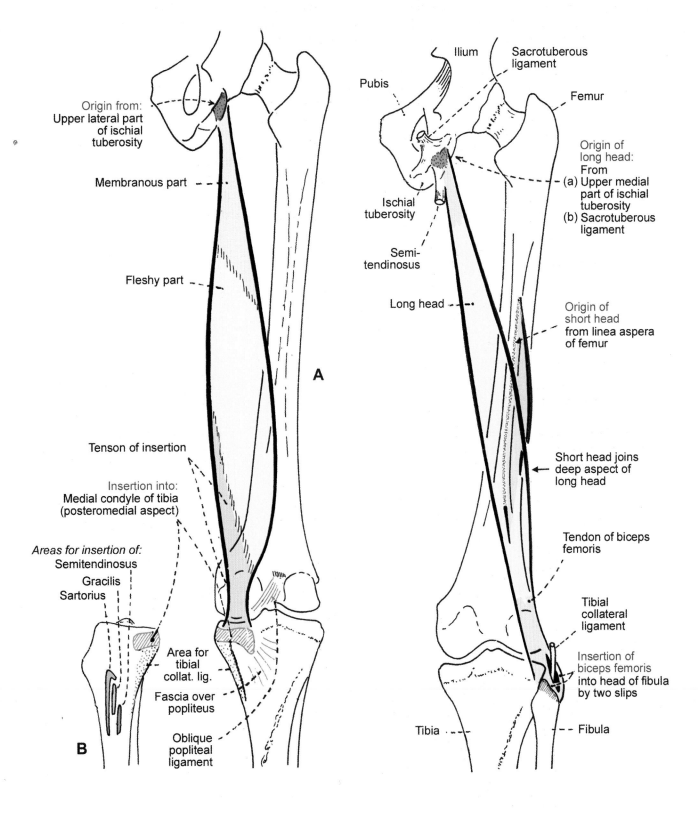

Origin from:
Upper lateral part
of ischial
tuberosity

Membranous part

Fleshy part

A

Tenson of insertion

Insertion into:
Medial condyle of tibia
(posteromedial aspect)

Areas for insertion of:
Semitendinosus
Gracilis
Sartorius

Area for
tibial
collat. lig.

Fascia over
popliteus

Oblique
popliteal
ligament

B

Ilium

Sacrotuberous
ligament

Pubis

Femur

Origin of
long head:
From
(a) Upper medial
part of ischial
tuberosity
(b) Sacrotuberous
ligament

Ischial
tuberosity

Semi-
tendinosus

Long head

Origin of
short head
from linea aspera
of femur

Short head joins
deep aspect of
long head

Tendon of biceps
femoris

Tibial
collateral
ligament

Insertion of
biceps femoris
into head of fibula
by two slips

Tibia

Fibula

Fig.29.21. Attachments of semimembranosus muscle.

Fig. 29.22. Attachments of biceps femoris muscle.

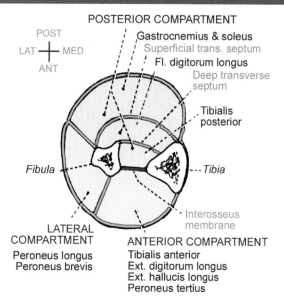

Fig. 29.23. Intermuscula septa and compartments of the leg.

Compartments of the leg

The leg is divided into anterior, lateral and posterior compartments by intermuscular septa (Fig. 29.23). These septa may be regarded as extensions of deep fascia.

The **anterior intermuscular septum** passes from deep fascia to the anterior border of the fibula. It separates the anterior and lateral compartments. The **posterior intermuscular septum** passes from deep fascia to the posterior border of the fibula. It separates the lateral and posterior compartments. The anterior and posterior compartments are separated from each other by the interosseous membrane (that stretches between the interosseous borders of the tibia and fibula). The posterior compartment of the leg is divided into superficial, middle and deep parts by **superficial and deep transverse septa**.

MUSCLES OF ANTERIOR COMPARTMENT OF LEG

Tibialis Anterior

Origin:

The muscle takes origin as follows (Fig. 29.24):

(a) The main origin is from the lateral surface of the shaft of the tibia (upper half to two thirds). The upper end of this area extends on to the lateral condyle.

(b) The muscle also arises from the adjoining part of the interosseous membrane.

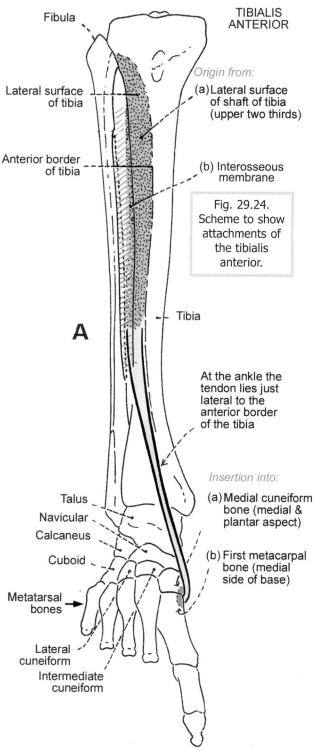

Fig. 29.24. Scheme to show attachments of the tibialis anterior.

The muscle ends in a tendon that runs across the front of the ankle.

Insertion:

The muscle is inserted into; **(a)** the medial cuneiform bone (medial and plantar aspect), and **(b)** the first metatarsal bone (medial side of base).

Nerve supply:

Deep peroneal nerve (L4, L5).

Actions:

The tibialis anterior takes part in:

(a) Dorsiflexion of the foot.

(b) Inversion of the foot.

(c) Helping to maintain the arches of the foot.

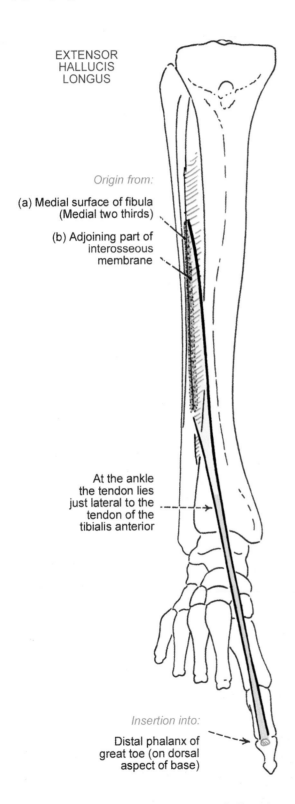

EXTENSOR
HALLUCIS
LONGUS

Origin from:

(a) Medial surface of fibula
(Medial two thirds)

(b) Adjoining part of
interosseous
membrane

At the ankle
the tendon lies
just lateral to the
tendon of the
tibialis anterior

Insertion into:

Distal phalanx of
great toe (on dorsal
aspect of base)

Fig. 29.25. Attachments of the extensor hallucis longus.

Extensor Hallucis Longus

Origin:

This muscle arises from the middle two-fourths of the medial surface of the fibula, and from the adjoining part of the interosseous membrane (Fig. 29.25).

The muscle ends in a tendon which runs downwards across the ankle.

Insertion:

Dorsal aspect of the base of the distal phalanx of the great toe.

Nerve supply :

The muscle is supplied by a branch from the deep peroneal nerve (L5, S1).

Actions:

(a) It extends the phalanges of the great toe.

(b) Continued action helps to dorsiflex the foot.

Extensor Digitorum Longus

Origin:

1. From the upper three-fourths of medial surface of the fibula (Fig. 29.26).

2. Interosseous membrane.

3. The uppermost part of the origin extends on to the lateral condyle of the tibia.

At the ankle the tendon passes deep to the extensor retinacula (Fig. 29.29) and then divides into four slips, one each for the 2nd, 3rd, 4th and 5th digits. The tendons for the 2nd, 3rd and 4th digits are joined (on their lateral sides) by a tendon of the extensor digitorum brevis (Figs. 29.26, 29.27).

Insertion:

The insertion is like that of the extensor digitorum in the hand. Over the proximal phalanx. the tendon (for that digit) divides into three slips: one intermediate, and two collateral. The intermediate slip is inserted into the base of the middle phalanx. The two collateral slips reunite over the middle phalanx and are inserted into the base of the distal phalanx.

Over the proximal phalanx the tendon is expanded into a triangular ***dorsal digital expansion***, which receives the insertions of interosseous and lumbrical muscles.

Nerve supply: Deep peroneal nerve (L5, S1).

Actions: The muscle helps in extension of the toes, and in dorsiflexion of the foot.

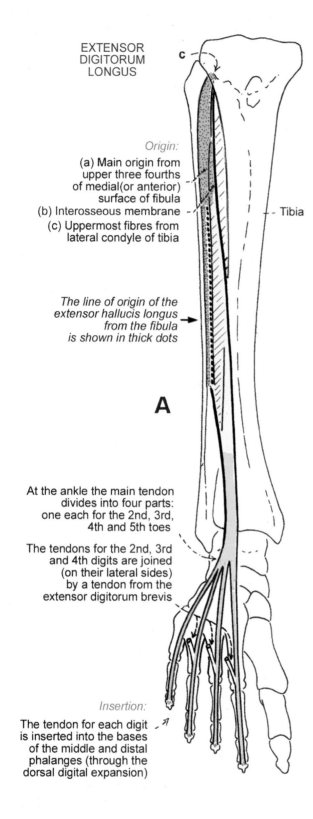

EXTENSOR DIGITORUM LONGUS

Origin:
(a) Main origin from upper three fourths of medial (or anterior) surface of fibula
(b) Interosseous membrane
(c) Uppermost fibres from lateral condyle of tibia

Tibia

The line of origin of the extensor hallucis longus from the fibula is shown in thick dots

A

At the ankle the main tendon divides into four parts: one each for the 2nd, 3rd, 4th and 5th toes

The tendons for the 2nd, 3rd and 4th digits are joined (on their lateral sides) by a tendon from the extensor digitorum brevis

Insertion:
The tendon for each digit is inserted into the bases of the middle and distal phalanges (through the dorsal digital expansion)

Fig. 29.26. Attachments of the extensor digitorum longus.

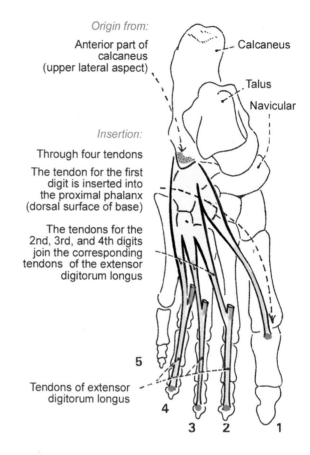

Origin from:
Anterior part of calcaneus (upper lateral aspect)

Calcaneus

Talus

Navicular

Insertion:
Through four tendons

The tendon for the first digit is inserted into the proximal phalanx (dorsal surface of base)

The tendons for the 2nd, 3rd, and 4th digits join the corresponding tendons of the extensor digitorum longus

5

Tendons of extensor digitorum longus

4

3   2   1

Fig. 29.27. Scheme to show attachments of extensor digitorum brevis.

Extensor Digitorum Brevis (Fig. 29.27)

Origin:
From anterior part of calcaneus.

Insertion:
The muscle ends in four tendons that pass to the first, second, third and fourth digits.

The tendons for the second, third and fourth digits end by joining the corresponding tendons of the extensor digitorum longus. The part of the muscle that gives origin to the tendon for the first digit is called the extensor hallucis brevis. Its tendon is inserted into the dorsal surface of the base of the proximal phalanx of the great toe.

Nerve supply:
Deep peroneal nerve (S1, 52).

Action:
The muscle helps the extensor digitorum longus to extend the phalanges of the foot. The extensor hallucis brevis extends the proximal phalanx of the great toe.

Peroneus Tertius

This muscle may be regarded as the lower separated part of the extensor digitorum longus

Origin:

The peroneus tertius arises from the medial (or anterior) surface of the shaft of the fibula, and from the adjoining part of the interosseous membrane below the level of the origin of the extensor digitorum longus.

Insertion:

The tendon is inserted into the fifth metatarsal bone, on the dorsal surface of its base.

Nerve supply: Deep peroneal nerve (L5, S1).

Actions: Dorsiflexion and eversion of the foot.

EXTENSOR AND PERONEAL RETINACULA

Extensor retinacula

The **superior extensor retinaculum** is attached **(a)** medially to the anterior border of the tibia, and **(b)** laterally to the anterior aspect of the fibula (Fig. 29.28).

The **inferior extensor retinaculum** is shaped like the letter 'Y' placed on its side; the stem of the 'Y' is directed laterally and the two limbs pass medially.

The stem of the 'Y' is attached to the upper surface of the calcaneus. The upper limb of the 'Y' is attached to the medial malleolus.

The lower limb of the 'Y' winds round the medial side of the foot to become continuous with the plantar aponeurosis,

Tendons passing under cover of extensor retinacula

The tendons passing under cover of the extensor retinacula are (from medial to lateral side (Fig. 29.29) those of the tibialis anterior, the extensor hallucis longus, the extensor digitorum longus, and the peroneus tertius,

As they pass under the retinacula the extensor tendons are surrounded by synovial sheaths. There is one sheath each for the tibialis anterior and for the extensor hallucis. The extensor digitorum and the peroneus tertius have a common sheath.

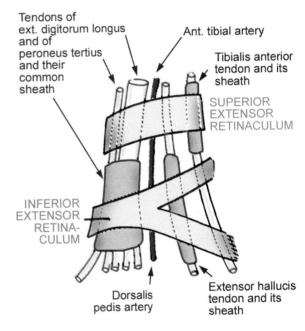

Fig. 29.29. Synovial sheaths of tendons on the front of the ankle and their relationship to the extensor retinacula.

Peroneal retinacula

The peroneal retinacula (Fig. 29.30) are present on the lateral aspect of the ankle. They keep the peroneal tendons (see below) in place.

The **superior peroneal retinaculum** is attached above to the lateral malleolus and below to the lateral surface of the calcaneus.

The **inferior peroneal retinaculum** is attached below to the lateral surface of the calcaneus. Above it becomes continuous with the inferior extensor retinaculum.

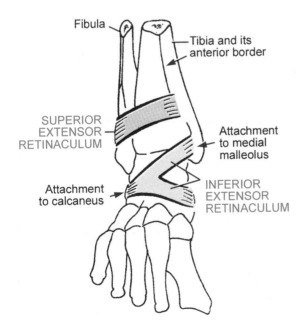

Fig. 29.28. Attachments of superior and inferior extensor retinacula.

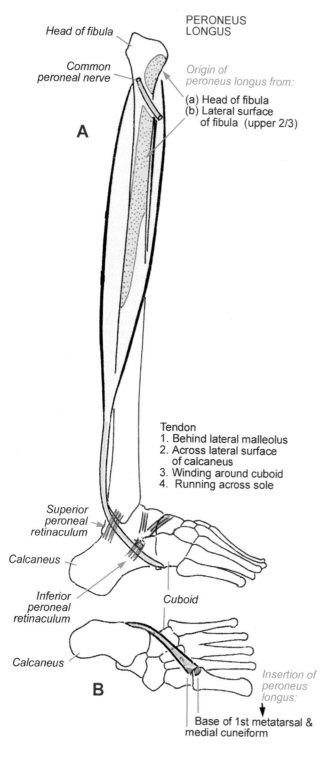

Head of fibula

Common
peroneal nerve

PERONEUS
LONGUS

A

Origin of
peroneus longus from:

(a) Head of fibula
(b) Lateral surface
of fibula (upper 2/3)

Tendon
1. Behind lateral malleolus
2. Across lateral surface
of calcaneus
3. Winding around cuboid
4. Running across sole

Superior
peroneal
retinaculum

Calcaneus

Inferior
peroneal
retinaculum

Calcaneus

B

Cuboid

Insertion of
peroneus
longus:

↓

Base of 1st metatarsal &
medial cuneiform

Fig. 29.30. Attachments of peroneus longus as seen from
the lateral side (a), and from below (b).

MUSCLES OF LATERAL COMPARTMENT OF LEG

Peroneus Longus (Fig. 29.30)

Origin:
  (a) Head of fibula, and
  (b) upper two-thirds of lateral surface of fibula. There is a gap between these two areas of origin: the common peroneal nerve passes through this gap.
  The muscle ends in a tendon which behind the lateral malleolus; here it is covered by the superior peroneal retinaculum. The tendon then runs along the lateral aspect of the calcaneus and then winds round the lateral side of the cuboid bone.

Insertion:
  Finally, the tendon runs medially across the sole to reach its insertion into **(a)** the lateral side of the base of the first metatarsal bone, and **(b)** the lateral side of the medial cuneiform bone.

Nerve supply:
  Superficial peroneal nerve (L5, S1, 52).

Actions:
  The muscle helps in:
  (a) Eversion of the foot.
  (b) Steadying the leg on the foot in standing.
  (c) Maintaining the arches of the foot (both longitudinal and transverse).

Peroneus Brevis

Origin:
  The muscle arises from the lower two thirds of the lateral surface of the shaft of the fibula (Fig. 29.31).
  At the ankle the tendon passes behind the lateral malleolus and then runs forwards on the lateral surface of the calcaneus.

Insertion:
  Lateral side of the base of the fifth metatarsal bone.

Nerve supply:
  Superficial peroneal nerve (L5, S1, S2).

Actions:
  I. Eversion of the foot.
  2. It helps to steady the foot on the leg.

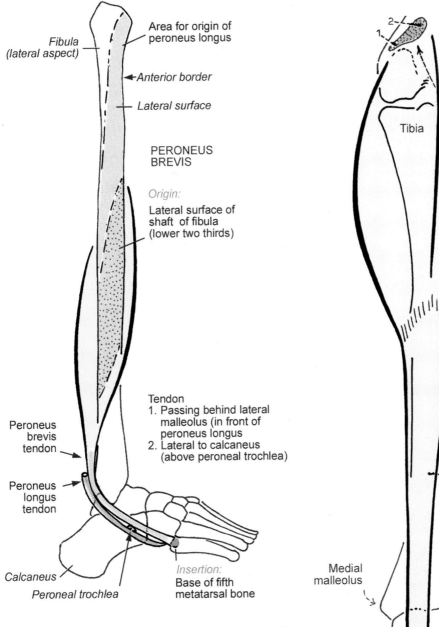

Fig. 29.31. Attachments of peroneus brevis (lateral view).

Synovial sheath of peroneal tendons

As the tendons of the peroneus longus and brevis run downwards and forwards lateral to the ankle, they are held in place by the superior and inferior peroneal retinacula. They are enclosed in a synovial sheath which is common to the two tendons.

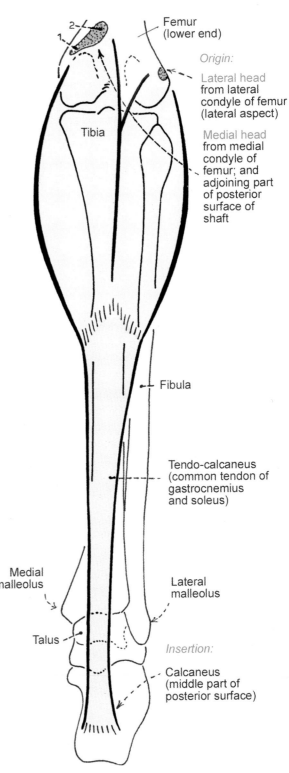

Fig. 29.32. Scheme to show the attachments of the gastrocnemius

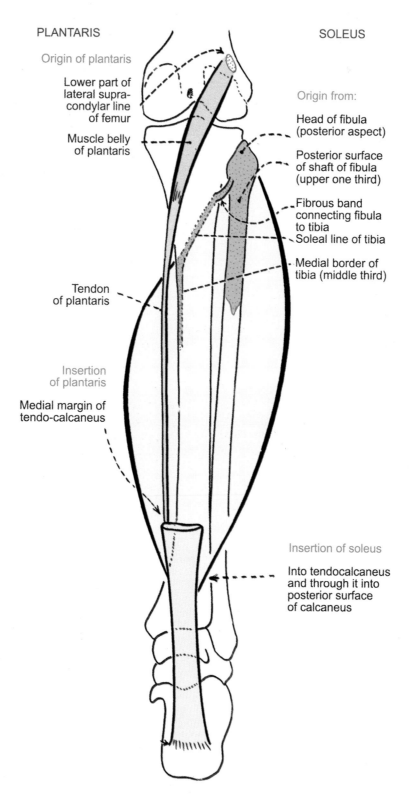

PLANTARIS

SOLEUS

Origin of plantaris

Lower part of
lateral supra-
condylar line
of femur

Muscle belly
of plantaris

Origin from:

Head of fibula
(posterior aspect)

Posterior surface
of shaft of fibula
(upper one third)

Fibrous band
connecting fibula
to tibia

Soleal line of tibia

Medial border of
tibia (middle third)

Tendon
of plantaris

Insertion
of plantaris

Medial margin of
tendo-calcaneus

Insertion of soleus

Into tendocalcaneus
and through it into
posterior surface
of calcaneus

Fig. 29.33. Scheme showing attachments of the soleus
and of the plantaris.

MUSCLES OF THE BACK OF THE LEG

Gastrocnemius

Origin:

The gastrocnemius arises from the femur by two heads (Fig. 29.32).

The ***medial head*** arises from the posterior aspect of the medial condyle (1), and from the adjoining part of the posterior surface (2). The ***lateral head*** arises from the lateral surface of the lateral condyle.

Insertion:

The ***tendocalcaneus*** is the common tendon of insertion of both the gastrocnemius and the soleus. It is the strongest tendon in the body. It is attached below to the middle of the posterior surface of the calcaneus.

Nerve supply: Tibial nerve (S1, S2).

Actions of gastrocnemius and soleus:

These are as follows:

(1) These muscles are strong plantar flexors of the foot. This movement provides the propelling force in walking, running or jumping.

(2) As the upper part of the muscle crosses the knee joint, it helps in flexion of that joint.

Notes:

(1) The gastrocnemius and the soleus are together called the ***triceps surae***.

(2) The uppermost parts of the medial and lateral heads of the gastrocnemius form the boundaries of the lower part of the popliteal fossa.

Plantaris

This is a small muscle lying deep to the gastrocnemius (Fig. 29.33).

Origin:

From lower part of lateral supracondylar line of femur.

Insertion:

Into the tendo-calcaneus.

Nerve supply: Tibial nerve (S1, S2).

Actions:

Because of its small size it is of little functional importance.

Soleus

This muscle lies deep to the gastrocnemius.

Origin:

It arises from the following (Fig. 29.33):

1. The posterior aspect of the head of the fibula.

2. The upper one fourth of the posterior surface of the fibula.

3. A fibrous band stretching from the head of the fibula to the tibia.

4. The soleal line of the tibia.

5. The middle one third of the medial border of the tibia.

Insertion:

Into tendocalcaneus and through it onto the posterior surface of the calcaneus.

Nerve supply: Tibial nerve (S1, S2).

Actions:

Described above with gastrocnemius.

Popliteus

This is a triangular muscle in the floor of the popliteal fossa.

Origin:

The muscle arises, by a tendon, from the lateral aspect of the lateral condyle of the femur. In this situation there is a prominent groove: the popliteus takes origin from the anterior part of the groove. The posterior part of the groove is occupied by the popliteus tendon in full flexion at the knee.

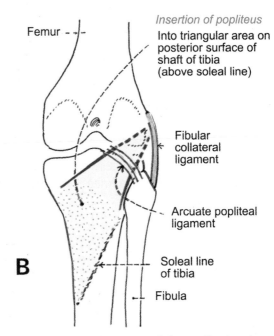

Fig. 29.34. Posterior aspect of the popliteal region to show the popliteus.

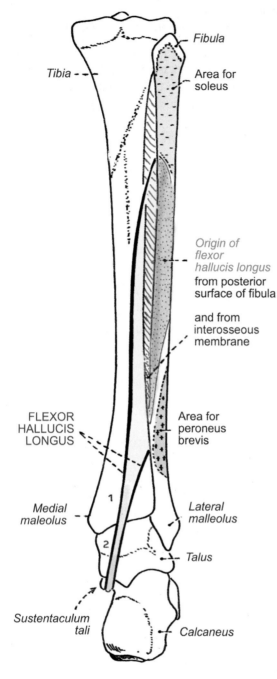

Fig. 29.35. Flexor hallucis muscle.

The origin lies within the capsule of the knee joint. The muscle emerges from the knee joint through an aperture in the capsule.

Insertion:

Into a triangular area on the posterior surface of the shaft of the tibia (Fig. 29.34).

Nerve supply :

Tibial nerve (L4, L5, S1).

Actions:

When the leg is off the ground, the popliteus rotates the tibia medially on the femur. When the leg is placed on the ground (thus fixing the tibia) the muscle rotates the femur laterally on the tibia. Because of this action the muscle can unlock the knee joint at the beginning of flexion.

Flexor Hallucis Longus

Origin:

The muscle takes origin from the lower two thirds of the posterior surface of the fibula (Fig. 29.35) and from the interosseous membrane.

The muscle ends in a tendon which runs across the lower part of the tibia (1) and the posterior aspect of the talus (2) to reach the calcaneus.

Here it turns forwards below the sustentaculum tali which serves as a pulley for it.

Insertion:

The tendon then runs forward in the sole to be inserted into the plantar aspect of the base of the distal phalanx (Fig. 29.36. Also see Fig. 29.33).

Nerve supply: Tibial nerve (S2, S3).

Actions.

These are as follows:

(a) Flexion of the distal phalanx of the great toe.

(b) Plantar flexion of the foot.

(c) The muscle helps to maintain the longitudinal arch of the foot.

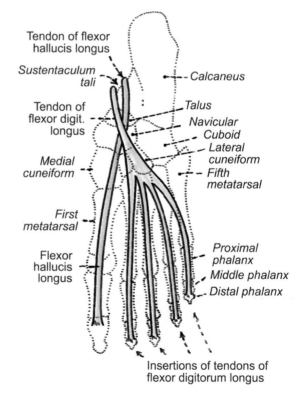

Fig. 29.36. Course and attachments of tendons of flexor hallucis longus and flexor digitorum longus in the sole.

Flexor Digitorum Longus

Origin:

From posterior surface of shaft of tibia (Fig. 29.37). The muscle ends in a tendon which passes behind the medial malleolus. It then turns laterally to enter the sole of the foot. In the sole the tendon divides into four slips, one each for the 2nd, 3rd, 4th and 5th digits. (Also see Fig. 29.36, 29.43).

Insertion:

Each slip is inserted into the distal phalanx (plantar surface of the base) of the digit concerned.

Nerve supply: Tibial nerve (S2, S3).

Actions:

The muscle causes plantar flexion of the distal phalanges. Its continued action helps in flexion of the middle and proximal phalanges, and in plantar flexion of the foot. It also helps to maintain the longitudinal arches of the foot.

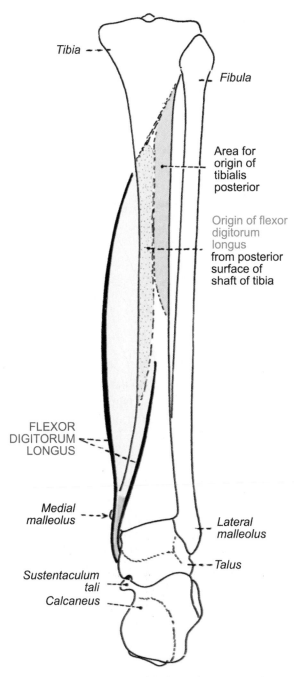

Fig. 29.37. Flexor digitorum longus muscle. Also see Fig. 29.36.

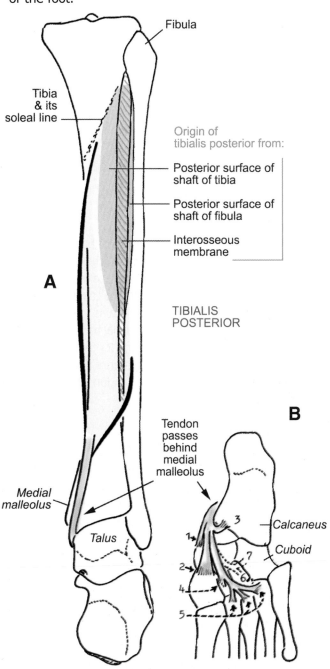

Insertion of tibialis posterior
Through a number of slips attached to
1. Tuberosity of navicular. 2. Medial cuneiform
3. Calcaneus. 4. Int. cuneiform. 5. Bases of 2nd, 3rd, 4th
metatarsals. 6. Lateral cuneiform. 7. Cuboid.

Fig. 29.38. A. Scheme to show the tibialis posterior muscle and its origin. B. Skeleton of foot seen from below to show insertion of tibialis posterior.

Tibialis Posterior

Origin:

This muscle arises from (Fig. 29.38A):

(a) Posterior surface of the shaft of the tibia below the soleal line.

(b) Posterior surface of the fibula.

(c) Interosseous membrane.

The tendon passes behind the medial malleolus to reach the sole of the foot.

Insertion:

The main insertions inserted into the tuberosity of the navicular bone, and the medial cuneiform bone. Some slips reach other bones of the foot.

Nerve supply: Tibial nerve (L4, L5).

Actions:

1. Inversion of the foot.
2. Maintains the longitudinal arches of the foot.

Flexor Retinaculum

The flexor retinaculum is a thickened band of deep fascia present on the medial side of the ankle (Fig. 29.39). It is attached above to the medial malleolus, and below to the medial surface of' the calcaneus. The structures passing under cover of it are as follows (from above downwards, and also from medial to lateral side): **(1)** tendon of the tibialis posterior, **(2)** tendon of the flexor digitorum longus, **(3)** the posterior tibial vessels, **(4)** the tibial nerve, and **(5)** the tendon of the flexor hallucis longus.

Synovial Sheaths

The three tendons passing deep to the flexor retinaculum are surrounded by synovial sheaths which

begin proximal to the retinaculum. The sheath for the tibialis posterior extends to the insertion of the muscle. The sheath for the flexor hallucis longus may end near the base of the first metatarsal, or may extend right up to the insertion into the terminal phalanx.

The sheath for the flexor digitorum longus expands to enclose the proximal parts of the tendons for the digits. The distal parts of the tendons for the 2nd, 3rd and 4th digits have independent synovial sheaths. The 5th digit has a similar sheath which is continuous proximally with the sheath for the tendon of the flexor digitorum longus.

MUSCLES AND RELATED STRUCTURES IN THE SOLE

Plantar Aponeurosis

Underlying the skin of the sole there is a thick layer of deep fascia which is given the name *plantar*

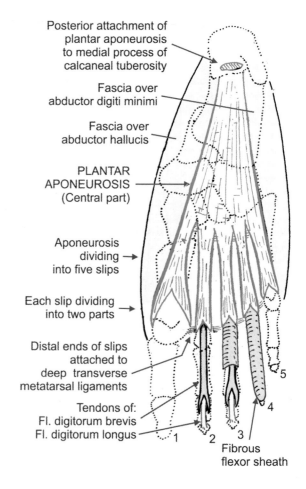

Fig. 29.40. Scheme to show the arrangement of the plantar aponeurosis.

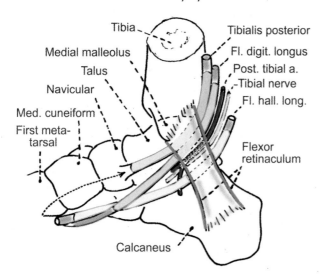

Fig. 29.39. Flexor retinaculum and structures passing deep to it. Note the extent of the tendon sheaths.

aponeurosis. It consists of central, medial and lateral parts. The central part is the thickest and strongest (Fig. 29.40). It overlies the flexor digitorum brevis. Traced distally the aponeurosis broadens and divides into five processes, one for each digit.

Fibrous Flexor Sheaths

Over each toe the deep fascia (which is thick) winds round the sides of the flexor tendons of the digit to get attached to the lateral margins of the phalanges. The fascia con-stitutes the ***fibrous flexor sheath***. The tendons are thus enclosed in an osseo-aponeurotic canal. This canal is lined by a synovial sheath to permit smooth movement of the tendons.

Flexor Digitorum Brevis

Origin:
From tuberosity of the calcaneus (medial process) (Fig. 29.41).
The muscle ends in four tendons, one each for the 2nd, 3rd, 4th and 5th digits.

Insertion:
The tendon for each digit divides into two slips that are inserted into the sides of the middle phalanx (Fig. 13.14).

Nerve supply: Medial plantar nerve (S2, S3).

Actions:
(a) Flexion of the middle and proximal phalanges.
(b) It helps to maintain the arches of the foot.

Abductor Hallucis

Origin:
The abductor hallucis arises from (Fig. 29.42):
(a) the medial process of the calcaneal tuberosity,
(b) the flexor retinaculum, and

Insertion:
Proximal phalanx of the great toe (medial side of base).

Nerve supply: Medial plantar nerve (S2, S3).

Action:
The abductor hallucis abducts and flexes the great toe.

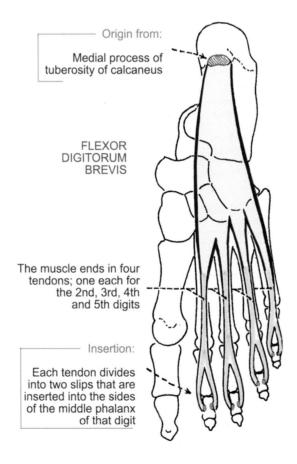

Origin from:
Medial process of tuberosity of calcaneus

FLEXOR DIGITORUM BREVIS

The muscle ends in four tendons; one each for the 2nd, 3rd, 4th and 5th digits

Insertion:
Each tendon divides into two slips that are inserted into the sides of the middle phalanx of that digit

Fig. 29.41. Attachments of the flexor digitorum brevis.

Fig. 29.42. Scheme to show attachments of the abductor hallucis and the abductor digiti minimi.

Abductor Digiti Minimi

Origin:
   Tuberosity of the calcaneus (lateral and medial processes)(Fig. 29.42).

Insertion: .
   Proximal phalanx of the fifth toe.

Nerve supply: Lateral plantar nerve (S2, S3).

Actions:
   The abductor digiti minimi abducts the fifth toe.

Flexor Digitorum Accessorius

Origin:
   From the calcaneus by two heads (Fig. 29.43). The **medial head** arises from the

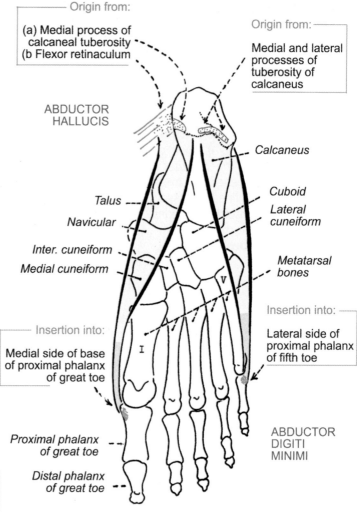

medial surface, and the **lateral head** from the lateral process of the tuberosity.

Insertion:
   Into tendon of flexor digitorum longus.

Nerve supply: Lateral plantar nerve (S2, S3).

Actions:
   This muscle straightens the oblique pull of the flexor digitorum longus.

Lumbrical Muscles of the Foot
   These are four slender muscles numbered from the medial to the lateral side (Fig. 29.43).

Origin:
   They take origin from the digital tendons of the flexor digitorum longus.

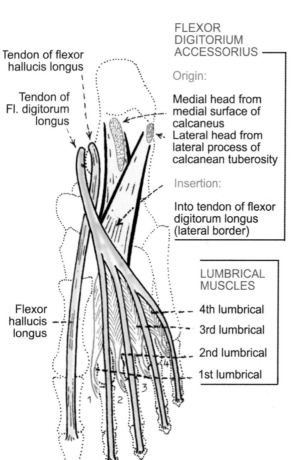

Fig. 29.43. Scheme to show the attachments of the flexor digitorum accessorius and the lumbrical muscles.

Insertion:

Each muscle ends in a tendon which curves round the medial side of the corresponding metatarsophalangeal joint. It is inserted partly into the base of the proximal phalanx, and partly into the extensor expansion.

Flexor Hallucis Brevis

Origin:

Mainly from the plantar surface of the cuboid bone (Fig. 29.44).

Insertion:

The muscle divides into two parts each of which ends in a tendon. The two tendons are inserted into the proximal phalanx of the great toe (corresponding side of the base).

Nerve supply: Medial plantar nerve (S2, S3).

Action:

Flexion of great toe.

Flexor Digiti Minimi Brevis

Origin:

From the base of the fifth metatarsal bone (plantar surface) (Fig. 29.44).

Insertion:

Into proximal phalanx of little toe (on the lateral side of its base).

Nerve supply: Lateral plantar nerve (S1, S2).

Action:

Flexion of little toe.

Adductor Hallucis

The adductor hallucis has two heads oblique and transverse.

Origin:

The **oblique head** arises from the bases of the 2nd, 3rd and 4th metatarsal bones.

The **transverse head** arises from the plantar aspect of the metatarsophalangeal joints of the 3rd, 4th and 5th toes.

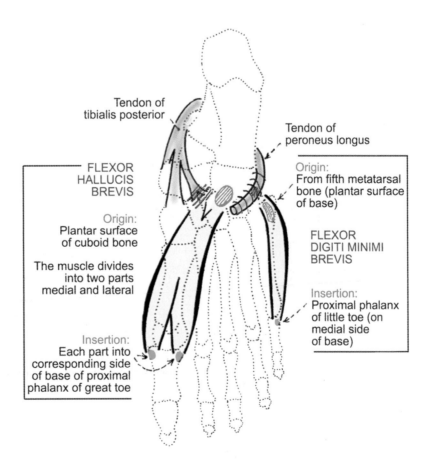

Fig. 29.44. Scheme to show the attachments of the flexor hallucis brevis and the flexor digiti minimi brevis.

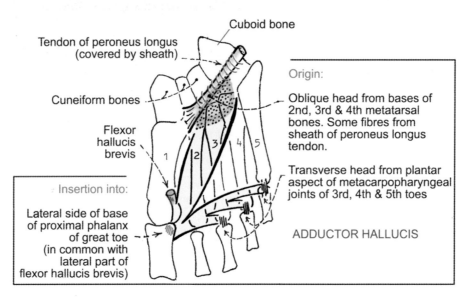

Fig. 29.45. Attachments of adductor hallucis.

Nerve supply: Lateral plantar nerve (S2, S3).

Insertion:

The two heads end in a common tendon which is inserted into the proximal phalanx of the great toe (lateral side of base).

Actions:

The muscle adducts the great toe.

Interosseous Muscles of ohe Foot

Introductory remarks

These are small muscles placed between the metatarsal bones. There are three plantar, and four dorsal, interossei. They are numbered from medial to lateral side.

Each plantar interosseous muscle arises from one metatarsal bone (from the plantar aspect of the shaft)

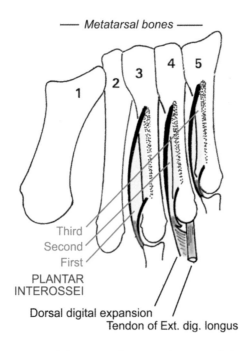

Fig. 29.46. Scheme to show attachments of plantar interossei of foot.

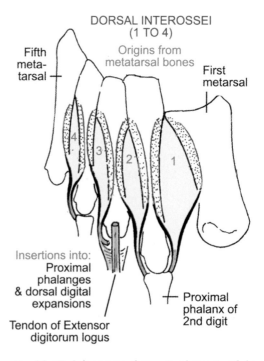

Fig. 29.47. Scheme to show attachments of dorsal interossei of foot.

(Fig. 29.46). It is inserted into the base of the proximal phalanx, and into the dorsal digital expansion of the corresponding digit.

Each dorsal interosseous muscle arises from the shafts of two adjoining metatarsal bone (Fig. 29.47). The dorsal interossei are inserted into the bases of the proximal phalanges, and into the dorsal digital expansions.

Details of the attachments of individual interosseous muscles are shown in Figs. 29.46 and 29.47.

Actions of interossei

The interossei adduct or abduct the toes with reference to an axis passing through the **second** digit. The plantar interossei are adductors. They pull the 3rd, 4th and 5th toes towards the second toe. The dorsal interossei are abductors of the 2nd, 3rd and 4th toes.

In addition to abduction and adduction, the interossei flex the metatarsophalangeal joints and extend the interphalangeal joints by virtue of their insertion into the dorsal digital expansions.

Nerve supply:

All the interossei are supplied by the lateral plantar nerve (S2, S3).

30

Nerves of the Lower Extremity

CUTANEOUS INNERVATION OF THE LOWER LIMB

Front of thigh

The cutaneous nerves that supply the front of thigh are shown in Fig. 30.1. Note that four longitudinal strips of skin are supplied (from lateral to medial side) by the *lateral cutaneous nerve of the thigh*, the *intermediate cutaneous nerve of the thigh*, the *medial cutaneous nerve of the thigh*, and by cutaneous branches of the *obturator nerve*. Three areas just below the inguinal ligament are supplied (from lateral to medial side) by the *subcostal* and *iliohypogastric* nerves, the femoral branch of the *genitofemoral nerve*, and the *ilioinguinal nerve*.

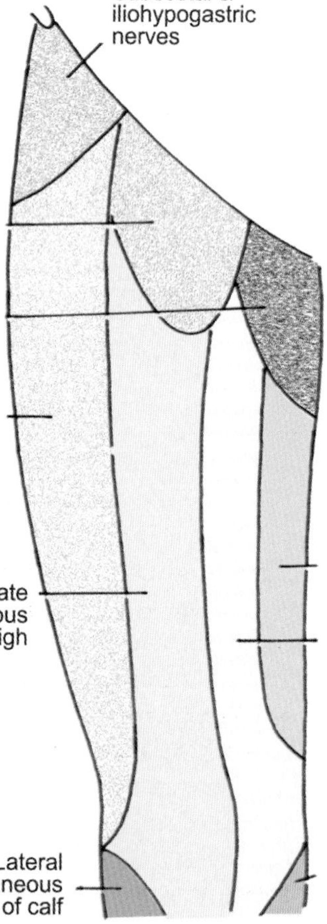

Front of leg and dorsum of foot

The cutaneous nerve supply of the front of the leg is shown in Fig. 30.2. The medial side of the front of the leg is supplied by the *saphenous nerve*. The lateral side of the leg is supplied, in its upper part, by the

Subcostal &
iliohypogastric
nerves

Femoral br.
of genito-
femoral n.

Ilioinguinal
nerve

Lateral
cutaneous
n. of thigh

Intermediate
cutaneous
n. of thigh

Obturator n.

Medial
cutaneous
n. of thigh

Lateral
cutaneous
n. of calf

Saphenous
nerve

Fig. 30.1. Cutaneous nerves supplying front of thigh.

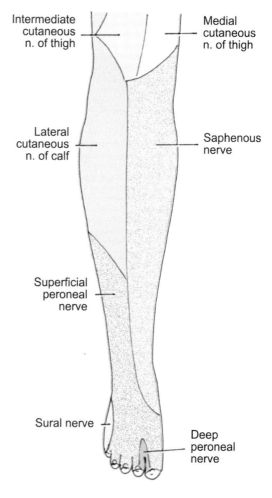

Intermediate
cutaneous
n. of thigh

Medial
cutaneous
n. of thigh

Lateral
cutaneous
n. of calf

Saphenous
nerve

Superficial
peroneal
nerve

Sural nerve

Deep
peroneal
nerve

Fig. 30.2. Cutaneous nerves on front of leg and dorsum of foot.

lateral cutaneous nerve of the calf and, lower down, by the *superficial peroneal nerve*.

The greater part of the dorsum of the foot, including most of the toes, is supplied by the *superficial peroneal nerve*. A triangular area of skin covering the adjoining sides of the big toe and the second toe is supplied by the *deep peroneal nerve*. A strip along the medial side of the foot is supplied by the *saphenous nerve*, but the area supplied does not reach the big toe. A strip along the lateral side of the foot is supplied by the *sural nerve*: the area reaches the little toe.

Gluteal region

The cutaneous nerves supplying the gluteal region are shown in Fig. 30.3. The first point to note is that whereas the predominant nerve supply of the entire lower limb is through *ventral rami* of spinal nerves, some areas of skin over the gluteal region are supplied by *dorsal rami*. An area over the sacrum is innervated by dorsal rami of spinal nerves S1, 2, 3. More laterally a wide area is innervated by dorsal rami of nerves L1, 2, 3. (All other areas are innervated by nerves derived from ventral rami).

The upper and lateral part of the gluteal region is supplied by lateral cutaneous branches of the *subcostal nerve*, and of the *iliohypogastric nerve*. The lower lateral part of the gluteal region receives a branch from the *lateral cutaneous nerve of the thigh*. Areas just above the fold of the buttock are supplied by the *perforating cutaneous nerve*, near the midline, and by the gluteal branch of the *posterior cutaneous nerve of the thigh*, more laterally.

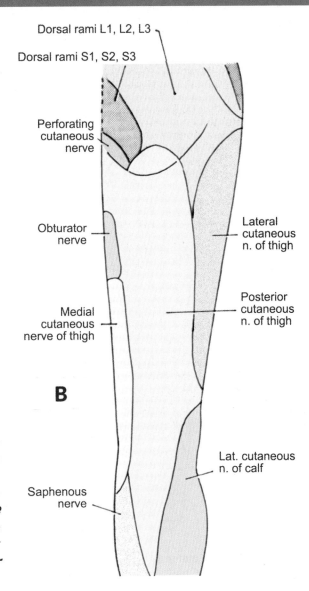

Fig. 30.4. Cutaneous nerves on back of thigh.

Back of thigh

The cutaneous nerve supply of the back of the thigh is shown in Fig. 30.4. Most of this aspect of the thigh is innervated by the *posterior cutaneous nerve of the thigh*. Note that this nerve also supplies the upper part of the back of the leg. Laterally and medially we can see some areas supplied by the same nerves that have already been seen from the front. These are the *obturator nerve* and the *medial cutaneous nerve of the thigh*, on the medial side, and the *lateral cutaneous nerve of the thigh* on the lateral side.

Back of leg

The cutaneous nerve supply of the back of the leg is shown in Fig. 30.5. On the medial and lateral sides we see the same nerves as seen from the front viz.,

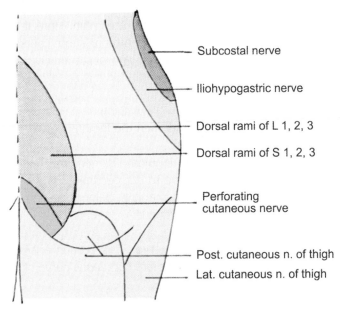

Fig. 30.3. Cutaneous nerves in gluteal region.

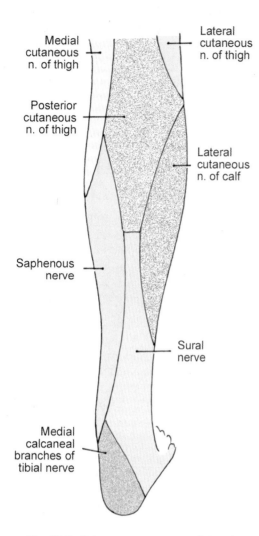

Fig. 30.7. Cutaneous nerves supplying the back of the leg.

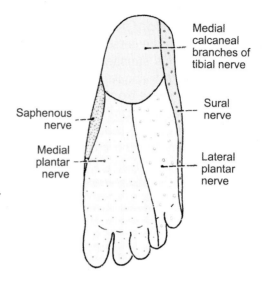

Fig. 30.6. Cutaneous nerves supply of the sole.

the medial side a strip is supplied by the **saphenous nerve**: this strip does not reach the big toe. Skin over the heel is supplied by medial calcaneal branches of the tibial nerve.

NERVES ON FRONT AND MEDIAL SIDE OF THIGH

THE FEMORAL NERVE

The femoral nerve arises, in the abdomen, from the lumbar plexus. The nerve is derived from the ventral rami of spinal nerves L2, L3 and L4. It passes behind the inguinal ligament to enter the thigh. Here it lies lateral to the femoral artery. After a short course it ends by dividing into anterior and posterior divisions. The distribution of the femoral nerve is as follows:

A. Muscular branches (Fig. 30.7):

1. While still in the abdomen the femoral nerve gives branches to the iliacus.

2. A little above the inguinal ligament the femoral nerve gives off the nerve to the pectineus. The nerve passes downwards and medially behind the femoral vessels to reach the pectineus.

3. The sartorius receives a branch from the anterior division of the femoral nerve. This branch arises in common with the intermediate cutaneous nerve of the thigh (see below).

the **saphenous nerve** medially, and the **lateral cutaneous nerve of the calf,** laterally. A strip along the middle of the back of the leg is innervated, in its upper part, by the **posterior cutaneous nerve of the thigh**, and in its lower part by the **sural nerve.** The skin over the heel is supplied by **medial calcaneal branches** of the tibial nerve.

Sole

The cutaneous innervation of the skin of the sole is shown in Fig. 30.6. The anterior part of the sole, including the medial 3½ digits, is supplied by the **medial plantar nerve**. The lateral part (including the lateral 1½ digits) is supplied through the **lateral plantar nerve**. Branches from these nerves also supply the dorsal aspect of the terminal parts of the toes including the nail beds. A strip of skin along the lateral margin of the sole (reaching up to the lateral surface of the little toe) is supplied by the **sural nerve**. On

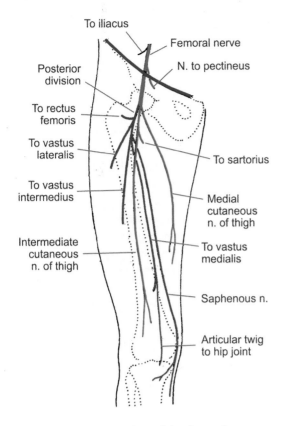

Fig. 30.7. Branches of the femoral nerve.

4. The rectus femoris, the vastus lateralis, the vastus medialis and the vastus intermedius receive branches from the posterior division of the femoral nerve.

B. Cutaneous branches (Fig. 30.7):

1. The intermediate cutaneous nerve of the thigh arises from the anterior division of the femoral nerve. The area of skin supplied by the nerve is shown in Fig. 30.1.

2. The medial cutaneous nerve of the thigh is a branch of the anterior division of the femoral nerve. It runs part of its course along the lateral side of the femoral artery which it crosses near the apex of the femoral triangle. It divides into branches that supply the skin of the medial side of the thigh: the area of skin supplied is shown in Fig. 30.1. The nerve takes part in forming the subsartorial plexus (along with branches of the saphenous and obturator nerves).

3. The saphenous nerve arises from the posterior division of the femoral nerve. It descends along the lateral side of the femoral artery. In the adductor canal the nerve crosses the artery from lateral to medial side. It leaves the adductor canal at its lower end and runs down along the medial side of the knee. Here it pierces the deep fascia and becomes subcutaneous. It then runs down the medial side of the leg (along side the

long saphenous vein). A branch extends along the medial side of the foot (but ends short of the great toe). The area of skin supplied by the nerve is shown in Fig. 30.1. The saphenous nerve takes part in forming the subsartorial plexus and the patellar plexus.

C. Articular branches:

(1) The posterior division of the femoral nerve sends fibres to the knee joint through the nerve to the vastus medialis.

(2) Some fibres reach the hip joint through the nerve to the rectus femoris.

D. Vascular branches

The femoral nerve gives some branches to the femoral artery and its branches.

THE OBTURATOR NERVE

This nerve arises from the lumbar plexus. It is formed by union of roots arising from L2, L3, and L4 (Fig. 30.8). For convenience of description its course can be considered in three parts. The first part runs downwards in the substance of the psoas major. The second part of the nerve lies in the lateral wall of the true pelvis. It leaves the lateral wall of the pelvis by passing through the upper part of the obturator foramen to enter the thigh. The third part of the nerve lies in the thigh. As it passes through the obturator foramen it divides into anterior and posterior divisions. The anterior division lies in front of the obturator externus (above) and the adductor brevis (below): it lies behind the pectineus (above) and the adductor longus (below). The posterior division lies in front of the obturator externus (above) and the adductor magnus (below). It is behind the pectineus (above) and the adductor brevis (below).

The obturator nerve is distributed as follows (Fig. 30.8):

A. Muscular branches:

(a) Branches arising from the anterior division supply the obturator externus, the adductor longus and the gracilis; and occasionally the pectineus and the adductor brevis.

(b) Branches of the posterior division supply the obturator externus, the adductor brevis and the adductor magnus.

B. Cutaneous branches:

After supplying the muscles named above the anterior division supplies the skin of the lower medial part of the thigh (Fig. 30.1).

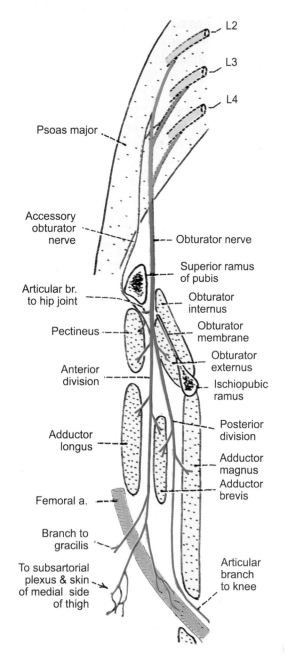

Fig. 30.8. Scheme to show the course and distribution of the obturator nerve.

C. Articular branches:

These are given off to the hip joint and to the knee joint.

D. Vascular branches:

The anterior division ends by supplying the femoral artery.

Accessory obturator nerve:

Occasionally some fibres of the obturator nerve arising from L2 and L3 follow a separate course and are termed the accessory obturator nerve.

Femoral branch of Genitofemoral nerve

The femoral branch descends on the lateral side of the external iliac artery. It passes deep to the inguinal ligament and comes to lie lateral to the femoral artery: here it lies within the femoral sheath. It becomes superficial by piercing the anterior wall of the sheath, and the deep fascia, and supplies an area of skin over the upper part of the femoral triangle (Fig. 30.1).

Lateral cutaneous nerve of thigh

The lateral cutaneous nerve of the thigh arises from the lumbar plexus. It is derived from the dorsal divisions of L2 and L3. Its initial part lies within the psoas major. Emerging from the lateral border of the muscle the nerve runs downwards, laterally and forwards over the iliacus muscle to reach the anterior superior iliac spine. It enters the thigh by passing behind the lateral end of the inguinal ligament. It divides into anterior and posterior branches through which it supplies the skin on the anterolateral part of the thigh right up to the knee (Fig. 30.1).

NERVES SEEN IN THE GLUTEAL REGION

Superior Gluteal Nerve (Fig. 30.9)

The superior gluteal nerve is derived from spinal nerves L4, L5 and S1. It passes from the pelvis to the gluteal region through the greater sciatic foramen, above the piriformis. It divides into superior and inferior branches. Both these branches run forwards deep to the gluteus medius. The superior branch supplies the gluteus medius, and (occasionally) the gluteus minimus. The inferior branch also supplies these two muscles: it ends by supplying the tensor fasciae latae.

Inferior Gluteal Nerve (Fig. 30.9)

The inferior gluteal nerve is derived from spinal nerves L5, S1 and S2. It passes from the pelvis to the gluteal region through the greater sciatic foramen, below the piriformis. It supplies the gluteus maximus.

Nerve to Quadratus Femoris (Fig. 30.9)

The nerve to the quadratus femoris is derived from spinal nerves L4, L5 and S1. It passes from the pelvis to the gluteal region through the greater sciatic foramen, below the piriformis. It runs downwards deep to the superior gemellus, the tendon of the obturator internus, and the inferior gemellus. After giving a branch

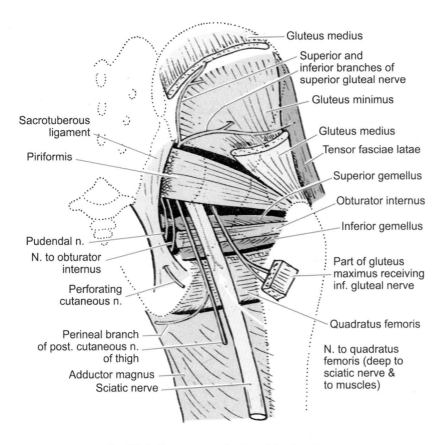

Fig. 30.9. Nerves seen in the gluteal region.

gluteal region (deep to the gluteus maximus) to enter the back of the thigh. Its lowest part extends into the upper part of the leg. It supplies an extensive area of skin including that over the lower part of the gluteal region, the perineum, the back of the thigh, and the back of the upper part of the leg.

Perforating Cutaneous Nerve (Fig. 30.9)

The perforating cutaneous nerve is derived from S2 and S3. It enters the gluteal region by piercing through the sacrotuberous ligament. It supplies the skin over the inferomedial part of the gluteus maximus (Fig. 30.3).

Pudendal Nerve (Fig. 30.9)

The pudendal nerve arises from the sacral plexus and derives its fibres from nerves S2, S3 and S4. The nerve passes from the pelvis to the gluteal region through the greater sciatic foramen. The nerve has a short course through the gluteal region. Emerging at the lower border of the piriformis it crosses the sacrospinous ligament and disappears into the lesser sciatic foramen.

The largest and most important nerve in the gluteal region is the sciatic nerve. It is considered below.

to the inferior gemellus it reaches the anterior (or deep) surface of the quadratus femoris and enters it to supply the muscle.

Nerve to Obturator Internus (Fig. 30.9)

The nerve to the obturator internus is derived from L5, S1 and S2. It passes from the pelvis to the gluteal region through the greater sciatic foramen passing below the piriformis.

It runs down posterior to the ischial spine and again enters the pelvis by passing through the lesser sciatic foramen. The nerve ends by supplying the obturator internus. Before passing through the lesser sciatic foramen it gives a branch to the superior gemellus.

Nerve to Piriformis

The nerve to the piriformis arises from S1 and S2. It is confined to the pelvis and ends by entering the anterior surface of the piriformis.

Posterior Cutaneous Nerve of Thigh

The posterior cutaneous nerve of the thigh is derived from S1, and S2 and S3. It passes from the pelvis to the gluteal region through the greater sciatic foramen, below the piriformis. It passes downwards through the

NERVES ON BACK OF THIGH

THE SCIATIC NERVE AND ITS RAMIFICATIONS

The sciatic nerve is the main continuation of the sacral plexus. It is the thickest nerve of the body. It receives fibres from spinal nerves L4 to S3. It passes from the pelvis to the gluteal region through the greater sciatic foramen, below the piriformis (Fig. 30.9). It descends through the gluteal region into the back of the thigh. At the junction of the middle and lower thirds of the thigh the sciatic nerve ends by dividing into the tibial and common peroneal nerves.

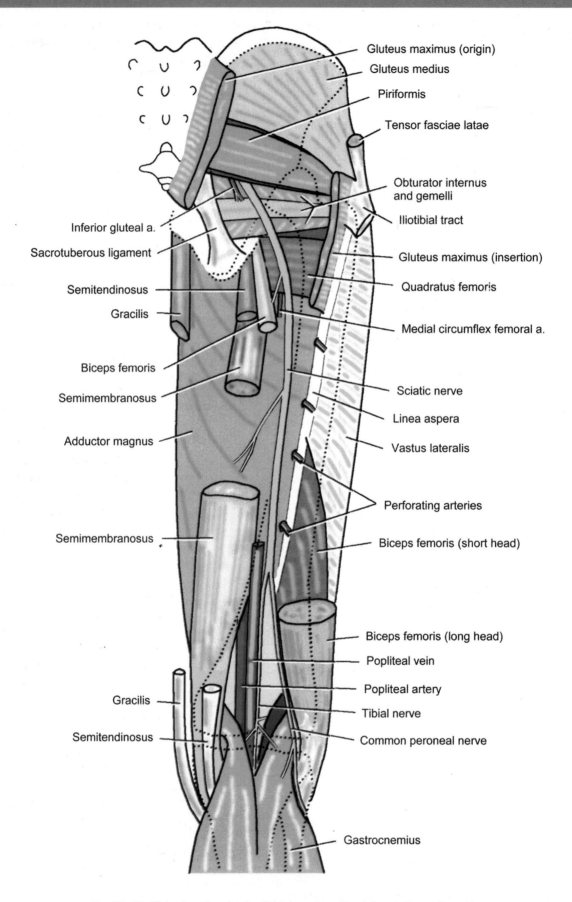

Fig. 30.10. Gluteal region, back of thigh and popliteal fossa. Deep dissection.

In its course through the gluteal region the nerve lies deep (or anterior) to the gluteus maximus. It lies successively on the posterior surface of the ischium, the superior gemellus, the obturator internus (tendon), the inferior gemellus and the quadratus femoris. In the thigh the nerve lies upon the adductor magnus, and is crossed superficially (i.e., posteriorly) by the long head of the biceps femoris.

Apart from its terminal branches the sciatic nerve gives the following branches.

(a) Branches arising from the tibial part of the nerve supply the hamstrings viz., the long head of the biceps femoris, the semitendinosus, the semimembranosus and the adductor magnus (part arising from the ischial tuberosity).

(b) The common peroneal part of the sciatic nerve gives a branch to the short head of the biceps femoris muscle.

(c) Articular branches are given off to the hip joint.

The nerves on the back of the thigh are the sciatic nerve, the tibial nerve and the common peroneal nerve. The sciatic nerve has already been described. The tibial nerve is distributed mainly in the leg and will will be considered in Chapter 13. The common peroneal nerve is described below.

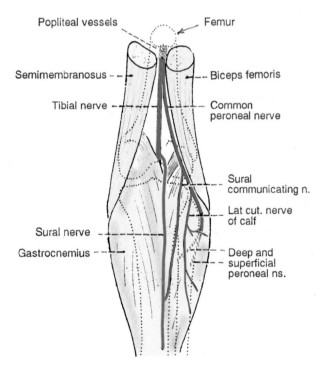

Fig. 30.11. Scheme to show the course and branches of the common peroneal nerve.

The Common Peroneal Nerve

This is also called the ***lateral popliteal nerve***. It is a terminal branch of the sciatic nerve. Its fibres are derived from the sacral plexus through roots L4, L5, S1 and S2. Starting at the bifurcation of the sciatic nerve it runs downwards and laterally along the lower part of the biceps femoris muscle to reach the head of the fibula (Fig. 30.10). It winds round the lateral side of the neck of the fibula and ends by dividing into its superficial and deep peroneal branches. Apart from these terminal branches the common peroneal nerve gives off the following branches (Fig. 30.11).

The ***lateral cutaneous nerve of the calf*** supplies the skin over the upper two thirds of the lateral side of the leg (Fig. 30.2).

The ***sural communicating branch*** arises near the upper end of the fibula. It joins the sural nerve and is distributed with it.

The Deep Peroneal Nerve

This is also called the anterior tibial nerve. It begins on the lateral side of the neck of the fibula, deep to the peroneus longus. It passes downwards and medially, enters the anterior compartment of the leg and descends in front of the interosseus membrane, and lower down on the anterior aspect of the shaft of the tibia. Accompanied by the anterior tibial artery it reaches the front of the ankle joint. It ends here by dividing into lateral and medial terminal branches.

The distribution of the deep peroneal nerve is as follows (Fig. 30.12):

A. *Muscular branches:*

(1) In the leg the nerve gives branches to muscles of the anterior compartment: these are the tibialis anterior, the extensor hallucis longus, the extensor digitorum longus, and the peroneus tertius.

(2) The lateral terminal branch supplies the extensor digitorum brevis.

B. *Cutaneous branches:*

The skin of part of the dorsum of the foot is supplied by the deep peroneal nerve through its medial terminal branch. This branch runs forwards on the dorsum of the foot along with the dorsalis pedis artery. It divides into two dorsal digital nerves which supply the adjacent sides of the great toe and the second toe (Fig. 30.2).

C. *Articular branches:*

These supply the ankle joint and some joints of the foot.

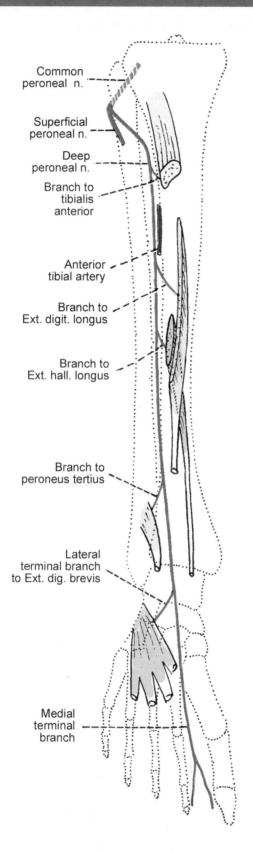

Fig. 30.12. Distribution of deep peroneal nerve.

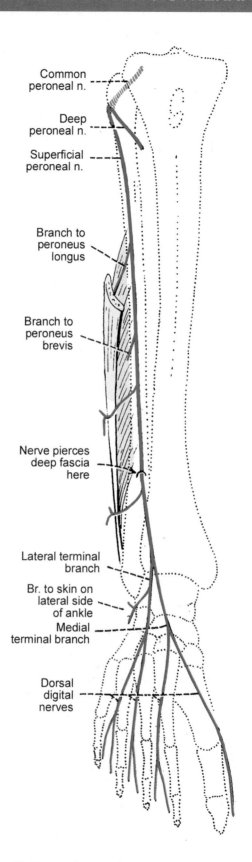

Fig. 30.13. Distribution of superficial peroneal nerve.

The Superficial Peroneal Nerve

This nerve is also called the ***musculocutaneous nerve***. It begins at the neck of the fibula deep to the peroneus longus (Fig. 30.13).

It is the nerve to muscles of the lateral compartment of the leg: these are the peroneus longus and the peroneus brevis. Reaching the lower part of the leg the nerve becomes superficial and supplies the skin on its lateral side (Fig. 30.2). It then divides into medial and lateral terminal branches which descend across the ankle to reach the dorsum of the foot.

Each terminal branch divides into two dorsal digital nerves. The medial branch gives one dorsal digital nerve to the medial side of the great toe; and another to the adjacent sides of the second and third toes. The lateral branch gives one dorsal digital nerve to the contiguous sides of the third and fourth toes and another to the adjacent sides of the fourth and fifth toes. The lateral terminal branch also supplies the skin on the lateral side of the ankle.

The Tibial Nerve

This is also called the medial popliteal nerve. It is a terminal branch of the sciatic nerve. It descends through the popliteal fossa, and the back of the leg. In the upper part of the popliteal fossa the nerve lies lateral to the popliteal artery and vein (Fig.30.10). In the lower part of the leg it ends midway between the medial malleolus and the tendocalcaneus by dividing into the medial and lateral plantar nerves.

The distribution of the tibial nerve (excluding that of its terminal branches) is as follows (Fig. 30.14):

A. Muscular branches:

(1) Branches given off in the lower part of the popliteal fossa supply the two heads of the gastrocnemius, the plantaris, the soleus and the popliteus. The ***nerve to the popliteus*** has an interesting course. After running down superficial (posterior) to this muscle the nerve turns round its lower border to reach its anterior surface which it enters.

(2) Branches arising in the leg supply the soleus, the tibialis posterior, the flexor digitorum longus and the flexor hallucis longus.

B. Cutaneous branches:

(1) The ***sural nerve*** is the main cutaneous branch. It arises in the popliteal fossa and runs down the back of the leg. The terminal part of the nerve runs forwards along the lateral margin of the foot reaching right up to the lateral side of the little toe. The nerve supplies

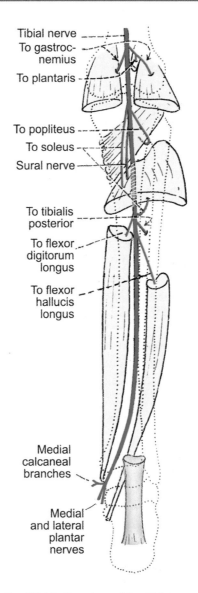

Fig. 30.14. Branches of the tibial nerve.

skin on the posterolateral part of the leg and along the lateral margin of the foot (Fig. 30.5).

(2) The ***medial calcaneal branches*** supply the skin over the heel (Figs. 30.5, 30.6).

C. Articular branches:

The tibial nerve gives branches to the knee joint and to the ankle joint.

Medial Plantar Nerve

The medial plantar nerve is a terminal branch of the tibial nerve. It begins on the posteromedial aspect of the ankle midway between the tendocalcaneus and the medial malleolus: here it lies under cover of the flexor retinaculum. The nerve passes forwards in the medial part of the sole. It is accompanied by the medial plantar artery. The nerve ends by dividing into one ***proper digital branch*** for the great toe, and three ***common plantar digital branches.*** The nerve is distributed as follows (Fig. 30.15):

A. Cutaneous branches:

(a) Branches arising from the trunk of the nerve supply the skin of the medial part of the sole.

(b) The skin on the medial side of the great toe is supplied by the proper digital branch to this digit.

(c) Each common plantar digital nerve divides into two ***proper digital nerves***. The first (most medial) common plantar digital nerve divides into the proper digital nerves that supply the skin on the adjacent sides of the great toe and second toe; the second into those that supply the second and third toes; and the third into those that supply the third and fourth toes.

B. Muscular branches:

(a) Branches arising from the trunk of the nerve supply the abductor hallucis, and the flexor digitorum brevis.

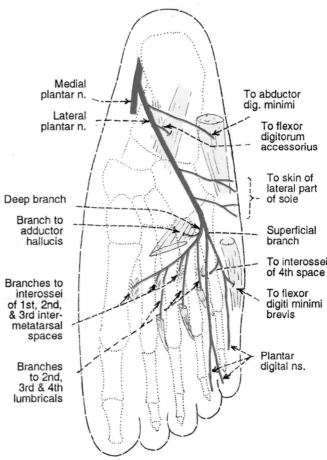

Fig. 30.16. Distribution of lateral plantar nerve.

(b) The flexor hallucis brevis receives a branch from the digital nerve to the great toe.

(c) The first lumbrical muscle is supplied by a branch from the first plantar digital nerve.

C. Articular branches:

These supply the tarsal, tarsometatarsal joints, metatarsophalangeal and interphalangeal joints.

The Lateral Plantar Nerve

The lateral plantar nerve is a terminal branch of the tibial nerve. It begins on the posteromedial aspect of the ankle midway between the tendocalcaneus and the medial malleolus. It passes forwards and laterally across the sole (Fig. 30.16). The nerve ends (near the tubercle of the fifth metatarsal bone) by dividing into superficial and deep branches.

The trunk of the lateral plantar nerve is accompanied by the lateral plantar artery.

The ***superficial branch*** runs distally and ends by dividing into two plantar digital nerves. The lateral of these runs along the lateral side of the fifth digit. The

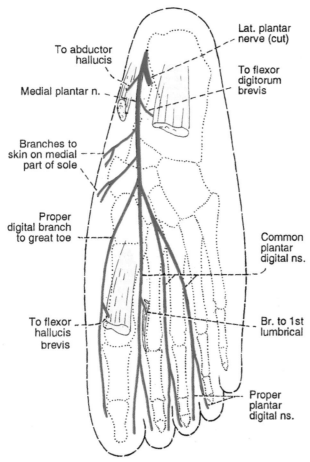

Fig. 30.15. Distribution of the medial plantar nerve.

medial one divides into two branches that supply the adjacent sides of the fourth and fifth digits (Fig. 30.16).

The **deep branch** begins near the tubercle of the fifth metatarsal bone. From here it runs medially deep to the flexor tendons and the adductor hallucis.

The distribution of the lateral plantar nerve and its terminal branches is as follows (Fig. 30.16).

A. Muscular branches:

(1) Branches arising from the trunk supply the flexor digitorum accessorius and the abductor digiti minimi.

(2) The flexor digiti minimi brevis is supplied by the digital branch for the lateral side of the fifth toe. This nerve also supplies the interosseus muscles that lie between the fourth and fifth metatarsal bones (i.e., the 3rd plantar and the fourth dorsal interosseus muscles).

(3) The deep branch supplies all interossei except those lying between the fourth and fifth metatarsals. It also supplies the 2nd, 3rd and 4th lumbrical muscles, and the adductor hallucis.

B. Cutaneous branches:

(1) Some branches arising from the trunk of the nerve supply the skin of the lateral part of the sole (Fig. 30.6).

(2) The skin on the lateral side of the little toe and the contiguous sides of the fourth and fifth toes is supplied by the corresponding digital branches.

31

Blood Supply of Lower Extremity

ARTERIES OF THE LOWER LIMB

THE FEMORAL ARTERY

The femoral artery is the continuation of the external iliac artery into the thigh. It begins at the midinguinal point (i.e., midway between the pubic symphysis and the anterior superior iliac spine). It descends first on the front of the thigh (upper third), and then on its medial side (middle third). It ends at the junction of the middle and lower thirds of the thigh. Here it passes through an aperture in the adductor magnus muscle to reach the back of the thigh where it becomes the *popliteal artery.*

The upper part of the femoral artery lies in the femoral triangle (Fig. 31.1). At the apex of the femoral triangle the artery passes into the adductor canal.

The femoral artery is accompanied by the femoral vein. Just below the inguinal ligament the vein is medial to the artery (Fig. 31.2). However, the vein gradually crosses to the lateral side posterior to artery.

The femoral nerve is lateral to the upper part of the artery (Fig. 31.3). Lower down the artery is related to the branches of the nerve, some of which cross it.

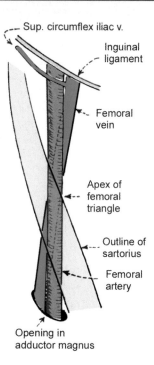

Fig. 31.2. Relationship of femoral artery to femoral vein.

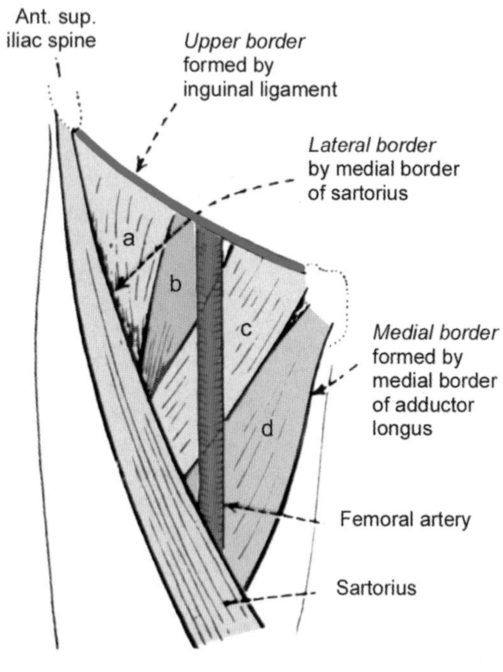

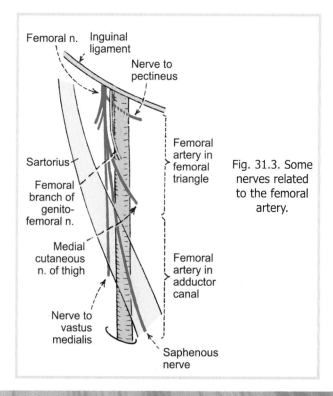

Fig. 31.1. Boundaries of the femoral triangle.

Fig. 31.3. Some nerves related to the femoral artery.

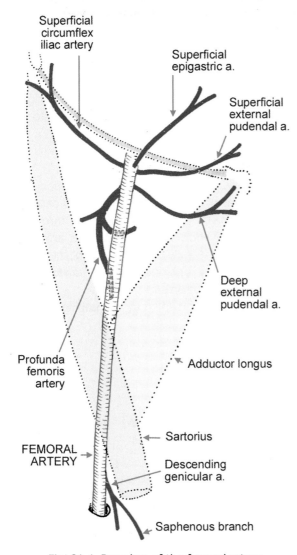

Fig. 31.4. Branches of the femoral artery.

The ***superficial external pudendal*** artery runs medially to supply the skin over the external genitalia and on the lower part of the abdomen.

The ***deep external pudendal*** artery runs medially and supplies the external genitalia.

The ***descending genicular*** artery arises from the femoral near its lower end. It gives numerous muscular branches, articular branches to the knee joint and a saphenous branch which accompanies the saphenous nerve (through the adductor canal) and supplies the skin over the upper and medial part of the leg.

Profunda femoris artery

The ***profunda femoris*** artery is the largest branch of the femoral artery (Fig. 31.5). It is the main artery of supply for the muscles of the thigh. It arises from the lateral side of the femoral artery, 3 to 4 cm below the inguinal ligament. It descends first lateral to the femoral vessels and then behind them. In the lower part of its course it is separated from the femoral artery by the adductor longus. It gives off several branches that are shown in Fig. 31.5. These are the ***medial and lateral circumflex femoral arteries,*** and three ***perforating arteries.*** The terminal part of the profunda femoris artery itself is called the fourth perforating artery.

The perforating branches pass through several muscles attached to the femur, at or near the linea aspera.

In the upper part of the femoral triangle the femoral artery and vein are enclosed in a funnel-like covering of fascia which is called the ***femoral sheath.*** The cavity within the femoral sheath is divisible into three parts. The lateral part contains the femoral artery. The middle part contains the femoral vein. The medial part is occupied only by some lymph nodes and some areolar tissue: this part is called the ***femoral canal.***

Branches of The Femoral Artery

These are shown in Fig. 31.4. The first three branches are superficial and the remaining are deep. The superficial branches arise from the femoral artery just below the inguinal ligament; and piercing the femoral sheath and the cribriform fascia they become subcutaneous. Their further course is given below.

The ***superficial epigastric*** artery ascends across the inguinal ligament and then runs upwards and medially towards the umbilicus.

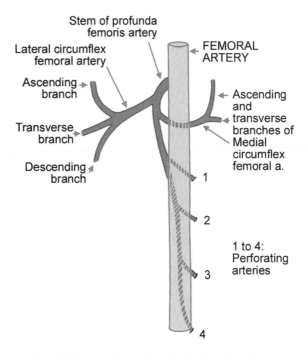

Fig. 31.5. Branches of profunda femoris artery.

Lateral circumflex artery (Fig. 31.5):

Its *ascending branch* passes laterally to the lateral side of the hip joint.

The *transverse branch* winds round the lateral side of the femur and takes part in forming the cruciate anastomosis (Fig. 31.6).

The *descending branch* runs downwards. Some of its branches reach the knee.

Medial circumflex artery (Fig. 31.5)

This artery winds round the medial side of the femur passing through muscles. It emerges on the back of the thigh. It then divides into transverse and ascending branches. The *transverse branch* takes part in forming the cruciate anastomosis. The *ascending branch* ascends to reach the trochanteric fossa. The medial circumflex artery also gives an *acetabular branch* to the hip joint.

Superior and Inferior Gluteal arteries

In Fig. 31.6 also observe some other arteries of the gluteal region. The superior and inferior gluteal arteries arise within the pelvis from the internal iliac artery. They enter the gluteal region through the greater sciatic foramen and supply muscles there. The inferior gluteal artery takes part in forming the cruciate anastomosis.

THE POPLITEAL ARTERY

The popliteal artery begins at the junction of middle and lower thirds of the thigh. It is continuous with the lower end of the femoral artery through the opening in the adductor magnus. The artery runs downwards and laterally over the floor of the popliteal fossa. It ends by dividing into the *anterior* and *posterior tibial arteries.*

The artery is accompanied by the popliteal vein and the tibial nerve.

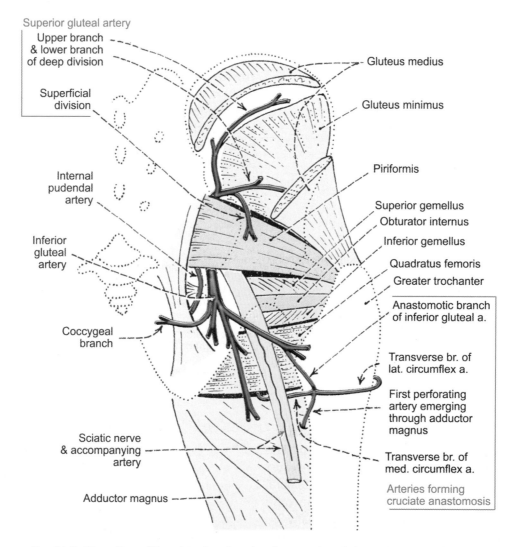

Fig. 31.6. Dissection of the gluteal region showing arteries of the region. Note the arteries taking part in the cruciate anastomosis.

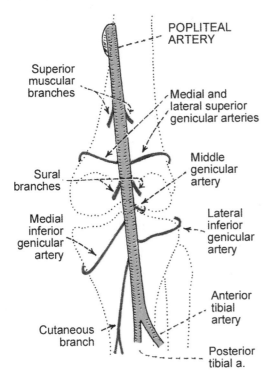

Fig. 31.7. Branches of popliteal artery.

Branches Of The Popliteal Artery

The popliteal artery terminates by dividing into the **anterior** and the **posterior tibial** arteries. Other branches are shown in Fig. 31.7.

Anastomoses around the knee joint

The knee is surrounded by complex arterial anastomoses as shown in Fig. 31.8.

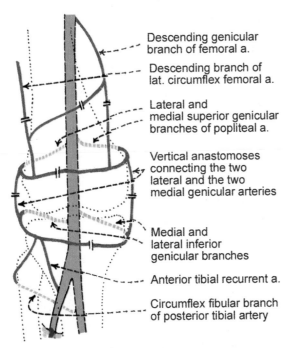

Fig. 31.8. Anastomoses around the knee joint.

THE ANTERIOR TIBIAL ARTERY

The anterior tibial artery begins as a terminal branch of the popliteal artery. Its origin is, therefore, situated in the upper part of the back of the leg. Almost immediately the artery turns forwards through the upper part of the interosseus membrane to enter the anterior compartment of the leg. It now descends over the anterior surface of the interosseus membrane and in front of the tibia. It terminates in front of the ankle joint, by becoming continuous with the **dorsalis pedis** artery.

The **branches of the anterior tibial artery** are shown in Fig. 31.9. They are as follows.

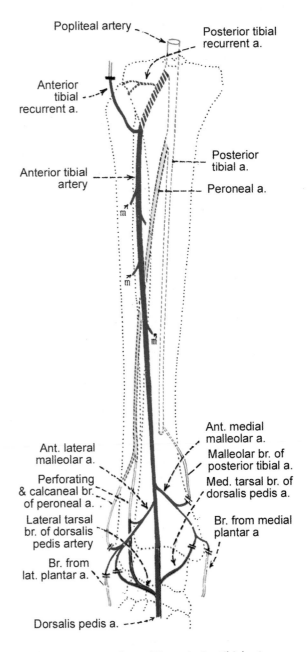

Fig. 31.9. Branches of the anterior tibial artery.

The **anterior tibial recurrent artery** ascends to take part in the anastomoses around the knee.

The **posterior tibial recurrent artery** arises from the uppermost part of the anterior tibial artery in the back of the leg. It supplies the superior tibiofibular joint.

Numerous muscular branches (m) supply muscles of the anterior compartment of the leg.

The **anterior lateral malleolar artery** arises near the ankle and runs to the lateral malleolus.

The **anterior medial malleolar artery** arises near the ankle and runs to the medial malleolus.

The Dorsalis Pedis Artery

This artery is also called the **dorsal artery of the foot**. It is the continuation of the anterior tibial artery. Beginning in front of the ankle it runs forwards, downwards and medially on the dorsum of the foot to reach the space between the first and second metatarsal bones. Here it turns downwards through the space to enter the sole of the foot.

The **branches of the dorsalis pedis artery** are shown in Fig. 31.10.

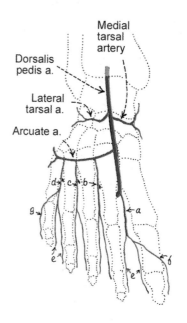

Fig. 31.10. Branches of dorsalis pedis artery.

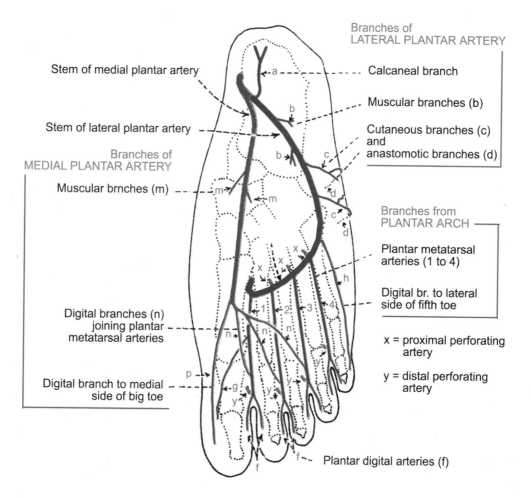

Fig. 31.11. Scheme to show branches of the medial and lateral plantar arteries.

MEDIAL PLANTAR ARTERY

The medial plantar artery is a terminal branch of the posterior tibial artery. It begins behind the medial malleolus, deep to the flexor retinaculum, and runs distally along the medial border of the sole of the foot. The branches of the artery are shown in Fig. 31.11.

LATERAL PLANTER ARTERY

This is the other terminal branch of the posterior tibial artery. It begins behind the medial malleolus deep to the flexor retinaculum. From here it runs obliquely across the sole to reach the base of the fifth metatarsal bone. The artery now turns medially and runs deep in the sole across the bases of the metatarsal bones. This part of the artery is called the **plantar arch**. It ends by joining the termination of the dorsalis pedis artery (in the interval between the bases of the first and second metatarsal bones).

The branches of the lateral plantar artery (including those of the plantar arch) are shown in Fig. 31.11.

VEINS OF THE LOWER LIMBS

The veins of the lower limbs can be divided into deep and superficial veins (like those of the upper limbs). The deep veins are placed subjacent to the deep fascia, and run along arteries. The superficial veins lie in the superficial fascia and many of them can be seen through the skin. The superficial veins drain into deep veins at their termination. They are also connected to deep veins through perforating veins that pass through deep fascia.

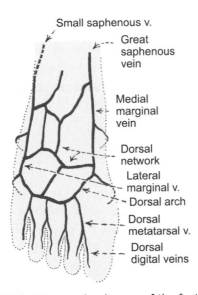

Small saphenous v.

Great saphenous vein

Medial marginal vein

Dorsal network

Lateral marginal v.

Dorsal arch

Dorsal metatarsal v.

Dorsal digital veins

Fig. 13.12. Veins on the dorsum of the foot.

Deep veins of lower limbs:

The deep veins are the femoral; the popliteal; the anterior and posterior tibial; medial and lateral plantar; the plantar venous arch; and metatarsal and digital veins. These veins accompany the corresponding arteries and (by and large) have tributaries corresponding to the branches of the arteries.

FEMORAL VEIN

The course of the femoral vein corresponds to that of the femoral artery. The relationship of the femoral vein to the femoral artery is shown in Fig. 31.2.

The chief tributaries of the femoral vein are the great saphenous vein, the profunda femoris vein; the medial and lateral circumflex femoral veins; and a number of muscular branches. Note that the medial and lateral circumflex veins generally open directly into the femoral vein and not through the profunda femoris vein. The veins accompanying the superficial branches of the femoral artery (viz., the superficial circumflex iliac, the superficial epigastric and the superficial external pudendal) end in the great saphenous vein and not directly into the femoral vein.

THE POPLITEAL VEIN

The course of the popliteal vein is similar to that of the popliteal artery. The chief tributaries of the popliteal vein are the anterior and posterior tibial veins, and the short saphenous vein. Smaller tributaries correspond to branches of the popliteal artery.

Superficial veins of the lower limbs:

The dorsal and plantar surfaces of the foot are covered by subcutaneous venous plexuses. On the dorsum of the foot a **dorsal venous arch** can be recognized (Fig. 31.12). Dorsal digital and dorsal metatarsal veins drain into this arch. Along the sides of the foot there are medial and lateral **marginal veins**) that communicate with both the plantar and dorsal venous networks. These veins are continued into two large superficial veins, the **great (or long) saphenous vein**, and the **small (or short) saphenous vein** respectively.

The **great saphenous vein** is a continuation of the medial marginal vein of the foot. It ascends into the leg a little in front of the medial malleolus. Ascending on the medial side of the leg it crosses the medial side of the knee joint, and ascends on the medial side of the thigh. In the upper part of the thigh it passes somewhat laterally and passes through an aperture in the deep fascia (saphenous opening) to end in the femoral vein (Fig. 31.13).

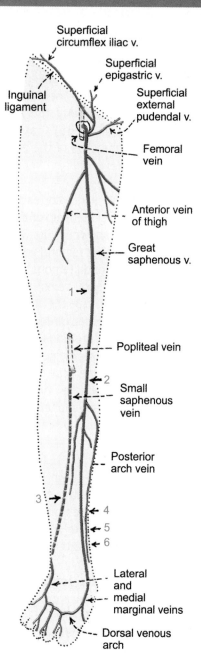

Fig. 31.13. Superficial veins of the lower limb. Numbered arrows indicate the position of perforating veins.

The great saphenous vein receives numerous tributaries. Just before it pierces the deep fascia it receives the superficial epigastric, superficial circumflex iliac and external pudendal veins: these veins accompany the corresponding arteries. It also receives the ***anterior cutaneous vein of the thigh*** which drains the lower part of the front of the thigh. Just below the knee it receives the ***anterior vein of the leg***, and the ***posterior arch vein***. Over the dorsum of the foot the great saphenous vein receives the ***medial marginal vein*** of the foot. The great saphenous vein is connected to the deep veins of the leg and thigh through a number of ***perforating veins*** that are mentioned below.

The ***small (or short) saphenous vein*** is a continuation of the lateral marginal vein of the foot. It ascends behind the lateral malleolus, and runs upwards along the middle of the back of the leg. Over the lower part of the popliteal fossa it perforates the deep fascia and ends in the popliteal vein a few centimeters above the knee joint (Fig. 31.13).

Perforating veins

The perforating veins (or perforators) are so called as they perforate through the deep fascia connect to connect the superficial veins to deep veins. Valves in them allow blood flow from superficial to deep veins, but not in the reverse direction. Similar communications with deep veins exist where the great and small saphenous veins end in deep veins.

PART SIX

THE
TRUNK

32

Bones of the Trunk

THE VERTEBRAL COLUMN

STRUCTURE OF A TYPICAL VERTEBRA

The parts of a typical vertebra are best seen by examining a vertebra from the mid-thoracic region. Such a vertebra is seen from above in Fig. 32.1 and from behind in Fig. 32.2. A lateral view of two such vertebrae is shown in Fig. 32.3. The following parts can be distinguished.

(**1**) The ***body*** lies anteriorly. It is shaped like a short cylinder, being rounded from side to side, and having flat upper and lower surfaces that are attached to those of adjoining vertebrae through ***intervertebral discs*** (Fig. 32.3).

(**2**) The ***pedicles*** (right and left) are short rounded bars that project backwards, and somewhat laterally, from the posterior part of the body.

(**3**) Each pedicle is continuous, postero-medially, with a vertical plate of bone called the ***lamina***. The laminae of the two sides pass backwards and medially to meet in the middle line. The pedicles and laminae together constitute the ***vertebral arch***.

(**4**) Bounded anteriorly by the posterior aspect of the body, on the sides by the pedicles, and behind by the laminae, there is a large ***vertebral foramen***. Each vertebral foramen forms a short segment of the ***vertebral canal*** that runs through the whole length of the vertebral column and transmits the spinal cord.

(**5**) Passing backwards (and usually downwards) from the junction of the two laminae, there is the ***spine*** (or ***spinous process***).

(**6**) Passing laterally (and usually somewhat downwards) from the junction of each pedicle and the corresponding lamina there is a ***transverse process***. The spinous and transverse processes serve as levers for muscles acting on the vertebral column.

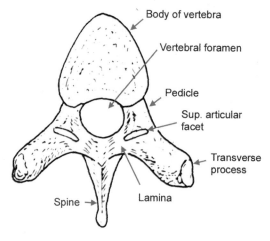

Fig. 32.1. Typical vertebra seen from above.

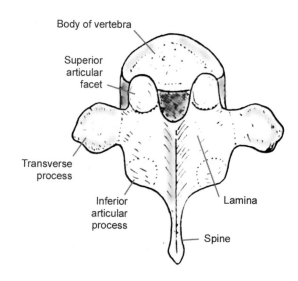

Fig. 32.2. Typical vertebra seen from behind.

When the vertebrae are viewed from the lateral side (Fig. 32.3) we see certain additional features.

(**7**) Projecting upwards from the junction of the pedicle and the laminae there is, on either side, a ***superior articular process***; and projecting downwards there is an ***inferior articular process***. Each process bears a smooth articular facet: the ***superior facet*** is directed

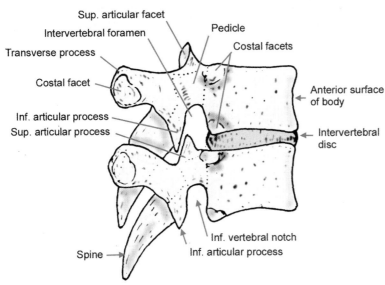

Fig. 32.3. Typical vertebrae seen from the lateral side. (Costal facets, for ribs, are shown on the bodies and transverses processes: they are present only in the thoracic region).

(**c**) A lumbar vertebra (Fig. 32.6) can be distinguished by the fact that it neither has foramina transversaria nor does it bear facets for ribs. It is also recognized by the large size of its body.

We may now consider additional differences between cervical, thoracic and lumbar vertebrae.

(**1**) The vertebral bodies progressively increase in size from above downwards. They are, therefore, smallest in the cervical vertebrae and largest in the lumbar vertebrae. In shape the body is oval in the cervical and lumbar regions and triangular or heart shaped in the thoracic region.

In the thoracic region the head of a typical rib articulates with the sides of the bodies of two vertebrae (Fig. 32.7).

posteriorly and somewhat laterally, and the ***inferior facet*** is directed forwards and some what medially.

The superior facet of one vertebra articulates with the inferior facet of the vertebra above it. Two adjoining vertebrae, therefore, articulate at three joints: two between the right and left articular processes and one between the bodies of the vertebrae (through the intervertebral disc).

(**8**) In Fig. 32.3 note that the pedicle is much narrower (in vertical diameter) than the body and is attached nearer its upper border. As a result there is a large ***inferior vertebral notch*** below the pedicle. The notch is bounded in front by the posterior surface of the body of the vertebra, and behind by the inferior articular process. Above the pedicle there is a much shallower ***superior vertebral notch***. The superior and inferior notches of adjoining vertebrae join to form the ***intervertebral foramina*** which give passage to spinal nerves emerging from the spinal cord.

Distinguishing features of Typical Cervical, Thoracic and Lumbar Vertebrae

The cervical, thoracic and lumbar vertebrae can be easily distinguished from one another because of the following characteristics.

(**a**) The transverse process of a cervical vertebra is pierced by a foramen called the ***foramen transversarium*** (Fig. 32.4).

(**b**) The thoracic vertebrae bear ***costal facets*** for articulation with ribs. These are present on the sides of the vertebral bodies and on the transverse processes (Fig. 32.3).

For this purpose each side of the body of a typical thoracic vertebra bears two costal facets, upper and lower, adjoining its upper and lower borders (Fig. 32.3). The upper facet is large and articulates with the

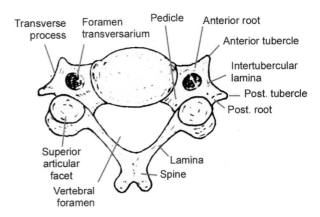

Fig. 32.4. Typical cervical vertebra seen from above.

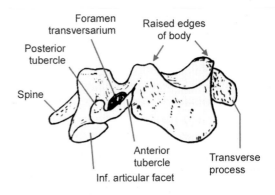

Fig. 32.5. Typical cervical vertebra seen from the anterolateral side.

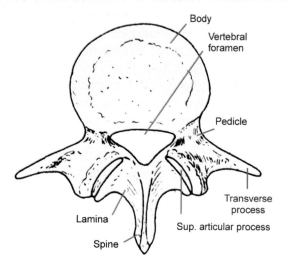

Fig. 32.6. Typical lumbar vertebra seen from above.

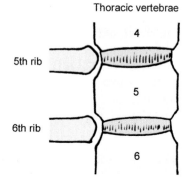

Fig. 32.7. Scheme showing the numerical relationship of thoracic vertebrae to ribs.

numerically corresponding rib. The lower, smaller facet articulates with the next lower rib.

(**2**) The vertebral foramen is triangular and large in cervical vertebrae (Fig. 32.4). In the lumbar vertebrae also it is triangular (Fig. 32.6), but in thoracic vertebrae it is small and circular or oval (Fig. 32.1). These variations in size correspond with those of the spinal cord which is largest (in diameter) in the cervical region.

(**3**) The pedicles are long and directed backwards and laterally in the cervical region (Fig. 32.4). In the thoracic region they pass almost directly backwards (Fig. 32.1). They are thick and short in the lumbar region and are directed backwards and somewhat laterally (Fig. 32.6).

(**4**) The laminae of cervical vertebrae are long (transversely) and narrow (vertically) (Fig. 32.4). In the thoracic region they are short (transversely) and so broad (vertically) that the laminae of adjacent vertebrae overlap (Figs. 32.1, 32.2). In the lumbar region also they are short and broad, but do not overlap (Fig. 32.6).

(**5**) The spinous processes are short and bifid in a typical cervical vertebra (Fig. 32.4). They are long and project downwards in the thoracic region (Fig. 32.3). In lumbar vertebrae they are large and quadrangular (Fig. 32.8).

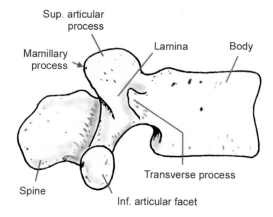

Fig. 32.8. Typical lumbar vertebra seen from the lateral side.

(**6**) The transverse processes of typical cervical vertebrae (Fig. 32.9A) are relatively short and, as mentioned earlier, they are pierced by foramina transversaria. The part of the process in front of the foramen is called the *anterior root*; and the part behind it is called the *posterior root*. The part lateral to the foramen is usually called the *costo-transverse bar*, but it is more correct to call it the *intertubercular bar*. The anterior and posterior roots end in thickenings called the *anterior and posterior tubercles* respectively. When viewed from the lateral side the transverse process is seen to be grooved (Fig. 32.5). The cervical nerves lie in these grooves after they pass out of the intervertebral foramina.

The transverse processes of a typical thoracic vertebra are large with solid blunt ends (Figs. 32.1, 32.3). They are directed backwards and laterally. Each process lies just behind the corresponding rib and bears a prominent facet for articulation with the rib.

The lumbar transverse processes are relatively small and often have tapering ends. (Fig. 32.9C).

(**7**) The direction of the articular facets is variable. It is shown diagramatically in Figs. 32.11 to 32.13.

In the cervical region the facets are flat. The superior facets are directed equally backwards and upwards (Also see Fig. 32.4). The inferior facets are directed forwards and downwards (Also see Fig. 32.5).

In the thoracic region again (Fig. 32.12) the facets are flat, and here they are almost vertical. The superior facets face backwards, slightly upwards and slightly laterally (Also see Fig. 32.2). The inferior facets face forwards, slightly downwards and slightly medially.

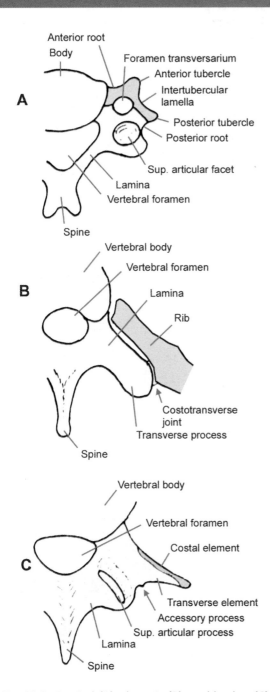

Fig. 32.9. Cervical (A), thoracic (B), and lumbar (C) transverse processes showing the parts derived from the costal elements (red shading).

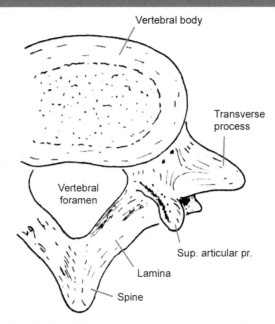

Fig. 32.10. Fifth lumbar vertebra seen from above.

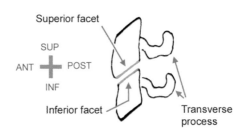

Fig. 32.11. Scheme to show the orientation of the articular facets of cervical vertebrae (lateral view).

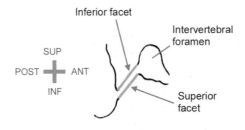

Fig. 32.12. Scheme to show the orientation of the articular facets of thoracic vertebrae (lateral view).

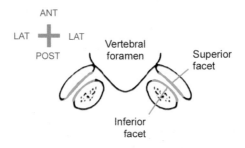

Fig. 32.13. Scheme to show the orientation of the articular facets of lumbar vertebrae. The facets are seen from above. The inferior processes are cut across.

In the lumbar region the facets are vertical. They are curved from side to side (Fig. 32.13). The superior facets are slightly concave (Also see Fig. 32.6) and are directed equally backwards and medially. The inferior facets are slightly convex, and are directed equally forwards and laterally (Also see Fig. 32.8). Each superior articular process of a lumbar vertebra bears a rough projection called the mamillary process, on its posterior border.

In the cervical region the superior and inferior articular processes form a solid *articular pillar* that helps to

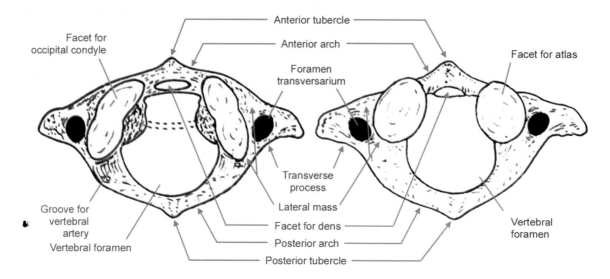

Fig. 32.14. The atlas (first cervical vertebra) seen from above.

Fig. 32.15. The atlas (first cervical vertebra) seen from below.

transmit some weight from one vertebra to the next lower one. This is not so in the thoracic and lumbar regions.

Joints between adjacent vertebrae are described in Chapter 33.

ATYPICAL CERVICAL VERTEBRAE

The Atlas (First Cervical) Vertebra

The first cervical vertebra is called the atlas. It looks very different from a typical cervical vertebra as it has no body, and no spine (Figs. 32.14, 32.15).

It consists of two **lateral masses** joined anteriorly by a short **anterior arch**, and posteriorly by a much longer **posterior arch**. The arches give the atlas a ring like appearance. A large transverse process, pierced by a foramen transversarium, projects laterally from the lateral mass. The superior aspect of each lateral mass shows an elongated concave facet which articulates with the corresponding condyle of the occipital bone (to form an **atlanto-occipital joint**). Nodding and lateral movements of the head take place at the two (right and left) atlanto-occipital joints. The inferior aspect of each lateral mass (Fig. 32.15) shows a large oval (almost circular) facet for articulation with the corresponding superior articular facet of the axis (second cervical vertebra) to form a **lateral atlanto-axial joint**. The medial side of the lateral mass shows a tubercle which gives attachment to the transverse ligament of the atlas (shown in dotted line in Fig. 32.14). This ligament divides the large foramen (bounded by the lateral masses and the arches) into anterior and

posterior parts. The posterior part corresponds to the vertebral foramen of a typical vertebra: the spinal cord passes through it. The anterior part is occupied by the dens (which is an upward projection from the body of the axis). The dens articulates with the posterior aspect of the anterior arch, which bears a circular facet for it. The dens also articulates with the transverse ligament, these two articulations collectively forming the **median atlanto-occipital joint**. In side to side movements of the head the atlas moves with the skull around the pivot formed by the dens.

The anterior arch bears a small midline projection called the anterior tubercle. The posterior arch bears a similar projection, the posterior tubercle, which may be regarded as a rudimentary spine.

The Axis (Second Cervical) Vertebra

The most conspicuous feature of the axis, which distinguishes it from all other vertebrae, is the presence of a thick finger like projection arising from the upper part of the body. This projection is called the **dens**, or **odontoid process**. We have already seen that the dens fits into the space between the anterior arch of the atlas and its transverse ligament to form the median atlanto-occipital joint. The anterior aspect of the dens bears a convex oval facet (Fig. 32.16) for articulation with the anterior arch. Its posterior aspect shows a transverse groove for the transverse ligament.

On either side of the dens the axis vertebra bears a large oval facet for articulation with the corresponding facet on the inferior aspect of the atlas. The transverse process of the axis lies lateral to this facet. It is small and ends in a single tubercle corresponding to the

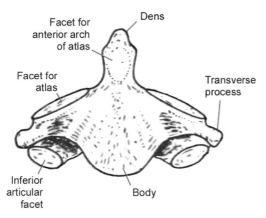

Fig. 32.16. The second cervical vertebra (axis) seen from the front.

posterior tubercle of a typical cervical vertebra. The transverse process is pierced by a foramen transversarium which runs upwards and laterally (to correspond with the lateral direction of the vertebral artery as it passes from the axis to the atlas).

OTHER ATYPICAL VERTEBRAE

First Thoracic Vertebra

This vertebra can be distinguished from a typical thoracic vertebra because of the following features (Figs. 32.17, 32.18). It has a small body similar in shape to that of a cervical vertebra. The superior costal facets

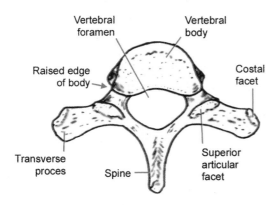

Fig. 32.17. First thoracic vertebra seen from above.

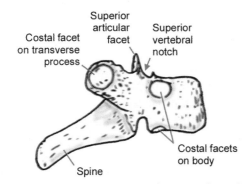

Fig. 32.18. First thoracic vertebra seen from the lateral side.

(on the body) are usually complete as the first rib articulates wholly with this vertebra. The spine is long and horizontal (Fig. 32.18).

Tenth, Eleventh & Twelfth Thoracic Vertebrae

These vertebrae tend to resemble the lumbar vertebrae in the shape and size of their bodies, of the vertebral foramina, and of the spines (Fig. 32.19). They can be distinguished from typical thoracic vertebrae by the fact that they have only one costal facet on each side of the body. The tenth vertebra (normally) has a costal facet on each transverse process. Facets on the transverse processes are absent in the eleventh and twelfth vertebrae.

Fifth Lumbar Vertebra

The fifth lumbar vertebra is the largest of lumbar vertebrae. We have seen that the transverse processes of typical lumbar vertebrae are small and tapering. In contrast the transverse processes of the fifth lumbar vertebra are very large: they form a distinguishing characteristic of this vertebra (Fig. 32.10).

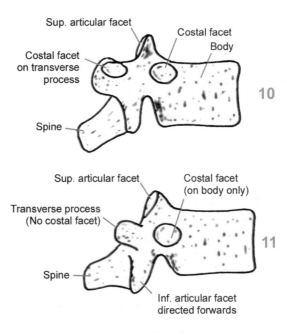

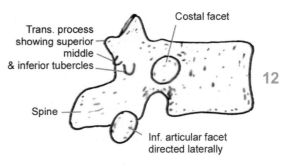

Fig. 32.19. Tenth, eleventh and twelfth thoracic vertebrae seen from the lateral side.

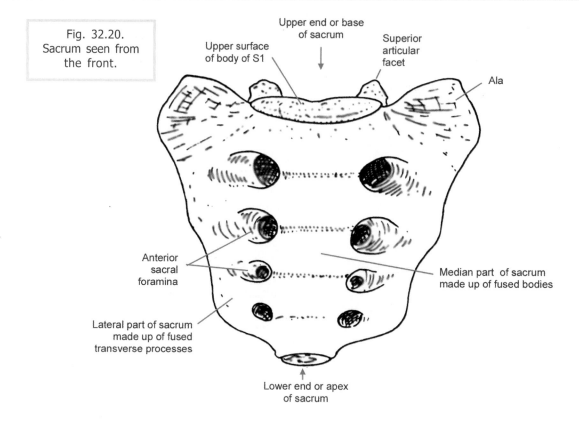

Fig. 32.20. Sacrum seen from the front.

THE SACRUM AND COCCYX

The Sacrum

The sacrum lies below the fifth lumbar vertebra. It is made up of five sacral vertebrae that are fused together (Figs. 32.20 to 32.24). It is wedged between the two hip bones and takes part in forming the pelvis. As a whole the bone is triangular. It has an upper end or *base* which articulates with the fifth lumbar vertebra; a lower end or *apex* which articulates with the coccyx; a concave *anterior (or pelvic) surface*; a convex *posterior or (dorsal) surface* (Fig. 32.22); and right

and left lateral surfaces that articulate with the ilium of the corresponding side (Fig. 32.23).

When viewed from the front (Fig. 32.20) the pelvic surface of the sacrum shows the presence of four pairs of *anterior sacral foramina*. The first foramen is the largest and the fourth the smallest.

The foramina separate the *medial part* of the bone from the *lateral part*. The medial part is formed by the fused bodies of the sacral vertebrae, while the lateral part represents the fused transverse processes, including the costal elements. The anterior sacral foramina, seen on the pelvic surface, are continued into the substance of the bone and become continuous posteriorly with the *posterior sacral foramina* that open on to the dorsal surface. The canals connecting the anterior and posterior foramina open medially into the *sacral canal* which is a downward continuation of the vertebral canal.

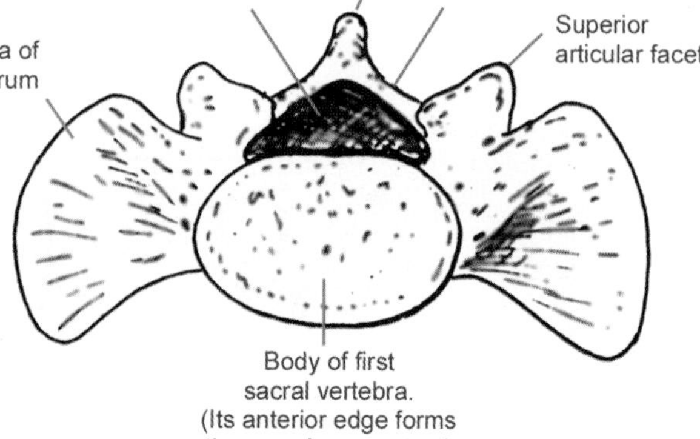

When viewed from above (Fig. 32.21) the base of the sacrum is seen to be formed by the first sacral vertebra in which we can recognize a large oval body that articulates with the body of the fifth lumbar vertebra. The body has a projecting anterior margin called the *sacral promontory*. Behind the body there is a triangular vertebral (or sacral) canal bounded by thick pedicles and laminae. Where the laminae meet there is a small tubercle representing the spine. Arising from the junction of the pedicles and laminae there are the

Fig. 32.21. Sacrum seen from above.

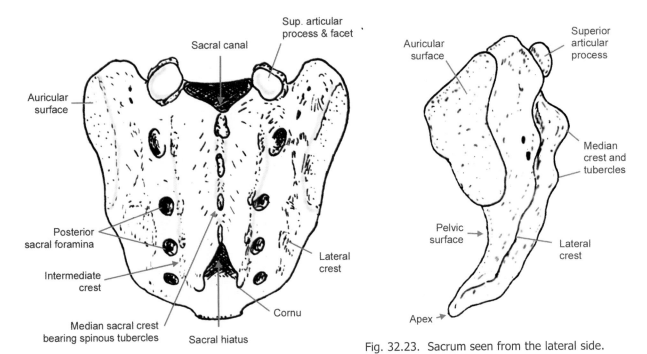

Fig. 32.22. Sacrum seen from behind.

Fig. 32.23. Sacrum seen from the lateral side.

superior articular facets that articulate with the inferior articular facets of the fifth lumbar vertebra. Lateral to the body we see the superior surface of the lateral part, that is also called the ala.

When the sacrum is viewed from behind (Fig. 32.22) we see the dorsal surface. We can again distinguish medial and lateral parts separated by four pairs of posterior sacral foramina. These foramina give passage to the dorsal rami of sacral nerves. The medial part of the dorsum of the sacrum is formed by the fused laminae of sacral vertebrae.

The laminae of the fifth sacral vertebra (sometimes also of the fourth) are deficient leaving an inverted U-shaped or V-shaped gap called the *sacral hiatus*. The midline is marked by a ridge called the *median sacral crest* on which four *spinous tubercles* (representing the spines) can be recognized. Just medial to the dorsal sacral foramina we see four small tubercles that represent fused articular processes: they collectively form the *intermediate crest*. Lateral to the foramina we see a prominent lateral sacral crest formed by the fused transverse processes. The crest is marked by tubercles which represent the tips of the transverse processes.

The lower end of the bone (apex) bears an oval facet for articulation with the coccyx. At the sides of the sacral hiatus we see two small downward projections called the *sacral cornua*. They represent the inferior articular processes of the fifth sacral vertebra. They are connected to the coccyx by ligaments.

When the sacrum is viewed from the side we see that the pelvic aspect of the bone is concave forwards, while the dorsal aspect is convex backwards. The lateral surface bears a large L-shaped *auricular area* (or facet) for articulation with the ilium. (It is so called because its shape resembles that of the auricle or pinna). It consists of a cranial limb present on the first sacral vertebra, and a caudal limb that lies on the second and third sacral vertebrae. The area behind the auricular surface is rough and gives attachment to strong ligaments that connect the sacrum to the ilium.

The Coccyx

The coccyx consists of four rudimentary vertebrae fused together (Fig. 32.24).

It has pelvic and dorsal surfaces. The base or upper end has an oval facet for articulation with the apex of the sacrum. Lateral to the facet there are two cornua

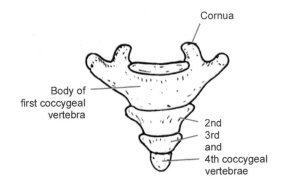

Fig. 32.24. Coccyx seen from the front.

that project upwards and are connected to the cornua of the sacrum by ligaments. The first coccygeal vertebra has rudimentary transverse processes. The remaining vertebrae are represented by nodules of bone.

THE SKULL

The skull consists of a large number of bones. The purpose of this section is to make the student familiar with their names. Detailed study of skull bones is not required.

The bone forming the lower jaw is called the **mandible** (Fig. 32.25). The other bones of the skull are firmly united to one another at joints called **sutures**: these bones collectively form the **cranium**. (Cranium = skull minus mandible).

The cranium consists of two main parts. Its upper and posterior part contains a large **cranial cavity** in which the brain lies. Anteriorly, and inferiorly, the cranium forms the skeleton of the face including the walls of the **orbits** (in which the eyeballs lie), the cavity of the nose, and the upper part of the cavity of the mouth. The upper dome-like part of the skull is called the **vault** or **skull cap**. It forms the upper, lateral, anterior and posterior walls of the cranial cavity. Note that its anterior wall forms the forehead. The part of the skull forming the floor of the cranial cavity is called the base.

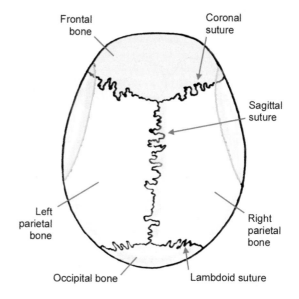

Fig. 32.26. Some features of the skull as seen from above.

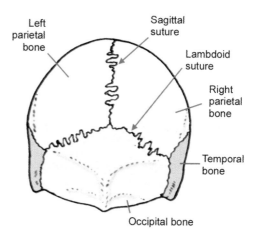

Fig. 32.27. Some features of the skull as seen from behind.

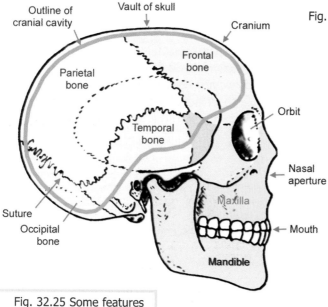

Fig. 32.25 Some features of the skull as seen from the lateral side.

With these preliminary remarks we can proceed to identify the individual bones of the skull.

Looking at the skull from above (Fig. 32.26) we see four bones. The bone forming the anterior part of the vault is the **frontal bone**. The greater part of the roof and side walls of the cranial cavity are formed by the right and left **parietal bones**. The two parietal bones meet in the midline at the **sagittal suture**. Their anterior margins join the frontal bone at the **coronal suture** which runs transversely across the vault. The posterior part of the vault is formed by the **occipital bone** which is better seen when the skull is viewed from behind (Fig. 32.27). The suture joining the occipital bone to the parietal bones is shaped like the Greek letter 'lambda' (which is like an inverted 'Y'). It is, therefore, called the **lambdoid**

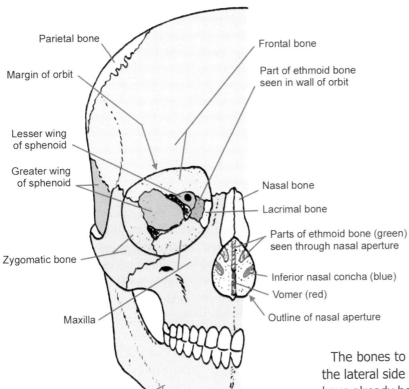

Fig. 32.28. Bones of the skull seen from the front.

aperture we see two large cavities, the right and left **orbits**, in which the eyeballs lie. The walls of the orbits receive contributions from the frontal, zygomatic, and ethmoid bones, from the maxilla, and from two bones not mentioned so far. One of these is a small bone, the **lacrimal**. The other is the **sphenoid**. The sphenoid is a large unpaired bone present in the base of the skull, and only a small part of it is seen in each orbit. A part of the sphenoid called the **greater wing** is also seen on the lateral surface of the skull. Lying in the area between the two orbits we see the right and left **nasal bones**. They lie just above the nasal aperture.

The bones to be seen when the skull is viewed from the lateral side are shown in Fig. 32.29. Many of these have already been seen from the front, from above, or from behind. These include the frontal, parietal, and occipital bones (in the vault), and the ethmoid, lacrimal, nasal and zygomatic bones (in the facial region). The maxilla, the mandible, and the greater wing of the sphenoid are also seen. Below the parietal bone the lateral wall of the cranium is formed by the squamous part of the **temporal bone**. Lower down the mastoid part of the same bone lies in relation to the base of skull. The temporal bone gives off a process that joins

suture. Lateral to the occipital bone we see a part of the temporal bone (which is better seen when the skull is viewed from the lateral side)(Fig. 32.29).

When the skull is viewed from the front (Fig. 32.28) the most conspicuous features are the **jaws** which bear the teeth. The bone forming the lower jaw is called the **mandible**. The upper jaw is formed by the right and left **maxillae**. The region of the forehead is formed by the frontal bone. The prominence of the cheek is formed by the **zygomatic bone**. Three large openings can be seen. A **median nasal aperture** is present between the two maxillae: it leads into the **nasal cavities**. In the depth of the aperture we can make out parts of three bones. These are the **ethmoid**, the **inferior nasal concha**, and the **vomer**. Above and lateral to the nasal

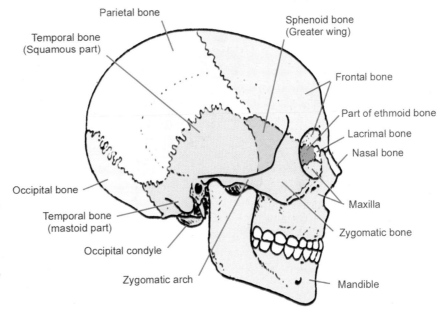

Fig. 32.29. Lateral view of the skull showing the position of individual bones.

(a process of) the zygomatic bone to form the **zygomatic arch**.

When the skull is viewed from below (Fig. 32.30) we see parts of several bones already identified. These are the maxilla, the sphenoid, the temporal and the occipital bone . We also see parts of the zygomatic bone and of the vomer; and the **palatine bone** which is seen for the first time.

The maxillae bear the upper teeth. Lateral to the teeth a part of the maxilla is seen articulating with the zygomatic bone. Medial to the teeth the maxilla forms the anterior part of the **bony palate**. The posterior part of the palate is formed by the right and left palatine bones. Above the posterior edge of the palate we see the posterior openings of the right and left nasal cavities which are separated by the vomer. Part of the vomer has been seen on the front of the skull through the anterior nasal aperture.

Behind the vomer we see the **sphenoid** which is an unpaired bone. It has a median part, the body. On either side of the body there is a greater wing (which is seen partly on the base of the skull and partly on the lateral wall: Fig. 32.29). Posteriorly, the body of the sphenoid is continuous with the basilar part of the occipital bone. Just behind the basilar part the occipital bone has a large foramen, the **foramen magnum** through which the cranial cavity communicates with the vertebral canal. Posterior to the foramen magnum the occipital bone forms a large part of the base of the skull.

The lateral part of the base of the skull is formed by the temporal bone which is wedged in between the sphenoid and occipital bones. It consists of a medial **petrous** (= stone like) **part**, a posterolateral **mastoid part**, and an anterolateral **squamous part** that is seen mainly on the lateral wall of the skull. The temporal bone gives off a process that joins the zygomatic bone to form the **zygomatic arch**. (Some other parts of the temporal bone will be identified later).

When the top of the skull (skull cap) is removed by a transverse cut we can view the floor of the cranial cavity (Fig. 32.31). It is seen to be divided into three depressions called the **cranial fossae**: anterior, middle (shaded with dots), and posterior. The floor of the **anterior cranial fossa** is formed mainly by the frontal bone, but near the midline, anteriorly, a small part is formed by the ethmoid. This bone lies mainly in the wall of the nasal cavity. A part of it has been seen in the wall of the orbit, and another part through the anterior nasal aperture. More posteriorly the median part of the floor of the anterior fossa is formed by a part of the body of the sphenoid; and the lateral parts by the lesser wings of the sphenoid.

The floor of each half of the anterior cranial fossa has a sharp posterior margin that separates

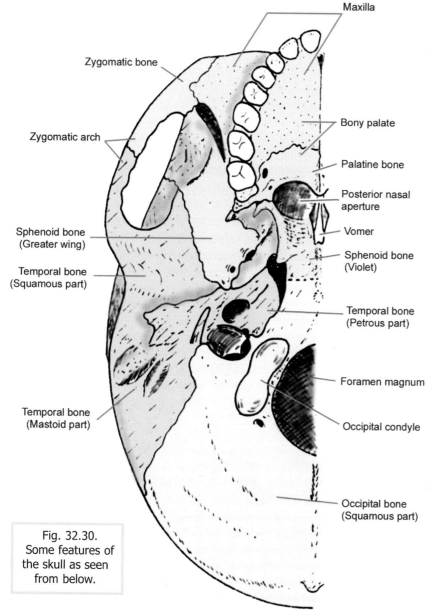

Maxilla

Zygomatic bone

Zygomatic arch

Sphenoid bone (Greater wing)

Temporal bone (Squamous part)

Temporal bone (Mastoid part)

Bony palate

Palatine bone

Posterior nasal aperture

Vomer

Sphenoid bone (Violet)

Temporal bone (Petrous part)

Foramen magnum

Occipital condyle

Occipital bone (Squamous part)

Fig. 32.30. Some features of the skull as seen from below.

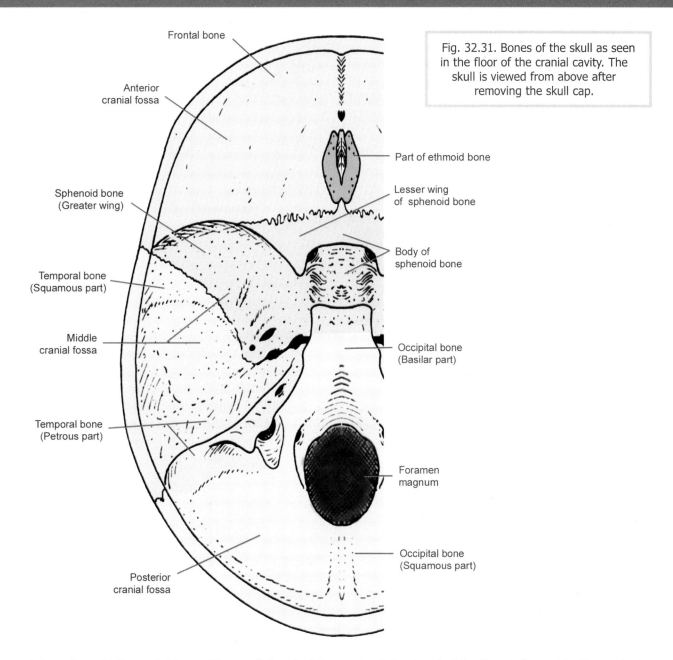

Fig. 32.31. Bones of the skull as seen in the floor of the cranial cavity. The skull is viewed from above after removing the skull cap.

Frontal bone

Anterior cranial fossa

Sphenoid bone (Greater wing)

Temporal bone (Squamous part)

Middle cranial fossa

Temporal bone (Petrous part)

Posterior cranial fossa

Part of ethmoid bone

Lesser wing of sphenoid bone

Body of sphenoid bone

Occipital bone (Basilar part)

Foramen magnum

Occipital bone (Squamous part)

it from the middle cranial fossa. The medial part of the margin is formed by the lesser wing of the sphenoid, and its lateral part by the frontal bone.

The floor of the *middle cranial fossa* is narrow (antero-posteriorly) in its median part, and broad laterally. The narrow median part is formed by the body of the sphenoid. The broad lateral part (which is also much deeper) is formed by the greater wing of the sphenoid, the squamous part of the temporal bone, and by the anterior surface of the petrous part of the same bone.

The greater part of the floor of the *posterior cranial fossa* is formed by the occipital bone. The foramen magnum is seen in the deepest part of the fossa. The

anterolateral part of the floor is formed by the posterior surface of the petrous temporal bone.

Most Important Foramina of the Skull

1. The *lower end of the medulla oblongata* passes through the *foramen magnum* to become continuous with the spinal cord.

2. The *internal carotid artery* enters the skull by passing through the *carotid canal*.

3. The junction of the upper end of the internal jugular vein with the *sigmoid sinus* lies in the *jugular foramen*.

4. Bundles of nerve fibres that constitute *the olfactory nerve* pass through minute apertures in the cribriform plate of the ethmoid bone. This plate

intervenes between the nasal cavity and the anterior cranial fossa.

5, The *optic nerve* passes from the middle cranial fossa into the orbit through the *optic canal*.

6. The *oculomotor, trochlear and abducent nerves* enter the orbit through the *superior orbital fissure*.

7. The trigeminal nerve has three divisions each of which leaves the middle cranial fossa through a different foramen. The *ophthalmic division* enters the orbit through the *superior orbital fissure*. The *maxillary division* passes into the *foramen rotundum*, while the *mandibular division* passes through the *foramen ovale* to reach the infratemporal region.

8. The *facial nerve* leaves the posterior cranial fossa by passing into the *internal acoustic meatus*. After a complicated course through the petrous part of the temporal bone, it emerges through the *stylomastoid foramen*.

9. The *vestibulocochlear nerve* leaves the posterior cranial fossa by passing through the *internal acoustic meatus*, to reach the internal ear which lies within the substance of the petrous part of the temporal bone.

10. The *glossopharyngeal, vagus* and *accessory nerves* leave the posterior cranial fossa through the *jugular foramen*, to enter the neck.

11. The *hypoglossal nerve* leaves the posterior cranial fossa through the *hypoglossal canal*.

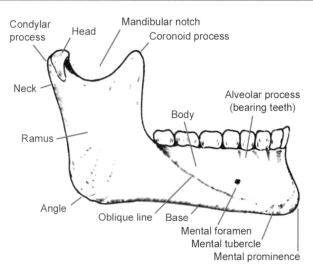

Fig. 32.33. Right half of mandible seen from the lateral side.

THE MANDIBLE

The mandible is the bone of the lower jaw and bears the lower teeth (Figs. 32.32 to 32.36). It consists of an anterior U-shaped *body*, and of two *rami* (right and left) that project upwards from the posterior part of the body. The bone has internal (or medial) and external (or lateral) surfaces. The body has an upper part that bears the teeth (*alveolar process*), and a lower border that is called the *base*. The ramus has a posterior border, a sharp anterior border, and a lower border that is continuous with the base of the body. The posterior and inferior borders of the ramus meet at the *angle* of the mandible. The anterior border of the ramus is continued downwards and forwards on the lateral surface of the body as the *oblique line*. This line ends anteriorly near the *mental tubercle* (see below). A little above the anterior part of the oblique line we see the *mental foramen* which lies vertically below the second premolar tooth. Just below the incisor teeth the external surface of the ramus shows a shallow *incisive fossa*.

Arising from the upper part of the ramus there are two processes. The anterior of these is the *coronoid process*. It is flat (from side to side) and triangular. The posterior or *condylar process* is separated from the coronoid process by the *mandibular notch*. The upper end of the condylar process is expanded to form the *head* of the mandible. The head is elongated transversely and is convex both transversely and in an anteroposterior direction. It bears a smooth articular surface that articulates with the mandibular fossa of the temporal bone to form the temporomandibular joint. The part immediately below the head is constricted and forms the *neck*. Its anterior surface has a rough depression called the *pterygoid fovea*.

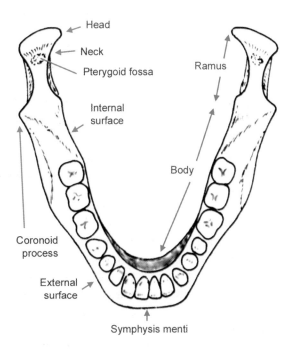

Fig. 32.32. The mandible seen from above.

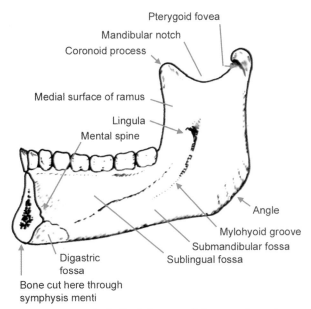

Fig. 32.34. Right half of the mandible seen from the medial side.

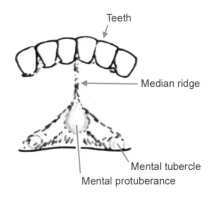

Fig. 32.35. Median part of the mandible, anterior aspect.

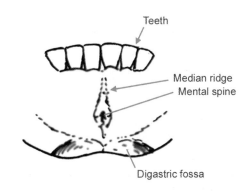

Fig. 32.36. Median part of mandible, posterior aspect.

In Fig. 32.34 the mandible is seen from the medial side. A little above the centre of the medial surface of the ramus we see the *mandibular foramen*. It leads into the mandibular canal which runs forwards in the substance of the mandible.

The medial margin of the foramen is formed by a projection called the *lingula*. Beginning just behind the lingula and running downwards and forwards we see the *mylohyoid groove*. A little above and anterior to the mylohyoid groove, the inner surface of the body of the mandible is marked by a ridge called the *mylohyoid line*. The posterior end of this line lies a little below and behind the third molar tooth. From here the line runs downwards and forwards to reach the symphysis menti (see below). The mylohyoid line divides the inner surface of the body into a *sublingual fossa* (lying above the line), and a *submandibular fossa* (lying below the line).

Just below the anterior end of the mylohyoid line the base of the mandible is marked by a deep *digastric fossa*. In the newborn the mandible consists of right and left halves that are joined to each other at the *symphysis menti*; but in later life the halves fuse to form one bone.

When viewed from the front (Fig. 32.35) the region of the symphysis menti is usually marked by a slight ridge. Inferiorly, the ridge expands to form a triangular raised area called the *mental protuberance*. The lateral angles of the protuberance are prominent and constitute the *mental tubercles*.

The posterior aspect of the symphysis menti also shows a median ridge (Fig. 32.36) the lower part of

which is enlarged and may be divided into upper and lower parts called the *mental spines* or *genial tubercles*.

THE STERNUM

The sternum lies in the anterior wall of the thorax, in the midline (Fig. 32.37). It is elongated vertically. It is flat and has anterior and posterior surfaces. Although it is (by convention) spoken of as a single bone it consists of three separate parts. From above downwards these are the *manubrium*, the *body*, and the *xiphoid process*.

The manubrium joins the body at the *manubriosternal joint*. The body joins the xiphoid process at the *xiphisternal joint*. The anterior ends of the upper seven costal cartilages are attached to the right and left margins of the sternum. The first costal cartilage is attached to the lateral margin of the manubrium. The second costal cartilage is attached partly to the manubrium, and partly to the upper end of the body. The third, fourth, fifth and sixth cartilages are attached to the lateral margin of the body. The

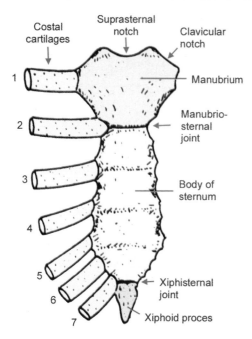

Fig. 32.37. Sternum and costal cartilages seen from the front.

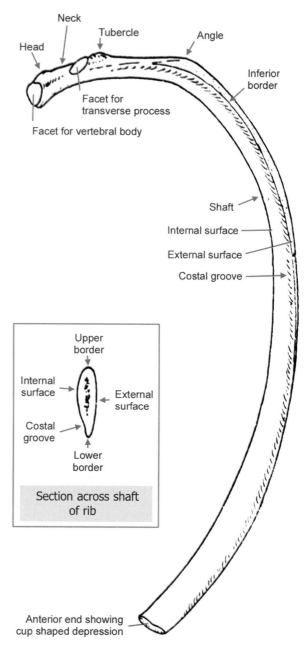

Fig. 32.38. A typical rib seen from below.

seventh costal cartilage is attached to the lateral side of the xiphisternal joint. The area of attachment of each cartilage is marked by a notch on the lateral margin of the sternum.

The upper border of the manubrium articulates, on either side, with the medial end of the clavicle to form the **sternoclavicular joint**. It bears prominent **clavicular notches** for this purpose. Between the right and left clavicular notches there is a median depression called the **jugular or suprasternal notch**. The manubrium and the body of the sternum lie at a slight angle to one another, and because of this fact the manubriosternal junction projects forwards. This projection forms a surface landmark and is often referred to as the **sternal angle**. The sternal angle forms a useful guide in identifying individual costal cartilages and ribs in the living subject.

The body of the sternum consists of four parts or **sternebrae** that are united by cartilage up to the age of puberty, but fuse thereafter to form a single bone. The lines of fusion can be seen on the anterior aspect of the bone.

The manubriosternal joint is a symphysis. The xiphoid process is cartilaginous in children, but undergoes ossification in the adult. After this happens the xiphisternal joint is said to be a symphysis. However, unlike a typical symphysis the joint disappears in old age and the xiphoid process and the body of the sternum become united by bone. The junction of the first costal cartilage with the manubrium is a synchondrosis. The other sternocostal joints usually have a joint cavity (i.e., they are synovial joints).

The posterior aspect of the manubrium is related to the arch of the aorta and its branches, and to the left brachiocephalic vein. Its lateral part is related to lungs and pleura. The body of the sternum is also related to lungs and pleura and to pericardium. The xiphoid process is related to the liver.

THE RIBS

TYPICAL RIBS

The ribs are curved long bones that form the side walls of the thorax (Fig. 32.38). There are twelve ribs on either side. They vary considerably in length: the seventh rib is the longest, those above and below it becoming progressively shorter. Adjacent ribs are separated by *intercostal spaces*.

The ribs are attached behind to the thoracic vertebrae. The anterior ends of the upper seven ribs are attached to bars of cartilage (*costal cartilages*) through which they gain attachment to the sternum. They are called *true ribs*. The anterior ends of the eighth, ninth and tenth ribs also end in costal cartilages. These cartilages do not reach the sternum, but end by gaining attachment to the next higher costal cartilage. They are, therefore, called *false ribs*. The anterior ends of the eleventh and twelfth ribs have small pieces of cartilage attached to their ends: these ends are free and these ribs are, therefore, called *floating ribs*.

At the posterior end of a typical rib we see a *head*, a *neck* and a *tubercle*. The head articulates partly with the superior costal facet on the body of the numerically corresponding vertebra; and partly with the inferior costal facet on the next higher vertebra. It is also attached to the intervertebral disc. The part of the rib immediately lateral to the head is called the neck. It lies in front of the transverse process of the numerically corresponding vertebra. It has a sharp upper border called the *crest* of the neck. Just lateral to the neck the posterior aspect of the rib presents an elevation called the tubercle. The tubercle has a medial articular part which bears a facet that articulates with the costal facet on the transverse process of the corresponding vertebra; and a lateral part that is rough for attachment of ligaments.

The anterior end of the rib shows a cup shaped depression for attachment of the costal cartilage.

The part of the rib between the anterior and posterior ends is called the shaft. It is curved like the letter 'C'. The shaft is flat: it has *inner and outer surfaces*, and *upper and lower borders*. The upper border is rounded. The lower border is sharp. The inner surface is concave. Just above the lower border the inner surface shows a *costal groove* running along the length of the shaft. The external surface of the shaft is convex. A short distance lateral to the tubercle it is marked by a rough line. At this point the rib appears to be bent: this point is, therefore, called the *angle*. The shaft is also somewhat twisted along its long axis. As a result the external surface faces somewhat downwards in the posterior part and somewhat upwards in its anterior part.

THE COSTAL CARTILAGES

These are bars of hyaline cartilage. A typical costal cartilage has medial and lateral ends, anterior and posterior surfaces, and upper and lower borders. The lateral end of each costal cartilage is attached to the anterior end of one rib. The medial ends of the upper seven costal cartilages are attached to the lateral margin of the sternum. The first costal cartilage is attached to the lateral margin of the manubrium sterni. The medial end of the second cartilage is attached partly to the manubrium and partly to the first sternebra. The 3rd, 4th and 5th cartilages gain attachment to the lateral edge of the sternum at the points of junction of sternebrae; the 6th on the fourth sternebra; and the 7th at the junction of the fourth sternebra and the xiphoid process.

The medial ends of the 8th, 9th and 10th costal cartilages are connected to the next higher costal cartilage. The cartilages of the 11th and 12th ribs are small and are attached to the tips of the ribs. Their lateral ends are free.

33

Joints of the Trunk

The joints of the trunk are intervertebral joints, other joints of the head and neck, joints of the pelvis and joints of the sternum and ribs.

INTERVERTEBRAL JOINTS

Adjoining vertebrae are connected to one another through three main joints. There is a median joint between the vertebral bodies, and two joints (right and left) between the articular processes.

The bodies, laminae, transverse processes and spinous processes of adjoining vertebrae are also united by a number of ligaments.

Joints between vertebral bodies

The lower surface of the body of one vertebra articulates with the superior surface of the body of the next vertebra. The surfaces are covered by thin layers of hyaline cartilage. The two plates of hyaline cartilage are united to each other by a thick **intervertebral disc** (Fig. 33.1).

Intervertebral discs

Intervertebral discs are the chief bonds of union between adjoining vertebrae. Each disc consists of an outer part called the **annulus fibrosus**, and an inner part the **nucleus pulposus**.

The superficial part of the annulus fibrosus is made up of collagen fibres. Its deeper part is of fibro-cartilage.

In the young the nucleus pulposus is soft and gelatinous, but this material is gradually replaced by fibrocartilage.

The intervertebral discs are very strong in the young. With advancing age, however, the annulus fibrosus becomes weak and it then becomes possible for the nucleus pulposus to burst through it. This is called **prolapse** of the disc. A prolapsed nucleus pulposus usually passes backwards and laterally and may press

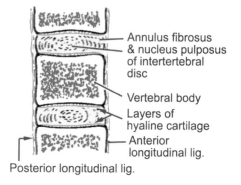

Annulus fibrosus
& nucleus pulposus
of intertebral
disc

Vertebral body

Layers of
hyaline cartilage

Anterior
longitudinal lig.

Posterior longitudinal lig.

Fig. 33.1, Schematic sagittal section across vertebral bodies and intervertebral discs.

upon nerve roots emerging from the spinal cord at that level. Prolapse results in local pain the back. When nerves are pressed upon there is shooting pain along the course of the nerve involved. Disc prolapse occurs most frequently in the lumbosacral region and results in pain shooting down the back of the thigh and leg. This is called **sciatica**. Prolapse is also frequently seen in the cervical region.

Intervertebral discs constitute about one fifth of the length of the vertebral column. They transmit weight, act as shock absorbers, and provide resilience to the spine.

Joints between vertebral articular processes

Each vertebra has four articular processes (or zygapophyses): right and left superior, and right and left inferior. Each process bears an articular facet. The inferior articular facets of one vertebra articulate with the superior articular facets of the next lower vertebra forming a series of **zygapophyseal joints**.

Ligaments connecting adjacent vertebrae

Adjoining vertebrae are connected by numerous ligaments. These are as follows (Fig. 33.2).

(1) The anterior longitudinal ligament passes from the anterior surface of the body of one vertebra to that of another.

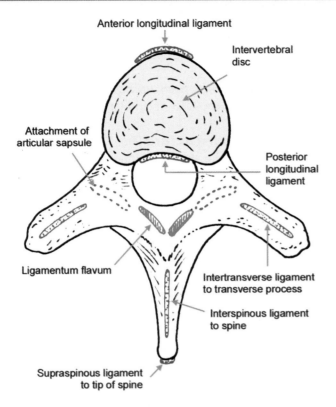

Fig. 33.2. Scheme to show ligaments connecting adjacent vertebrae.

(2) The posterior longitudinal ligament passes from the posterior surface of the body of one vertebra to that of another. This ligament lies within the vertebral canal.

(3) **Intertransverse ligaments** interconnect adjacent transverse processes.

(4) **Interspinous ligaments** connect adjacent spinous processes.

(5) **Supraspinous ligaments** connect the tips of spinous processes.

(6) The **ligamenta flava** (= yellow ligaments) are made up of elastic tissue. They pass from the lower border of the lamina of one vertebra to the upper border of the lamina of the next lower vertebra.

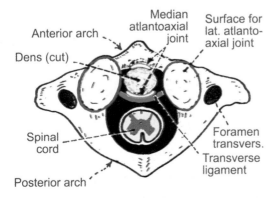

Fig. 33.3. Schematic view of the inferior aspect of the atlas to show the atlantoaxial joints.

JOINTS OF THE HEAD AND NECK

The joints to be seen in the head and neck are as follows.

1. *Joints between bones of the skull*

Adjacent edges of bones of the skull are united to each other by fibrous joints called ***sutures***. The sutures are fibrous joints. The names of some sutures have been mentioned while describing the skull.

The bodies of the occipital and sphenoid bones are united by a ***synchondrosis***. A synchondrosis is also present between the body of the sphenoid and the apex of the petrous temporal bone. A synchondrosis is a primary cartilaginous joint. At such a joint the two articulating surfaces are united by a plate of hyaline cartilage. As age increases the cartilage is gradually invaded by bone and the union becomes bony.

2. *The temporomandibular joint*

At this joint the head of the mandible articulates with the articular fossa present on the temporal bone. This joint is described later in this chapter.

3. *The atlanto-occipital joints*

These are the joints between the occipital bone and the atlas. They are described below.

4. *Joints between cervical vertebrae.*

Of these the joints between the atlas and axis vertebrae are atypical, and are described below. The remaining intervertebral joints are similar to typical intervertebral joints described earlier in this chapter.

The Atlantoaxial Joints

The atlas and axis vertebrae articulate with each other at three joints, one median, and two lateral.

The ***median atlantoaxial joint*** is a synovial joint of the pivot variety. The dens of the axis (the pivot) lies in the ring formed by the anterior arch of the atlas and its transverse ligament. In this situation there are really two synovial joints with independent capsules: one between the anterior surface of the dens and the posterior aspect of the anterior arch, and the other between the posterior surface of the dens and the transverse ligament. The transverse ligament is attached at each end to the medial surface of the lateral mass of the atlas.

The ***lateral atlantoaxial joints*** are synovial joints of the plane variety.

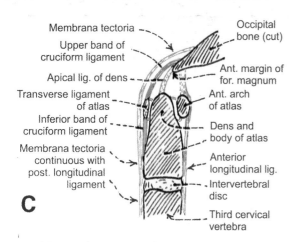

Fig. 33.4. Median section through atlantoaxial joints.

The ligaments connecting the atlas and axis, and the movements at the atlanto-axial joints are considered below along with those of the atlanto-occipital joints.

The Atlanto-Occipital Joints

There are two atlanto-occipital joints, right and left. At each joint the occipital condyle articulates with a facet on the upper surface of the lateral mass of the atlas (Fig. 33.3).

The occipital condyles lie on either side of the foramen magnum. They are large. The long axis of each condyle is directed forwards and medially. The condyle is convex both anteroposteriorly and from side to side. The facet on the upper surface of the atlas is concave and corresponds in size and direction to the occipital condyle.

These articular surfaces are enclosed in capsules to form synovial joints. From a functional point of view the right and left atlanto-occipital joints together form an ellipsoid joint.

Ligaments uniting the Atlas the Axis and the Occipital Bone

Apart from their capsules the atlas and axis are united to each other and to the occipital bone by a number of ligaments that are considered below.

(**1**) The *anterior longitudinal ligament* (continued upwards from lower vertebrae) is attached to the front of the body of the axis; to the anterior arch of the atlas; and to the basilar part of the occipital bone.

(**2**) Between the atlas and the occipital bone, the anterior longitudinal ligament is incorporated in the *anterior atlanto-occipital membrane*. This membrane is attached below to the upper border of the anterior arch of the atlas, and above to the anterior part of the margin of the foramen magnum.

(**3**) The *posterior atlanto-occipital membrane* is attached above to the posterior margin of the foramen magnum, and below to the upper border of the posterior arch of the atlas.

(**4**) The highest *ligamentum flavum* connects the posterior arch of the atlas to the laminae of the axis vertebra.

(**5**) The *membrana tectoria* (Fig. 33.4) is an upward continuation of the posterior longitudinal ligament (which connects the posterior surfaces of the bodies of adjacent vertebrae).

(**6**) The dens (of the axis) is connected to the occipital bone by the following:

   a) The *apical ligament* passes upwards from the tip of the dens to the anterior margin of the foramen magnum (Fig. 33.4).

   b) The right and left *alar ligaments* are attached below to the upper part of the dens lateral to the apical ligament, and above to the occipital bone.

(**7**) The *transverse ligament of the atlas* stretches between the two lateral masses of the bone, behind the dens of the axis (Fig. 33.4).

Movements at the Atlanto-occipital and Atlantoaxial Joints

Being a pivot joint the median atlantoaxial joint allows the atlas (and with it the skull) to rotate around the axis provided by the dens. This is accompanied by gliding movements at the lateral atlantoaxial joints. From a functional point of view the two atlanto-occipital joints together form an ellipsoid joint. The main movements allowed by it are those of flexion and extension (of the head) as in nodding. Slight lateral movements are also allowed, but no rotation in possible.

THE TEMPOROMANDIBULAR JOINT

This is a synovial joint of the condylar variety. Its cavity is divided into upper and lower parts by an intra-articular disc.

The *upper articular surface* of the joint is formed by the mandibular fossa of the temporal bone. Anteriorly, the surface extends onto the articular tubercle. The posterior part of the surface is, therefore, concave downwards; and the anterior part is convex.

The *inferior articular surface* is formed by the head of the mandible which is markedly convex anteroposteriorly, and more gently convex from side to side.

The *articular disc* is made of fibrocartilage. Its upper surface is concavoconvex to fit the upper articular surface of the joint. Its lower surface is concave, the head of the mandible fitting into the concavity.

The **capsule** of the joint is attached to the margins of the articular surfaces. The inside of the capsule is lined by synovial membrane. The lateral part of the capsule is strengthened by the **lateral temporomandibular ligament**. In addition the joint has two accessory ligaments (that are independent of the capsule and lie some distance away from it). The **sphenomandibular ligament** is attached above to the spine of the sphenoid, and below to the lingula of the mandible. The **stylomandibular ligament** extends from the apex of the styloid process to the angle and posterior border of the ramus of the mandible.

Movements at the temporomandibular joint

The movements at the joint can be divided into those between the upper articular surface and the articular disc, and those between the disc and the head of the mandible. Most movements occur simultaneously at the right and left temporomandibular joints. In forward movement or **protraction** of the mandible the articular disc glides forwards over the upper articular surface, the head of the mandible moving with it. The reversal of this movement is called **retraction**. In slight opening of the mouth (depression of the mandible) the head of the mandible moves on the under-surface of the disc like a hinge. In wide opening of the mouth, this hinge like movement is followed by a forward gliding of the disc along with the head of the mandible. These movements are reversed in closing the mouth (or **elevation** of the mandible). **Chewing movements** involve side to side movements of the mandible.

JOINTS AND LIGAMENTS OF THE PELVIS

Pubic Symphysis

The two pubic bones are united in front at the **pubic symphysis**. This joint corresponds in structure to that of a secondary cartilaginous joint. Each bone end is covered by a thin layer of hyaline cartilage. The two layers of hyaline cartilage are united by fibrocartilage.

Sacroiliac joints

The sacrum articulates on each side with the corresponding ilium forming the right and left sacroiliac joints. These are synovial joints. The iliac and sacral articular surfaces are shown in Figs.33.5 and 33.6. They are both shaped like the auricle (pinna) and are, therefore, called **auricular surfaces**.

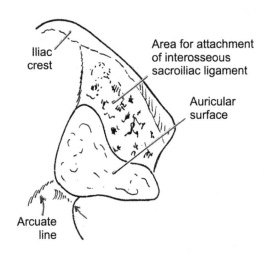

Fig. 33.5. Posterior part of ilium viewed from the medial side to show the auricular surface that articulates with the sacrum.

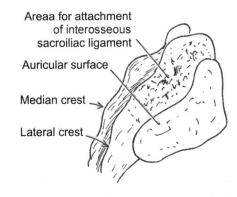

Fig. 33.6. Upper part of the lateral surface of the sacrum showing the auricular surface that articulates with the ilium.

The surfaces are covered by cartilage, but because of the presence of a number of raised and depressed areas the joint allows little movement. The capsule of the joint is attached around the margins of the articular surfaces. It is thickened in its anterior part to form the **ventral sacroiliac ligament**. The main bond of union between the sacrum and ilium is, however, the **interosseous sacroiliac ligament** that is attached to rough areas above and behind the auricular surfaces of the two bones. The posterior aspects of the sacrum and ilium are connected by a strong **dorsal sacroiliac ligament** which covers the interosseus ligament from behind.

The stability of the sacroiliac joints is important as body weight is transmitted from the sacrum to the lower limbs through them.

Two other ligaments that connect the sacrum to the hip bone are the sacrotuberous and the sacrospinous ligaments that have been encountered in the gluteal region (Fig. 33.7).

The **sacrotuberous ligament** is large and strong. It has a broad upper medial end and a narrower lower lateral end. The upper end is attached (from above downwards) to the posterior superior and posterior inferior iliac spines, the lower part of the posterior surface of the sacrum and the lateral margin of the lower part of the sacrum and the upper part of the coccyx. Its lower end is attached to the medial margin of the ischial tuberosity.

The **sacrospinous ligament** is attached medially to the sacrum and coccyx and laterally to the ischial spine.

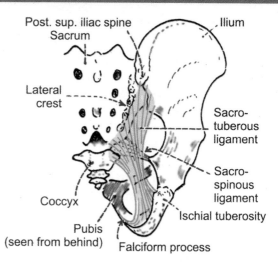

Fig. 33.7. Posterior aspect of the pelvis showing the attachments of the sacrotuberous and sacrospinous ligaments.

JOINTS OF THE THORAX

The joints between the bones of the thorax are:

(1) *Intervertebral joints* connecting adjacent vertebrae. These have already been described.

(2) *Sternal joints* between different parts of the sternum.

(3) *Costovertebral joints* between ribs and vertebrae.

(4) *Costochondral joints* between ribs and costal cartilages.

(5) *Sternocostal joints* or *chondrosternal joints* between costal cartilages and the sternum.

(6) *Interchondral joints* amongst the lower costal cartilages.

JOINTS OF THE STERNUM

We have seen that the sternum consists of three parts, the manubrium, the body, and the xiphoid process. These three elements are connected by joints.

Manubriosternal joint

The lower end of the manubrium is attached to the body of the sternum at the manubriosternal joint. This joint is a symphysis. The bony surfaces are covered by thin layers of hyaline cartilage that are connected to each other by fibrocartilage. Bony union between the two bones takes place in many individuals after the age of 30.

Xiphisternal joint

This joint is a symphysis, but the two bones generally undergo bony union by the age of 40 years.

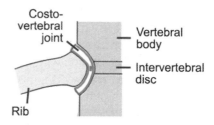

Fig. 33.8. Schematic coronal section across a costovertebral joint.

JOINTS OF RIBS WITH VERTEBRAL COLUMN

Costovertebral joints

These joints (also called **costocorporeal joints**) unite the heads of ribs to the sides of the vertebral column (Fig. 33.9, 33.10). The head of a rib bears a facet that is divided into upper and lower parts by a ridge. The lower part of the facet articulates with the demifacet on the superior border of the body of the numerically corresponding vertebra. The upper part of the facet articulates with the lower demifacet on the next higher vertebra. The ridge separating the facets is attached to the intervertebral disc through an **intra-articular ligament** which divides the joint cavity into upper and lower parts.

The joint is enclosed in a capsule which is strengthened in front by fibres that radiate from the head of the rib to the two vertebrae and to the intervertebral disc. These fibres constitute the **radiate ligament** (or triradiate ligament).

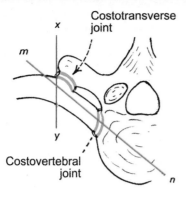

Fig. 33.9. Schematic section across the posterior part of a rib to show costovertebral and costotransverse joints.

Costovertebral joints of the 1st, 10th, 11th and 12th ribs are atypical in that these ribs articulate only with the corresponding vertebrae.

Costotransverse joint

A short distance lateral to the head, each rib bears a tubercle which is divisible into a medial articular part and a lateral non-articular part. The medial part bears a facet which articulates with a facet on the front of the transverse process of the corresponding vertebra. The joint surfaces are enclosed in a capsule. The joint is strengthened by a number of ligaments.

JOINTS BETWEEN RIBS, COSTAL CARTILAGES AND STERNUM

Costochondral joints

The anterior end of each rib bears a depression into which the rounded lateral end of a costal cartilage is fixed.

Chondrosternal joints

These are joints between the (medial ends of) the 1st to 7th costal cartilages and the sternum. The first costal cartilage is united to the manubrium through a plate of *fibrocartilage*.

The joints between the 2nd to 7th costal cartilages and the sternum are synovial joints.

Interchondral joints

The 6th to 9th costal cartilages come into contact with one another and form a number of small interchondral synovial joints.

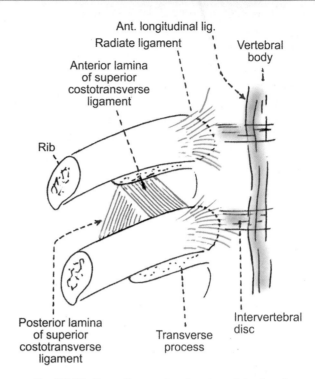

Fig. 33.10. Some ligaments of costovertebral and costotransverse joints seen from the front.

MOVEMENTS OF RIBS

The movements taking place at the joints of the thorax allow for rhythmic expansion and contraction of the thoracic wall during respiration. The precise nature of the movements is complex and differs in different ribs, but the two fundamental movements to be understood are as follows.

(**a**) The anterior ends of the ribs can move up or down by rotation at the costovertebral and costotransverse joints. During inspiration the anterior end moves upwards in an arc. This increases the anteroposterior diameter of the thorax.

(**b**) The second movement of the ribs occurs on an axis that is roughly anteroposterior. In expiration the middle of the rib is lower than its ends. In inspiration it is raised (like a bucket handle). This increases the transverse diameter of the thorax.

During quiet breathing the movements of the ribs described above are produced by intercostal muscles. Other muscles attached to the ribs come into play in deep inspiration. Remember that the most important role in respiration is that of the diaphragm.

34

Muscles of the Trunk

The trunk contains a very large number of muscles. However, only a few of these are of interest to the physiotherapist. Superficially, many parts of the trunk are covered by muscles that belong to the limbs (for example the trapezius and the latissimus behind the trunk, and the pectoral muscles in front of the chest). These have already been considered. We will now consider those muscles that come into view when the muscles of the limbs are removed.

DEEP MUSCLES OF THE BACK

Deep muscles of the back and their layout

The deep muscles of the back are arranged in layers (from superficial to deep) as follows (Fig. 34.1):

(**a**) The **splenius** group is confined to the upper thoracic and cervical region. It consists of the **splenius capitis** and the **splenius cervicis**.

(**b**) Deep to the splenius group we have the **erector spinae**, a large muscle mass extending vertically from the back of the sacrum and ilium up to the skull; and

transversely from the spines of the vertebrae to the angles of the ribs.

It is subdivided longitudinally into three parts as follows (Fig. 34.4):

(1) The **spinalis** is most medial;

(2) the **longissimus** is intermediate in position; and

(3) the **iliocostocervicalis** is most lateral.

(**c**) Deep to the erector spinae we have a group of muscles that are collectively called the **transversospinalis**. They occupy the interval between the spines and transverse processes of the vertebrae.

The transversospinalis is made up of three sub-groups placed one over the other. These (from superficial to deep) are as follows (Figs. 34.1, 34.2):

(1) The **semispinalis** group (consisting of semispinalis thoracis, cervicis and capitis) is most superficial.

(2) The **multifidus** is intermediate in position.

(3) The **rotatores** are deepest.

A good idea of the relative depth at which the various muscle groups mentioned above lie can be had by examining a transverse section (Fig. 34.1). The vertical extend of the various muscles is shown in Figs. 34.2 in

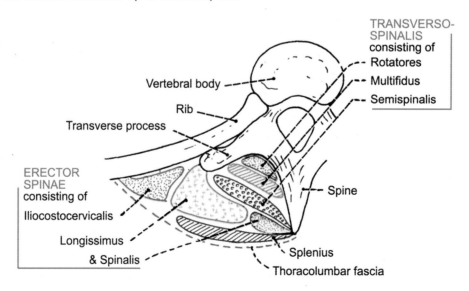

Fig. 34.1. Schematic transverse section to show the arrangement of deep muscles of the back.

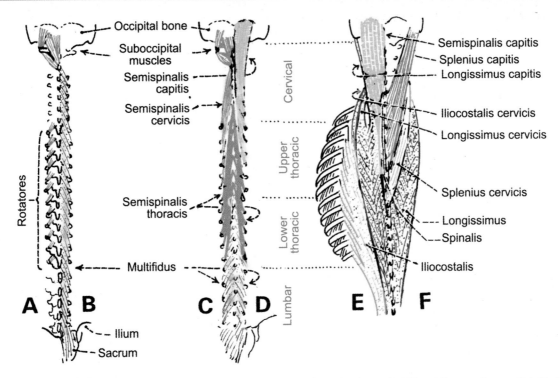

Fig. 34.2 A to F. Deep muscles of the back. The deepest layer is shown in 'A' and the most superficial in 'F'.

which the deepest level is shown in 'A' and progressively more superficial layers are shown in 'B' to 'F'.

In the descriptions that follow we will consider only three muscles in detail. These are the splenius capitis, the erector spinae and the semispinalis capitis. The remaining muscles will be mentioned briefly.

Splenius Group

This group consists of the splenius capitis and the splenius cervicis. The fibres of the muscles of this group arise from vertebral spines and pass upwards and laterally.

Splenius Capitis

Origin:

The splenius capitis arises from the

(**a**) lower half of the ligamentum nuchae, and

(**b**) spines of vertebrae C7, T1, T2, T3 (and sometimes T4). From this origin the fibres pass upwards and laterally (Fig. 34.3).

Insertion:

The muscle is inserted into the back of the skull. The area of insertion is on the back of the mastoid process (temporal bone) and on the occipital bone below the lateral one third of the superior nuchal line.

The splenius capitis forms the (upper and posterior part of the) floor of the posterior triangle of the neck.

Splenius Cervicis

The splenius cervicis arises from spines T3 to T6 and is inserted into the transverse processes of upper cervical vertebrae (C1, C2 and sometimes C3).

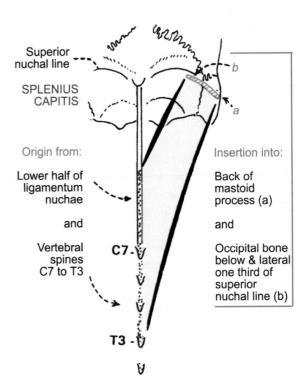

Fig. 34.3. Attachments of the splenius capitis muscle.

Nerve Supply and Actions of Splenius Muscles:

The splenius capitis and cervicis are supplied by dorsal rami of cervical nerves.

When the splenius capitis and cervicis of both sides contract the head is pulled backwards. When the muscles of one side contract the face is rotated to the same side.

The Erector Spinae

The erector spinae is deep to the splenius group and superficial to the semispinalis group. It consists of a lateral part, the *iliocosto-cervicalis;* an intermediate part called the *longissimus;* and a small medial part, the *spinalis.*

Origin:

The main origin of the muscle is from the back of the sacrum through a U-shaped tendon attached to the median and lateral sacral crests. The medial limb of the 'U' extends upwards to the lumbar and lower thoracic spines. The lateral limb extends on to the dorsal part of the iliac crest and the sacrotuberous and sacroiliac ligaments. (The origin is indicated by thick interrupted line in the lower part of Fig. 34.4).

The muscle mass passes upwards and divides into three main parts.

The *spinalis* part is most medial and least developed. Its fibres pass from *spines to spines.* It is subdivided into the following:

(**a**) The *spinalis thoracis* passes from the upper lumbar and lower thoracic spines to the upper thoracic spines.

(**b**) The *spinalis cervicis* passes from the ligamentum nuchae and upper thoracic spines to the spine of the axis vertebra.

(**c**) The *spinalis capitis* passes from the lower cervical spines to the occipital bone (along with the semispinalis capitus).

The *longissimus* is the largest division of the erector spinae. It is subdivided into the following:

(**a**) The fibres of the *longissimus thoracis* arise mainly from the sacrum. They are inserted into the transverse processes of lumbar and thoracic vertebrae, and into the ribs.

(**b**) The *longissimus cervicis* arises from the upper thoracic transverse processes (and upper ribs) and is inserted into the transverse processes of the cervical vertebrae.

(**c**) The *longissimus capitis* arises from the transverse processes of the upper thoracic vertebrae, and from the articular processes of the lower cervical vertebrae. It is inserted into the mastoid process deep to the splenius capitis.

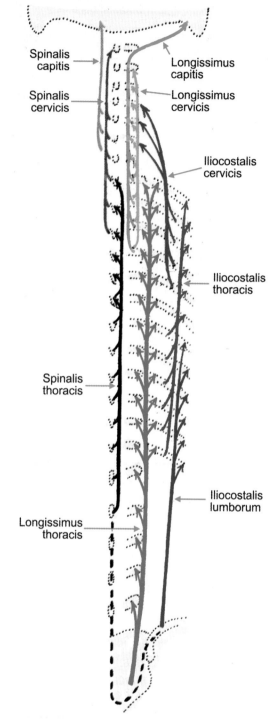

Fig. 34.4. Scheme to show the components of the erector spinae muscle.

The *iliocostocervicalis* lies lateral to the longissimus and consists of:

(**a**) the *iliocostalis lumborum* which arises mainly from the ilium and is inserted into the lower ribs;

(**b**) the *iliocostalis thoracis* which passes from the lower ribs to the upper ribs; and

(**c**) the *iliocostalis cervicis* which passes from the upper ribs to the lower cervical transverse processes.

Note that out of the large muscle mass of the erector spinae only three slender slips (namely the *iliocostalis cervicis, longissimus cervicis* and *longissimus capitis*) reach the neck.

Nerve Supply and Actions of Erector Spinae:

The erector spinae is supplied by **dorsal** primary rami of spinal nerves.

As a whole the erector spinae is an extensor and lateral flexor of the vertebral column. The longissimus capitis turns the face to its own side.

The erector spinae is a very important postural muscle. In persons who lead a sedentary life, and with old age, the muscle becomes weak. The vertebral column then tends to bend forwards. This puts excessive strain on ligaments of the vertebral column and also predisposes to prolapse of intervertebral discs. These are common causes of back ache. Tone in the erector spinae can be maintained by exercises and also by brisk walking.

Semispinalis Group

This group consists of the semispinalis capitis, semispinalis cervicis, and semispinalis thoracis.

The **semispinalis thoracis** arises from the transverse processes of lower thoracic vertebrae and is inserted into the spines of upper thoracic and lower cervical vertebrae.

The **semispinalis cervicis** arises from the transverse processes of upper thoracic vertebrae and is inserted into the (2nd and 5th) cervical spines.

Semispinalis Capitis

Origin:

The semispinalis capitis arises from:

(**a**) the transverse processes of the upper thoracic and seventh cervical vertebrae; and

(**b**) the articular processes of the fourth, fifth and sixth cervical vertebrae.

Insertion:

The muscle is inserted into the occipital bone on the medial part of the area between the superior and inferior nuchal lines. (Also see Figs. 34.5).

The muscle forms the roof of the suboccipital triangle.

Nerve Supply and Actions:

The semispinalis group is supplied by dorsal rami of cervical and thoracic spinal nerves.

The main action of the semispinalis capitis is to extend the head. It also has a slight rotatory action turning the face to the opposite side.

Multifidus and Rotatores

The **multifidus** extends from the sacrum to the axis vertebra. It consists of numerous short oblique slips each arising from a transverse process and passing to the spines of higher vertebrae.

The **rotatores** are well formed only in the thoracic region. Each muscle consists of a slip that arises from the transverse process of one thoracic vertebra and is inserted into the lamina of the vertebra next above it.

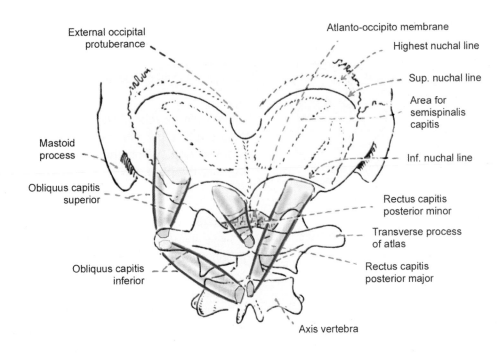

Fig. 34.5. Schematic diagram to show the attachments of the suboccipital muscles.

The rotatores, multifidus and semispinalis are rotators of the vertebral column. The multifidus and semispinalis are, in addition, extensors and lateral flexors. However, their main function is postural.

Other muscles in the back

Apart from the deep muscles of the back described above there are small muscles that bridge the intervals between adjacent spines (*interspinales*) and between adjacent transverse processes (*intertransversarii*).

The *suboccipital muscles* are considered below.

Suboccipital Muscles

This is a group of small muscles placed in the uppermost part of the back of the neck, deep to the semispinalis capitis. They form the boundaries of the suboccipital triangle (Fig. 34.5).

The *rectus capitis posterior minor* arises from the posterior arch of the atlas. Its fibres pass upwards to be inserted into the occipital bone in the medial part of the area below the inferior nuchal line (i.e., between the line and the foramen magnum).

The *rectus capitis posterior major* arises from the spine of the axis vertebra. It is inserted into the lateral part of the area below the inferior nuchal line.

The *obliquus capitis inferior* arises from the spine of the axis vertebra. It is inserted into the transverse process of the atlas vertebra.

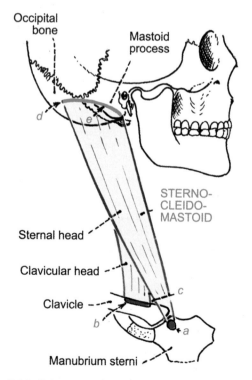

Fig. 34.6. Scheme to show the attachments of the sternocleidomastoid muscle.

The *obliquus capitis superior* arises from the transverse process of the atlas. It inserted into the lateral part of the area between the superior and inferior nuchal lines.

Nerve Supply and Actions:

The suboccipital muscles are supplied by the dorsal ramus of the first cervical nerve.

The main action of the suboccipital muscles is to maintain the posture of the head. Note that the head tends to fall forwards due to gravity. This is resisted by the two recti and the superior oblique which extend it. They can rotate the head and tilt it laterally.

OTHER MUSCLES OF THE NECK

STERNOCLEIDOMASTOID

Origin:

The muscle arises by two heads (Fig. 34.6).

(a) The *sternal head* arises from the anterior surface of the manubrium sterni.

(b) The *clavicular head* arises from the upper surface of the medial part of the clavicle.

Insertion:

The muscle is inserted into the:

(a) lateral half of the superior nuchal line; and

(b) the lateral surface of the mastoid process.

Nerve Supply:

Accessory nerve (spinal part) and by branches from the ventral rami of spinal nerves C2, C3.

Actions:

When the muscle of one side contracts the head is tilted to the same side, and the face is rotated to the opposite side. When the muscles of both sides act together the head and neck are flexed.

SUPRAHYOID MUSCLES

These are the digastric, stylohyoid, mylohyoid and geniohyoid muscles (Fig. 34.7).

Digastric muscle

The digastric muscle has two bellies, anterior and posterior, united by an intermediate tendon. The posterior belly arises from the base of the skull just deep to the mastoid process. The anterior belly is

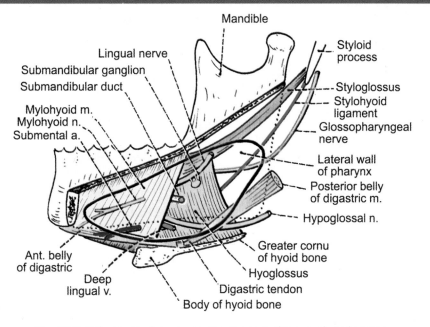

Fig. 34.7. Scheme to show some structures in the suprahyoid region.

attached to the anterior part of the base of the mandible near the midline.

The digastric can elevate the hyoid bone. Acting along with other muscles attached to the hyoid bone it can fix the bone.

Stylohyoid muscle

The stylohyoid muscle arises from the posterior aspect of the styloid process. The tendon is inserted into the hyoid bone. It elevates the hyoid bone and retracts it.

Geniohyoid muscle

The geniohyoid arises from the posterior aspect of the symphysis menti and runs backwards to be inserted into the anterior aspect of the hyoid bone.

Mylohyoid muscle

Oral diaphragm

The mylohyoid muscles of the two sides bridge the gap between the two halves of the mandible. In the median plane the two muscles become continuous with each other at a median raphe. In this way the right and left muscles form the floor of the mouth. This floor is called the oral diaphragm (Fig. 34.8). This diaphragm is strengthened above by the geniohyoid muscle; and below by the anterior belly of the digastric muscle.

On each side the mylohyoid muscle arises from the mylohyoid line on the medial surface of the body of the mandible. Most of the fibres fibres are inserted into a median fibrous raphe extending from the hyoid bone to the mandible.

The muscle helps in deglutition by raising the floor of the mouth.

MUSCLES OF THE TONGUE

The *extrinsic muscles* of the tongue (Fig. 34.9) enter it from the outside. They are the styloglossus, the palatoglossus, the genioglossus, and the hyoglossus. The *intrinsic muscles* lie within the substance of the tongue.

The styloglossus arises from the styloid process. The palatoglossus muscle arises from the soft palate. The genioglossus arises from the mandible (posterior surface of the symphysis menti). The hyoglossus arises from the hyoid bone. All these muscles converge to be inserted into the tongue.

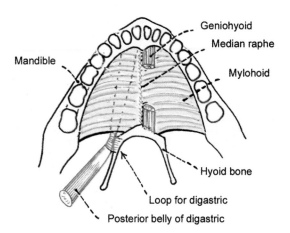

Fig. 34.8. Schematic diagram of floor of mouth seen from above. Note the layout of the mylohyoid and geniohyoid muscles.

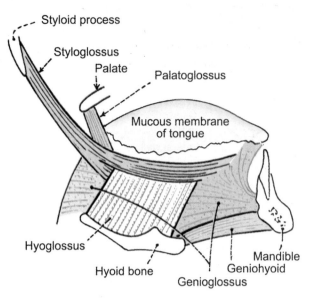

Fig. 34.9. Drawing to show the extrinsic muscles of the tongue.

The muscles of the tongue are important in chewing and swallowing of food, and in speech.

All muscles of the tongue are supplied by the hypoglossal nerve except the palatoglossus which is supplied by the cranial part of the accessory nerve.

INFRAHYOID MUSCLES

These are the sternohyoid, the sternothyroid, the thyrohyoid and the omohyoid muscles. Their main attachments are evident from their names. Identify them in Fig. 34.10.

The omohyoid has two bellies, superior and inferior, joined by an intermediate tendon.

Nerve supply of infrahyoid muscles:

All the infrahyoid muscles are supplied by branches from the ansa cervicalis except the thyrohyoid which is supplied by fibres of the first cervical nerve that travel through the hypoglossal nerve.

Actions of infrahyoid muscles:

The sternohyoid, the omohyoid and the thyrohyoid depress the hyoid bone. The sternothyroid pulls the larynx downwards, whereas the thyrohyoid can raise it when the hyoid bone is fixed.

THE LATERAL VERTEBRAL MUSCLES

These are the *scalenus anterior*, the *scalenus medius*, the *scalenus posterior* and the *scalenus minimus*. Each muscle is attached at one end to the transverse processes of one or more cervical vertebrae,

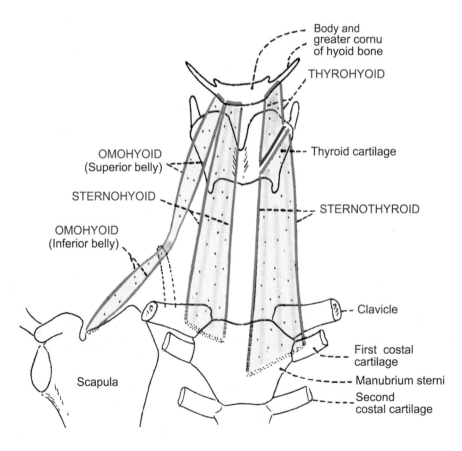

Fig. 34.10. Scheme to show the attachments of the infrahyoid muscles.

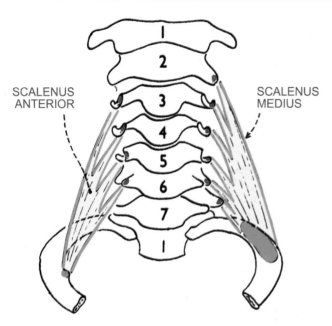

Fig. 34.11. Attachments of the scalenus anterior and scalenus medius muscles.

and at the other end to the first or second rib. The first two muscles are shown in Fig. 34.11.

Scalenus Anterior

The scalenus anterior arises from the transverse processes of vertebrae C3 to C6 (Fig. 34.11). It is inserted into the inner border of the first rib.

Nerve supply and action

It is supplied by the ventral rami of spinal nerves C4, C5, and C6. It bends the neck forwards and laterally.

Scalenus Medius

The scalenus medius takes origin from the transverse process of the axis, and from the transverse processes of vertebrae C3 to C7 (Fig. 34.11). The muscle is inserted into the upper surface of the first rib.

*Nerve supply :*Ventral rami of spinal nerves C3 to C8.

Action

The muscle bends the cervical spine to its own side.

Scalenus Posterior

The scalenus posterior takes origin from the transverse processes of vertebrae C4, C5, C6. It is inserted into the outer surface of the second rib.

Nerve supply and action

The scalenus posterior is supplied by the ventral rami of spinal nerves C6, C7, C8. It bends the cervical spine to the same side.

ANTERIOR VERTEBRAL MUSCLES (PREVERTEBRAL MUSCLES)

These are **(a)** the *rectus capitis anterior*, **(b)** the *rectus capitis lateralis*, **(c)** the *longus capitis*, and **(d)** the *longus colli*. The rectus capitis anterior and lateralis are short muscles passing from the atlas vertebra to the base of the skull. The longus capitis passes from cervical transverse processes to the base of the skull. The longus colli lies over the anterior aspect of the cervical and upper thoracic vertebrae. For further details see Fig. 34.12.

TRIANGLES OF THE NECK

THE POSTERIOR TRIANGLE

Boundaries:

The posterior triangle is bounded anteriorly by the posterior border of the sternocleidomastoid, posteriorly by the anterior border of the trapezius, and inferiorly (base) by the clavicle (Fig. 34.13).

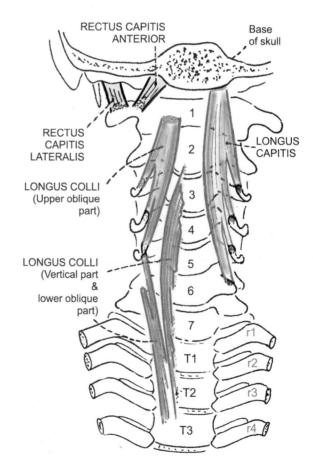

Fig. 34.12. The prevertebral muscles.

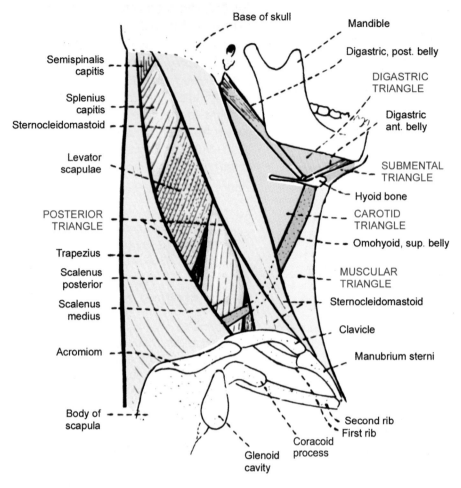

Fig. 34.13. Triangles of the neck.

Floor:

The floor of this triangle is formed mainly by the splenius capitis, the levator scapulae, and the scalenus medius.

The lower part of the posterior triangle is crossed by the inferior belly of the omohyoid muscle which divides the triangle into an upper part (also called the ***occipital triangle***), and a lower part (also called the ***supraclavicular triangle***).

SUBDIVISIONS OF THE ANTERIOR TRIANGLE

The part of the neck anterior to the sternocleidomastoid muscle is called the anterior triangle. It is subdivided as follows.

Submental Triangle

Above and laterally, this triangle is bounded by the anterior belly of the digastric muscle. The third side of the triangle (base) is formed by the hyoid bone. The floor of the triangle is formed by the mylohyoid muscle.

Digastric Triangle

This triangle is bounded above by the base of the mandible, and below by the anterior and posterior bellies of the digastric muscle. The main content of this triangle is the submandibular gland.

Carotid Triangle

This triangle is bounded posteriorly by the anterior margin of the sternocleidomastoid muscle, superiorly by the posterior belly of the digastric muscle, and anteroinferiorly by the superior belly of the omohyoid muscle.

The carotid triangle contains several important blood vessels and nerves including the following.
1. Common carotid artery.
2. Internal carotid artery.
3. External carotid artery and branches arising from it.
4. Internal jugular vein
5. Vagus, spinal accessory, and hypoglossal nerves and the sympathetic trunk.

Muscular Triangle

This triangle is bounded posteroinferiorly by the sternocleidomastoid muscle, posterosuperiorly by the superior belly of the omohyoid muscle, and anteriorly (or medially) by the anterior middle line of the neck.

The triangle contains the infrahyoid muscles. Deep to these muscles it contains the thyroid gland, the larynx and the trachea. On either side of the trachea we see the carotid sheath and its contents.

SUBOCCIPITAL TRIANGLE

The suboccipital muscles form the boundaries of the suboccipital triangle as shown in Fig. 34.5.

SOME OTHER MUSCLES OF THE HEAD AND NECK

1. In the face there are a large number of **facial muscles** responsible for facial expressions.

2. In relation to the eyeball there are several **extraocular muscles** that move the eyeball.

3. In relation to the ramus of the mandible there are a number of muscles that are responsible for chewing movements. These are the **muscles of mastication**. They include the masseter, the temporalis and the medial and lateral pterygoid muscles.

4. In relation to the tongue there are several muscles that move it (Fig. 34.9).

5. Many other muscles are present.

MUSCLES OF THE THORAX

There are several muscles in the thoracic wall. The most important are the intercostal muscles and the diaphragm, and we will consider these only.

Intercostal Muscles

The **intercostal muscles** fill the intervals between adjacent ribs. They are arranged in three layers: **external, internal** and **innermost** (Fig. 34.14)). There being twelve ribs on either side, and eleven intercostal spaces between them, we have eleven sets of external and internal intercostal muscles.

The internal intercostal muscles do not extend over the entire length of the intercostal space. Anteriorly they extend right up to the sternum, but posteriorly they end at the level of the angles of the ribs beyond which they are replaced by the **posterior intercostal membranes.** The external intercostals are deficient in front. Between the costal cartilages they are replaced by the **anterior intercostal membranes.**

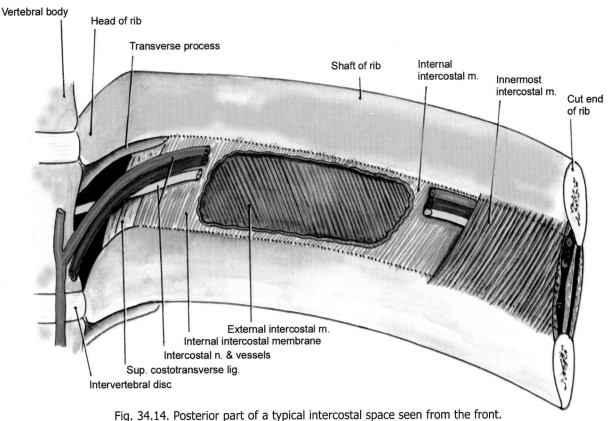

Fig. 34.14. Posterior part of a typical intercostal space seen from the front.

The intercostal nerves and vessels run between the muscles of the second and third layer. They supply all the muscles mentioned above.

Attachments of intercostal muscles:

Each **external intercostal** muscle arises from the lower border of the rib above, and is inserted into the upper border of the rib below. The fibres of the muscle run obliquely from one rib to the other, the upper attachment being nearer the vertebra and the lower attachment nearer the sternum.

Each **internal intercostal** muscle arises from the costal groove of the rib above and is inserted into the upper border of the rib below. Its fibres run at right angles to those of the external intercostal.

The **innermost intercostal muscles** are attached both above and below to the inner surfaces of adjoining ribs. The direction of their fibres of is the same as that of the internal intercostal. They are separated from the internal intercostals by the intercostal nerves and vessels.

Actions of intercostal muscles:

The external intercostal muscles are generally regarded as elevators of ribs, and the internal intercostal muscles as depressors. However, their main importance is to provide strong, but elastic, supports that prevent the thoracic wall from bulging inwards or outwards as a result of pressure changes associated with inspiration or expiration.

Nerve Supply:

The intercostal and subcostal muscles are supplied by the intercostal nerves of the spaces concerned.

THE DIAPHRAGM

The diaphragm is a large muscle that forms a partition between the cavities of the thorax and the abdomen.

Attachments of the diaphragm:

The diaphragm has a more or less circular origin from the thoracic outlet (Fig. 34.15). The origin of the diaphragm can be divided into sternal, costal and vertebral parts. The **sternal part** consists of two slips, right and left, that arise from the back of the xiphoid process. The **costal part** consists of broad slips one from the inner surface of each of the lower six ribs and their costal cartilages.

The **lumbar part** consists of two crura (right and left) that arise from the bodies of lumbar vertebrae; and of fibres that arise (on either side) from two tendinous arches called the lateral and medial arcuate ligaments (Fig. 34.15). The medial margins of the two crura are joined to each other (at the level of the lower border of vertebra T12) to form the **median arcuate ligament.** The descending aorta passes from thorax to abdomen under cover of this ligament. The **lateral arcuate ligament** represents a thickened band of the fascia over the quadratus lumborum (a muscle in the posterior wall of the abdomen). The **medial arcuate**

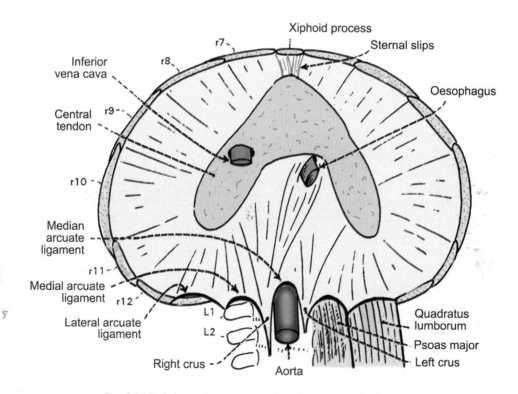

Fig. 34.15. Scheme to show attachments of the diaphragm.

ligament is a thickened band of the fascia covering the psoas major.

From its extensive origin, described above, the muscular fibres of the diaphragm run upwards and converge to be inserted on the margins of a large, flat, *central tendon* which is located just below the pericardium and heart.

The upper convex part of the diaphragm is called its *dome*. The central part of the dome is formed by the central tendon and lies at the level of the xiphisternal joint. It is placed somewhat lower than the right and left muscular convexities (or *cupolae*). The right cupola is slightly higher than the left because of the presence of the liver below it. The level of the dome rises and falls with expiration and inspiration respectively. It is also influenced by posture; being highest when the body is supine, intermediate while standing and lowest while sitting.

The upper surface of the diaphragm is related to thoracic contents including the heart and pericardium in the middle and the lungs and pleura on the sides.

The inferior surface is related to abdominal contents including the peritoneum, the liver, the stomach, the spleen, the right and left kidneys and the right and left suprarenal glands.

Apertures in the diaphragm:

Many structures passing from thorax to abdomen (or *vice versa*) pass through apertures in (or around) the diaphragm. They can be fully understood only after the study of the thorax and abdomen has been completed. However, they are listed here for completeness.

There are three large apertures, one each for the aorta, the oesophagus and the inferior vena cava, and several smaller ones.

(**1**) The *aortic aperture* lies behind the median arcuate ligament, and in front of the disc between vertebrae T12 and L1.

(**2**) The *aperture for the oesophagus* is situated at the level of the tenth thoracic vertebra. It is formed by splitting of the fibres of the right crus a little below their attachment to the central tendon. Because the oesophagus is surrounded by muscle it is compressed during expiration: this prevents regurgitation of the contents of the stomach.

(**3**) The *opening for the inferior vena cava* lies in the central tendon at the level of the eighth thoracic vertebra (lower border). The wall of the vena cava is adherent to the opening. This helps to expand the vessel during inspiration and facilitates venous return through the vessel.

Actions of the Diaphragm:

The diaphragm is the chief muscle of respiration. There are two phases of its action. In the first phase it acts from its origin (the ribs being fixed by other muscles). As a result the central tendon is pulled downwards increasing the vertical diameter of the thorax. In the second phase, the central tendon is fixed as described above. The lower ribs are now drawn upwards. Through them the sternum is pushed forwards. As a result the transverse and anteroposterior diameters of the thorax are also increased.

Acting along with the muscles of the anterior abdominal wall, the diaphragm helps to increase intra-abdominal pressure during acts like urination, defaecation or vomiting. Acts requiring forcible expulsion of air from the lungs like sneezing or laughing are preceded by a deep inspiration (diaphragm) followed by contraction of the expiratory muscles.

Nerve supply:

The diaphragm receives a double nerve supply. Motor innervation is through the right and left phrenic nerves. The diaphragm is also supplied by the lower six intercostal nerves which provide a sensory supply to the peripheral part of the muscle.

MUSCLES OF THE ABDOMEN AND PELVIS

MUSCLES OF ANTERIOR ABDOMINAL WALL

Preliminary considerations

In considering the muscles of the anterior abdominal wall reference has to be made to a number of structures. These are briefly considered here because some of the attachments of the muscles of the abdominal wall cannot be understood unless the student has a clear idea about them.

1. The hip bone has been described in Chapter 27. Refer to that description and make sure that you understand the terms pubic symphysis, pubic crest, and pubic tubercle.

2. The *linea alba* is a tendinous raphe present in the midline of the anterior abdominal wall. It is attached above to the xiphoid process and below to the symphysis pubis.

3. The *inguinal ligament* is a thick curved band of fibres which lies at the junction of the abdomen and

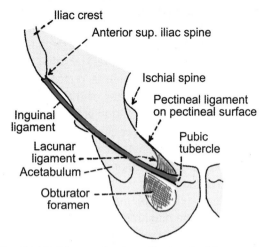

Fig. 34.16. Diagram to show the inguinal ligament and some related structures.

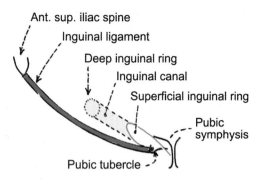

Fig. 34.17. Diagram to show the position of the inguinal canal.

the front of the thigh. It is attached medially to the pubic tubercle and laterally to the anterior superior iliac spine (Fig. 34.16). It represents the lower border of the aponeurosis of the external oblique muscle, which is folded on itself.

4. The *lacunar ligament* is also called the *pectineal part of the inguinal ligament.* It is a triangular membrane placed horizontally, behind the medial most part of the inguinal ligament (Fig. 34.16).

5. Just above the medial part of the inguinal ligament there is an aperture in the aponeurosis of the external oblique muscle called the *superficial inguinal ring* (Fig. 34.17). The so called ring is really an obtuse angled triangle. The base of the triangle is formed by the pubic crest. The two sides of the triangle form the lateral (or lower) and the medial (or upper) margins of the opening: these are referred to as crura. The lateral crus is nothing but the medial part of the inguinal ligament. The medial crus is attached to the front of the symphysis pubis.

5. The *transversalis fascia* is a thin layer of connective tissue that lines the inner surface of the transversus abdominis muscle.

The inguinal canal

This is an oblique passage through the anterior abdominal wall placed a little above the medial part of the inguinal ligament (Fig. 34.17). It begins at the deep inguinal ring which is situated in the trasversalis fascia (see below). The canal passes downwards and medially to reach the superficial inguinal ring. The canal gives passage to the spermatic cord in the male, and the round ligament of the uterus in the female.

The importance of the inguinal canal is that abdominal contents can pass through it to reach the scrotum. This is called inguinal hernia.

The conjoint tendon (or falx inguinalis)

This is made up of some fibres of the aponeuroses of the internal oblique and transversus abdominis muscles that join together and descend to be attached to the pubic crest. The conjoint tendon lies behind the superficial inguinal ring.

Thoracolumbar fascia

This fascia is present in relation to the posterior abdominal wall. The thoracolumbar fascia has three layers (anterior, middle and posterior). The anterior and posterior layers meet at the lateral edge of the quadratus lumborum muscle and the fused layers give attachment to the transversus abdominis and the internal oblique muscles.

Obliquus Externus Abdominis (Fig. 34.18)

Origin:

The muscle arises from the lower eight ribs (i.e., 5th to 12th).

Insertion:

The fibres of the muscle run downwards and forwards and end in an extensive aponeurosis. The aponeurosis is inserted as follows:

(**a**) The upper margin of the aponeurosis passes horizontally to reach the xiphoid process (a in Fig. 34.18).

(b) Succeeding fibres are inserted into the entire length of the linea alba, the lowest ones reaching the pubic symphysis.

(c) The next fibres have a bony attachment to the pubic crest and tubercle.

(d) Lateral to the pubic tubercle the aponeurosis has a free lower border that forms the inguinal ligament; it is attached laterally to the anterior superior iliac spine (d in Fig. 34.18).

The muscle fibres arising from the 11th and 12th ribs are inserted into the anterior half of the iliac crest.

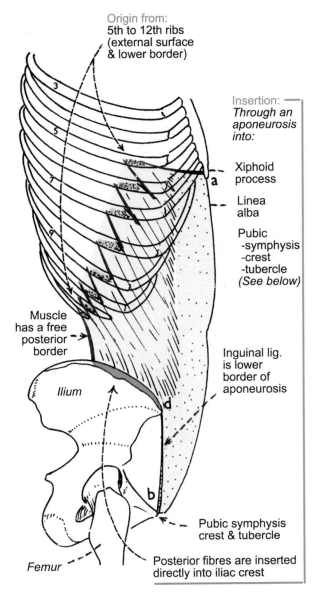

Origin from:
5th to 12th ribs
(external surface
& lower border)

Insertion: ——
*Through an
aponeurosis
into:*

Xiphoid
process

Linea
alba

Pubic
-symphysis
-crest
-tubercle
(See below)

Muscle
has a free
posterior
border

Inguinal lig.
is lower
border of
aponeurosis

Ilium

Femur

Pubic symphysis
crest & tubercle

Posterior fibres are inserted
directly into iliac crest

Fig. 34.18. Lateral view of the trunk to show
the attachments of the external oblique muscle
of the abdomen.

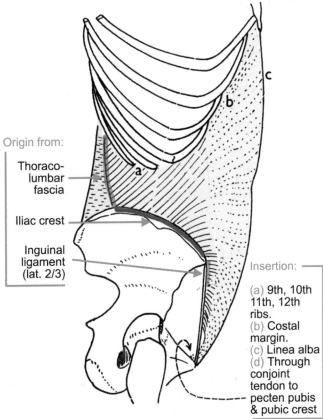

Origin from:

Thoraco-
lumbar
fascia

Iliac crest

Inguinal
ligament
(lat. 2/3)

Insertion: ——

(a) 9th, 10th
11th, 12th
ribs.
(b) Costal
margin.
(c) Linea alba
(d) Through
conjoint
tendon to
pecten pubis
& pubic crest

Fig. 34.19. Lateral view of the trunk to show
attachments of the internal oblique muscle
of the abdomen.

Obliquus Internus Abdominis

The internal oblique muscle of the abdomen lies between the external oblique and the transversus abdominis muscles (Fig. 34.19). The muscle has an origin behind and below, from which the fibres pass forwards and upwards to their insertion. The direction of the fibres is thus at right angles to that of the external oblique.

Origin:

(**a**) The uppermost fibres arise from the thoracolumbar fascia at the lateral border of the quadratus lumborum.

(**b**) The middle fibres arise from the iliac crest (anterior two thirds).

(**c**) The lowest fibres arise from the lateral 2/3 of the inguinal ligament.

Insertion:

The fibres are inserted as follows from above downwards.

(**a**) The fibres arising from the lumbar fascia and the posterior part of the iliac crest are inserted into the lower borders of the 10th, 11th and 12th ribs (a in Fig. 34.19).

(**b**) The fibres from the anterior part of the iliac crest and from the lateral part of the inguinal ligament fan out and end in an aponeurosis. Its upper part is attached to the costal margin (b in Fig. 34.19). Its lower part is attached to the entire length of the linea alba (c in Fig. 34.19).

(**c**) The fibres arising from the middle one third of the inguinal ligament are closely related to the inguinal canal. (They form its anterior wall and its roof). The fibres join some fibres of the transversus abdominis to form the conjoint tendon through which they are attached to the pubic crest and the pecten pubis.

Transversus Abdominis

The transversus abdominis is the deepest muscle of the anterolateral part of the abdominal wall (Fig. 34.20). It has its origin posteriorly. From the origin the fibres run horizontally forwards around the abdominal wall to their insertion.

Origin:

The origin can be divided into four parts from above downwards.

(**a**) The upper fibres arise from the lower six costal cartilages.

(**b**) The middle fibres arise from the thoracolumbar fascia.

(**c**) The lower fibres arise from the ventral segment of the iliac crest (anterior two thirds).

(**d**) The lowest fibres arise from the lateral one third of the inguinal ligament.

Insertion:

The fibres end in an aponeurosis which is inserted chiefly into the linea alba. The lowest part of the aponeurosis joins that of the internal oblique to form the conjoint tendon through which it is inserted into the pecten pubis and the pubic crest.

The aponeurosis of the transversus abdominis muscle takes part in forming the sheath for the rectus abdominis muscle along with those of the external and internal oblique muscles.

Nerve supply of anterolateral muscles of abdomen

The external oblique, the internal oblique and the transversus abdominis muscles are all supplied by the lower six thoracic spinal nerves. The internal oblique and transversus abdominis are also supplied by the first lumbar nerve.

Actions of anterolateral muscles of abdomen

The actions of these muscles are as follows:

(**a**) They support the abdominal viscera, counteracting the effect of gravity specially in the sitting or standing position.

(**b**) By active contraction they increase the intra-abdominal pressure which pushes up the diaphragm during expiration: and helps to expel contents of abdominal viscera in defaecation, micturition, vomiting and in child birth.

Rectus Abdominis

The rectus abdominis runs vertically in the anterior abdominal wall next to the midline (Fig. 34.21). The muscles of the two sides are separated by the linea

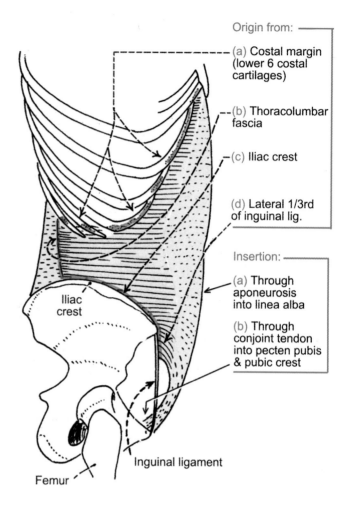

Origin from:
(a) Costal margin (lower 6 costal cartilages)
(b) Thoracolumbar fascia
(c) Iliac crest
(d) Lateral 1/3rd of inguinal lig.

Insertion:
(a) Through aponeurosis into linea alba
(b) Through conjoint tendon into pecten pubis & pubic crest

Iliac crest

Inguinal ligament

Femur

Fig. 34.20. Lateral view of the trunk to show the attachments of the transversus abdominis muscle.

alba. The origin of the muscle lies at its lower end, and the insertion at its upper end.

At its lower end the muscle is attached to the pubis. Its upper end is attached to the 5th, 6th and 7th costal cartilages.

Nerve supply:

The rectus abdominis is supplied by the lower six or seven thoracic nerves.

Actions:

The rectus abdominis can bend the trunk forwards. It assists the anterolateral muscles in supporting the abdominal viscera and in increasing intraabdominal pressure.

The lateral border of the rectus abdominis can be made out on the surface of the living as a groove called the linea semilunaris.

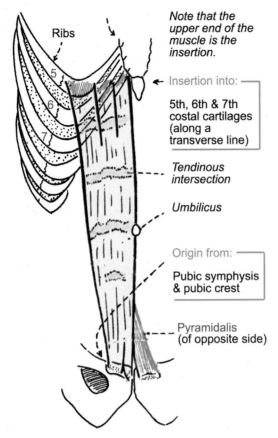

Note that the upper end of the muscle is the insertion.

Ribs

Insertion into:

5th, 6th & 7th costal cartilages (along a transverse line)

Tendinous intersection

Umbilicus

Origin from:

Pubic symphysis & pubic crest

Pyramidalis (of opposite side)

Fig. 34.21. Scheme to show the attachments of the rectus abdominis.

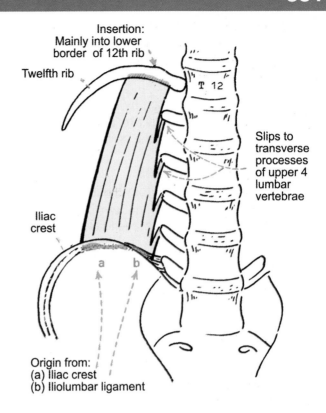

Insertion: Mainly into lower border of 12th rib

Twelfth rib

T 12

Slips to transverse processes of upper 4 lumbar vertebrae

Iliac crest

a   b

Origin from:
(a) Iliac crest
(b) Iliolumbar ligament

Fig. 34.22. Scheme to show attachments of the quadratus lumborum muscle.

MUSCLES OF POSTERIOR ABDOMINAL WALL

The muscles of the posterior abdominal wall are the psoas major and minor, the iliacus and the quadratus lumborum. The attachments of the psoas muscles and of the iliacus have been described in Chapter 29. The quadratus lumborum is described below.

The Quadratus Lumborum

The quadratus lumborum is so called because of its quadrilateral shape. It forms the posterior abdominal wall between the psoas major medially, and the transversus abdominis laterally. It is enclosed between the anterior and middle layers of the thoracolumbar fascia.

Origin:

The origin of the muscle lies inferiorly (Fig. 34.22). It arises laterally, from the iliac crest (posterior one third); and medially from the iliolumbar ligament. This ligament stretches from the transverse process of the 5th lumbar vertebra to the iliac crest .

Insertion:

The muscle is inserted chiefly into the lower border of the twelfth rib (medial half).

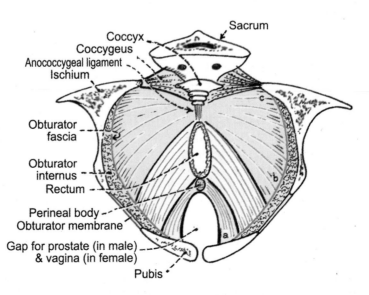

Sacrum

Coccyx
Coccygeus
Anococcygeal ligament
Ischium

Obturator fascia

Obturator internus

Rectum

Perineal body
Obturator membrane

Gap for prostate (in male) & vagina (in female)

Pubis

Fig. 34.23. Scheme to show the arrangement of the levator ani and coccygeus muscles.

Nerve Supply:

It is supplied by the ventral rami of the twelfth thoracic and upper lumbar nerves.

Actions:

The muscle aids respiration by fixing the twelfth rib allowing the diaphragm to act to better advantage. It can cause lateral flexion of the vertebral column.

MUSCLES OF THE PELVIS

The pelvic muscles arise from the inner wall of the bony pelvis. Two of them, the *piriformis*, and the *obturator internus*, have been considered in the lower extremity.

The other pelvic muscles are the *levator ani* and the *coccygeus*. Their subdivisions and attachments are shown in Fig. 34.23. The muscles of the two sides form the *pelvic diaphragm*.

Present in relation to pelvic muscles (and viscera) there are layers of fascia that are collectively referred to as *pelvic fascia*.

Pelvic diaphragm

The levator ani and the coccygeus form a transverse partition across the pelvis which is called the pelvic diaphragm. This diaphragm separates the pelvic viscera (above) from structures in the perineum and the ischiorectal fossa. The pelvic diaphragm is pierced by the rectum, the urethra, and in the female by the vagina. The diaphragm supports the pelvic viscera. It acts as a sphincter for the rectum and the vagina.

35

Nerves of the Trunk

The trunk contains a large number of nerves. The purpose of this section is to give students a general idea of these nerves. For details please a consult the authors *Textbook of Anatomy*.

The nerves of the trunk can be divided into two major categories.

1. Some of them are similar to nerves studied in the limbs are concerned with the supply of skeletal muscles and skin.

2. Others are concerned with the supply of viscera. They provide a sensory supply to viscera, innervate smooth muscle in their walls, and give a secretomotor supply to glands. These nerves belong to the autonomic nervous system. Parts of the autonomic nervous system are to be seen throughout the trunk. We will, therefore, first consider this system.

THE AUTONOMIC NERVOUS SYSTEM

The autonomic nervous system is responsible for the nerve supply of viscera and blood vessels. It is subdivided into two main parts. These are the **sympathetic** and **parasympathetic** nervous systems. Both these divisions contain efferent as well as afferent fibres. The basic arrangement of sympathetic and parasympathetic neurons is shown in Fig. 35.1

The efferent fibres supply smooth muscle throughout the body. The influence of these nerves may be either to cause contraction or relaxation. In a given situation the sympathetic and parasympathetic nerves generally produce opposite effects. For example, sympathetic stimulation causes dilatation of the pupil, whereas parasympathetic stimulation causes constriction. In addition to the supply of smooth muscle, autonomic nerves supply glands: such nerves are described as **secretomotor**. The secretomotor nerves to almost all glands are parasympathetic. The only exception are the sweat glands which have a sympathetic supply.

In the thorax, the parasympathetic nervous system is represented by the vagus nerve; and the sympathetic nervous system by the right and left sympathetic trunks and their branches. Autonomic fibres pass

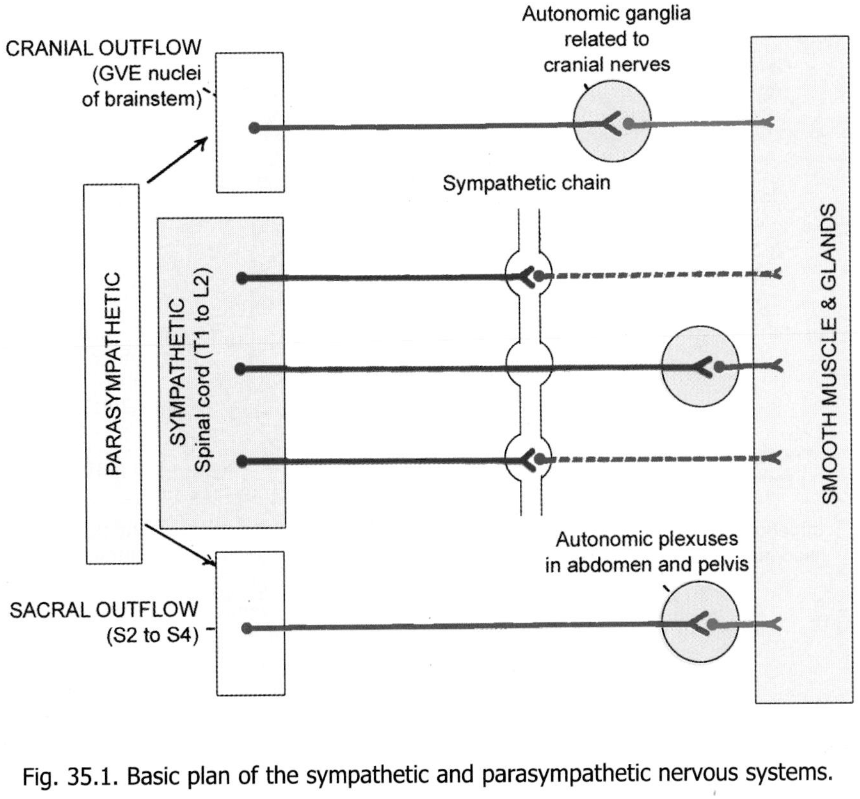

Fig. 35.1. Basic plan of the sympathetic and parasympathetic nervous systems.

through a number of plexuses. These include cardiac and oesophageal plexuses present in the thorax, and numerous plexuses present in the abdomen and pelvis.

The Sympathetic Trunk

There are two sympathetic trunks, right and left. Each trunk is a long nerve cord placed on either side of the vertebral column and extending from the base of the skull above, to the coccyx below. The trunk bears a number of sympathetic ganglia along its length. The ganglia contain sympathetic neurons (Fig. 35.3).

Basically there is one ganglion corresponding to each spinal nerve, but in many situations the ganglia of adjoining segments fuse so that they appear to be fewer in number than the spinal nerves. The ventral primary ramus of each spinal nerve receives fibres from a sympathetic ganglion through a delicate communication called the **_grey ramus communicans_**. In the case of spinal nerves T1 to L2 (or L3) there is, in addition to the grey ramus, a **_white ramus communicans_** through which fibres pass from the spinal nerve to the ganglion. Some sympathetic neurons are also present in autonomic plexuses.

Sympathetic neurons supply:
1. Sweat glands and some smooth muscle present in the skin.
2. Blood vessels.
3. Viscera.

NERVES OF THE HEAD AND NECK

The nerves of the head and neck are cranial nerves arising from the brain, and spinal nerves arising from the spinal cord. Spinal nerves of the head and neck are cervical nerves.

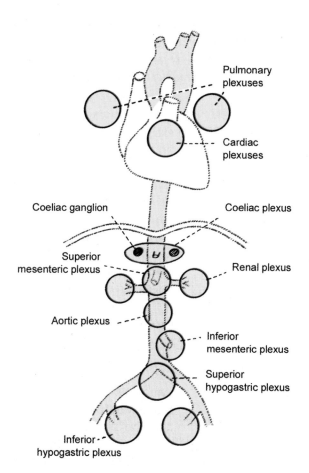

Fig. 35.2. Schematic presentation of the location of important autonomic plexuses in the thorax and abdomen.

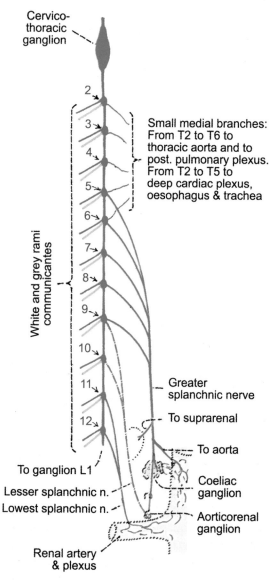

Fig. 35.3. Thoracic part of the sympathetic trunk. Note the ganglia and the numerous branches.

CERVICAL NERVES

In the thoracic, lumbar and sacral regions the number of spinal nerves corresponds to that of vertebrae, each nerve lying **below** the numerically corresponding vertebra. However, in the neck we have seven cervical vertebrae, and eight cervical nerves. The reason for this will be clear from Fig. 35.4. Note that the upper seven cervical nerves lie above the numerically corresponding vertebrae. The eighth cervical nerve lies below vertebra C7.

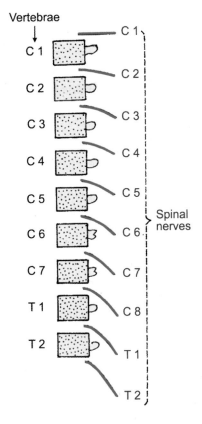

Fig. 35.4. Scheme to show the relationship of cervical and upper thoracic nerves to vertebrae.

Dorsal rami of cervical nerves

The dorsal ramus of a typical spinal nerve is smaller than the ventral ramus. It divides into branches which supply the deep muscles and skin of the back. The area of skin supplied by dorsal rami is shown in Fig. 35.5. This is all that needs to be known about the dorsal rami of most spinal nerves.

The dorsal ramus of the first cervical nerve is seen the suboccipital triangle. It supplies the rectus capitis posterior major and minor, the superior and inferior oblique muscles and the semispinalis capitis

The dorsal ramus of the second cervical nerve is large. It reaches the suboccipital region and its main continuation forms the **greater occipital nerve**.

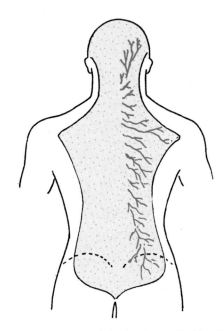

Fig. 35.5. Area of skin of the back supplied by dorsal rami of spinal nerves.

THE VENTRAL RAMI OF CERVICAL NERVES

The ventral rami of the first, second, third and fourth cervical nerves unite with each other to form the **cervical plexus**. The ventral rami of the fifth, sixth, seventh and eighth cervical nerves, and the greater part of the ventral ramus of the first thoracic nerve, join one another to form the brachial plexus. The brachial plexus has been described in Chapter 25. The cervical plexus is described below.

THE CERVICAL PLEXUS AND ITS BRANCHES

The cervical plexus is formed by the ventral rami of the first, second, third and fourth cervical nerves. as shown in Fig. 35.6.

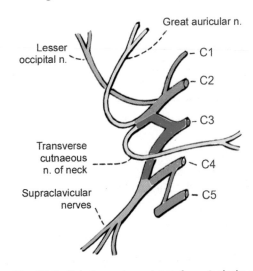

Fig. 35.6. Cutaneous branches of cervical plexus.

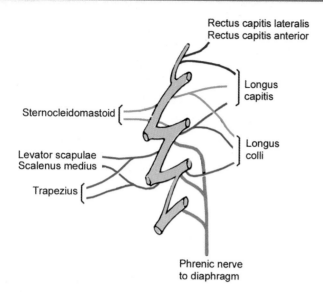

Fig. 35.7. Scheme to show the muscular branches of the cervical plexus.

The cervical plexus gives off a large number of branches. The **cutaneous branches** are shown in Fig. 35.6 and are as follows. The **lesser occipital** nerve arises from the second cervical nerve. The **greater auricular** nerve and the **transverse cutaneous nerve of the neck** arise from the second and third nerves. The **supraclavicular** nerves arise from the third and fourth nerves. The **muscular branches** of the cervical plexus are shown in Fig. 35.7. The most important of these is the phrenic nerve.

The Phrenic Nerve

The phrenic nerve is important as it is the only motor supply to the diaphragm.

This nerve arises from the (ventral rami of) spinal nerves C3, C4 and C5. The nerve descends vertically through the lower part of the neck, and then through the thorax to reach the diaphragm..

THE CRANIAL NERVES

There are twelve pairs of cranial nerves that emerge from the surface of the brain. They are identified by number (in cranio-caudal sequence) and also bear names as follows.

The **first** cranial nerve is called the **olfactory** nerve. It is the nerve of smell (Olfaction = smell). The pathway for smell has been considered in Chapter 21.

The **second** cranial nerve is called the **optic** nerve. It is the nerve of sight (Optics = science of formation of images). The

pathway for sight has been considered in Chapter 21

The **third** cranial nerve is called the **oculomotor** nerve as it supplies several muscles that move the eyeball (Ocular = pertaining to the eye). This nerve also carries fibres that supply the sphincter pupillae, and the ciliaris muscles (responsible for accomodation of vision).

The **fourth** cranial nerve is called the **trochlear** nerve. It is so called because it supplies a muscle (superior oblique) that passes through a pulley (trochlea = pulley).

The **sixth** cranial nerve is called the **abducent** nerve because it supplies a muscle (lateral rectus) which 'abducts' the eyeball.

Note that the oculomotor, trochlear and abducent nerves are together reesponsible for movements of the eyeball.

The Trigeminal nerve

The trigeminal nerve is so called because it consists of three main divisions. These are the **ophthalmic nerve**, the **maxillary nerve** and the **mandibular nerve**.(Fig. 35.8). The trigeminal nerve contains both afferent and efferent fibres. Afferent fibres are distributed through all three divisions of the nerve. They carry sensations from the skin of the face, the mucous membrane of the mouth, and the mucous membrane of the nose. The ophthalmic nerve is distributed to structures in the orbit. The maxillary nerve is distributed to structures present in relation to the upper jaw. The

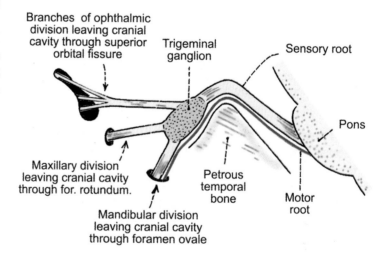

Fig. 35.8. Roots and divisions of the trigeminal nerve.

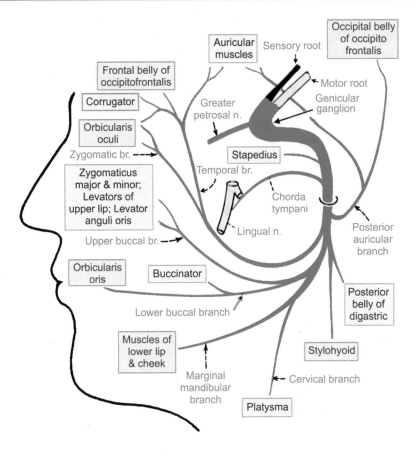

Fig. 35.9. Scheme to show the branches of the facial nerve.

mandibular nerve is distributed to structures in the region of the mandible. These include the muscles of mastication. One of its branches (the lingual nerve) supplies the tongue.

The Facial nerve

The *facial* nerve is the *seventh* cranial nerve. It gives of several branches that supply the muscles in the face, in the scalp and some in the neck (Fig. 35.9). It also carries secretomotor fibres for the lacrimal gland, the submandibular and sublingual salivary glands. The facial nerve also carries fibres of taste from the anterior part of the tongue. Many of the secretomotor and taste fibres travel for part of their course through a branch of the facial nerve called the *chorda tympani*. The exact pathways concerned are very complex and we will not go into them.

The *eighth* cranial nerve is called the *vestibulo-cochlear* nerve because it supplies structures in the vestibular and cochlear parts of the internal ear. The pathway for hearing has been considered in Chapter 21. The *ninth* cranial nerve is called the *glossopharyngeal* nerve as it is distributed to the

pharynx and to part of the tongue (glossal = pertaining to the tongue). It carries fibres of taste from the posterior part of the tongue, and secretomotor fibres for the parotid gland.

The Vagus nerve

The *tenth* cranial nerve is called the *vagus*. It has an extensive course through the neck, the thorax and the abdomen. (The word vagus may be correlated with 'vagrant' = wandering from place to place). *The fibres of the vagus nerve are parasympathetic*. They are distributed to numerous organs in the thorax and abdomen. These include the heart, the respiratory system, and the greater part of the alimentary canal. Fibres of the vagus nerve take part in the formation of many plexuses present in close relation to these organs.

The Accessory nerve

The *eleventh* cranial nerve is called the *accessory* nerve because it appears to be a part of the vagus nerve (or 'accessory' to the vagus). It divides into cranial and spinal branches. The cranial branch joins the vagus nerve and is distributed through branches of the latter to the pharynx and larynx. The spinal branch supplies the sternocleidomastoid and trapezius muscles.

The *twelfth* cranial nerve is called the *hypoglossal* nerve (because it runs part of its course below the tongue before supplying the muscles in it (hypo = below; glossal = pertaining to tongue).

Attachment of cranial nerves to the brain

The olfactory and optic nerves are connected to the cerebral hemispheres. The third and fourth nerves emerge from the surface of the midbrain; and the fifth from the pons. The sixth, seventh and eighth nerves emerge at the junction of the pons and medulla. The ninth, tenth, eleventh and twelfth cranial nerves emerge from the surface of the medulla.

Relevant Foramina of Skull

The foramina through which cranial nerves enter or leave the skull are given in Chapter 32.

NERVES OF THORACIC WALL

VENTRAL RAMI OF THORACIC NERVES

There are twelve pairs of thoracic nerves, each pair emerging from the vertebral canal below the corresponding vertebra. Each nerve divides into a dorsal ramus and a ventral ramus. The dorsal rami pass backwards and divide into medial and lateral branches

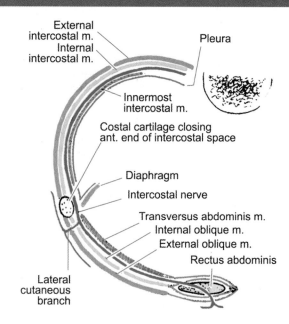

Fig. 35.11. Scheme to show the course of one of the lower intercostal nerves. The intercostal space and the abdominal wall are cut along the course of the nerve.

that supply muscles and skin of the back. The ventral rami are considered below.

Typical Intercostal Nerves

The ventral rami of the thoracic nerves run into the thoracic wall as the intercostal and subcostal nerves (Fig. 35.10). There being twelve ribs on either side, there are eleven intercostal spaces, and each space has one intercostal nerve. The intercostal nerves are numbered from above downwards. The twelfth pair of nerves lie below the twelfth ribs and are called the *subcostal nerves.*

Typical intercostal nerves are distributed to both muscles and skin through a number of branches. Each intercostal nerve gives several branches that supply the intercostal muscles.

The initial parts of the seventh, eighth, ninth, tenth and eleventh intercostal nerves resemble those of typical intercostal nerves described above. However, on reaching the anterior end of the intercostal space concerned each nerve passes deep to the costal margin to enter the abdominal wall (Fig. 35.11).

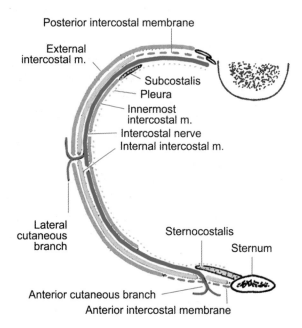

Fig. 35.10. Course and relations of a typical intercostal nerve.

NERVES OF ANTERIOR ABDOMINAL WALL

The nerves that take part in supplying the anterior abdominal wall are:

1. Seventh, eighth, ninth, tenth and eleventh intercostal nerves.

2. The subcostal nerve.

3. The iliohypogastric nerve (derived from the first lumbar nerve).

4. The ilioinguinal nerve (also from L1).

These nerves supply muscles of the anterior abdominal wall and overlying skin.

Autonomic Innervation of the gut

We have already seen that the parasympathetic nerve supply to the greater part of the gastrointestinal tract (from pharynx to the right two thirds of the transverse colon) is through the vagus.

The left one third of the transverse colon, the descending colon, the sigmoid colon, the rectum and the upper part of the anal canal are supplied by the sacral part of the parasympathetic system. These fibres travel through sacral nerves.

As a rule, parasympathetic nerves stimulate intestinal movement and inhibit the sphincters. They are also secretomotor to the glands in the mucosa. Sympathetic fibres are distributed chiefly to blood vessels.

LUMBAR NERVES AND LUMBAR PLEXUS

There are five lumbar nerves. After emerging from the intervertebral foramina they divide into dorsal and ventral rami. Each dorsal ramus gives branches that supply deep muscles of the back (erector spinae). Some branches supply a strip of skin of the back near the middle line.

The ventral rami of the upper four lumbar nerves join each other to form the *lumbar plexus* which is shown

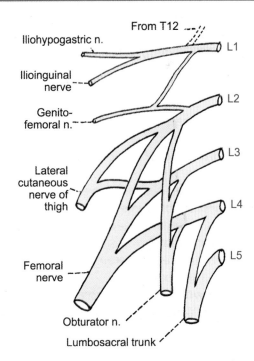

Fig. 35.12. Scheme to show the lumbar plexus and its branches.

in Fig. 35.12. Note that part of the fourth lumbar nerve joins the fifth lumbar to form the lumbosacral trunk which takes part in forming the sacral plexus.

The greater part of the first lumbar nerve is continued into a nerve trunk that divides into the *iliohypogastric* and *ilioinguinal* nerves. The rest of the first lumbar nerve is joined by a branch from the second lumbar to form the *genitofemoral* nerve.

The second, third and the greater part of the fourth lumbar nerve divide into *anterior and posterior divisions*.

The posterior divisions (which are large) from the *femoral nerve*. The posterior divisions of L2 and L3 also give rise to the *lateral cutaneous nerve of the thigh*. The anterior divisions unite to form the *obturator nerve*. Some other branches are shown in Fig. 35.12

Coeliac ganglion

The *coeliac ganglion* (right or left) is the largest autonomic ganglion in the body. Fibres passing from one ganglion to the other (across the aorta and around the origin of the coeliac trunk) form the *coeliac plexus*.

NERVES OF THE PELVIS

The nerves to be seen in relation to the pelvic wall are as follows.

1. The **genitofemoral nerve** divides into genital and femoral branches.

2. The **obturator nerve** is a branch of the lumbar plexus. It supplies structures in the medial side of the thigh and has been described in Chapter 30.

3. The **lumbosacral trunk** is derived from the fourth and fifth lumbar nerves. It descends into the true pelvis. to join the sacral plexus.

4. **Sacral ventral rami** and **sacral plexus**: Lying in front of the sacrum, just behind the lumbosacral trunk we see the ventral rami of sacral nerves. The roots S1, S2 and S3 are large and that of S4 is much smaller. These roots take part in forming the sacral plexus which is described below. The main continuation of the sacral plexus is the **sciatic nerve** which passes out of the pelvis (into the gluteal region) through the greater sciatic foramen.

5. The **pudendal nerve** is a branch of the sacral plexus. It receives contributions from nerves S2, S3 and S4. Along with the internal pudendal artery the nerve passes through the greater sciatic foramen to enter the gluteal region. After a short course in this region the nerve passes through the lesser sciatic foramen to reach the lateral wall of the ischiorectal fossa. The nerve is distributed mainly to the perineum.

The lower sacral rami (S4, S5) join the coccygeal nerve to form the **coccygeal plexus** which lies over the pelvic surface of the coccygeus muscle.

SACRAL PLEXUS

The sacral plexus is formed by the upper four sacral nerves along with the lumbosacral trunk (derived from L4 and L5). Nerves L4, L5, S1 and S2 each divide into anterior and posterior divisions. The posterior divisions of these nerves unite to form the common peroneal part of the sciatic nerve. The anterior divisions of these nerves, and S3 (which does not divide into anterior

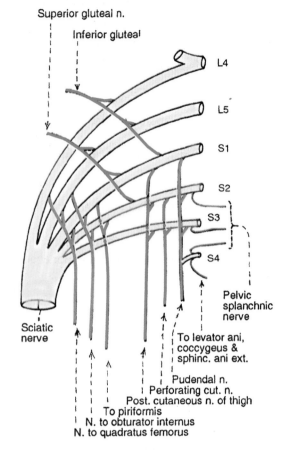

Fig. 35.13. Simplified plan of the sacral plexus.

and posterior divisions) unite to form the tibial part of the sciatic nerve (Fig. 35.13).

Part of nerve S4 joins branches from the ventral divisions of S2 and S3 to form the pudendal nerve.

Apart from the sciatic and pudendal nerves and sacral plexus gives off several branches that are shown in Fig. 31.6. These are as follows:

The branches arising from the posterior divisions are the superior gluteal (L4, L5, S1), the inferior gluteal (L5, S1, S2), the nerve to the piriformis (S1, S2), and the perforating cutaneous nerve (S2, S3). The posterior cutaneous nerve of the thigh receives contributions from both the posterior divisions (S2, S3) and anterior divisions (S1, S2).

The branches arising from the anterior divisions are the nerve to the quadratus femoris (L4, L5, S1); and the nerve to the obturator internus (L5, S1, S2). Nerve S4 gives branches to the levator ani, the coccygeus and the sphincter ani externus. Branches to pelvic viscera (**pelvic splanchnic nerves**) arise from S2, S3 and S4.

36

Main Blood Vessels of the Trunk

The arteries and veins of the body belong to two distinct circulations, pulmonary and systemic (Fig.36.1).

THE PULMONARY CIRCULATION

The vessels of the pulmonary circulation are concerned only with transport of deoxygenated blood to the lungs, and its return to the heart after oxygenation. Even though they carry deoxygenated blood , vessels going from the heart to the lungs are called arteries; and vessels bringing this blood back are called veins. The vessels of the pulmonary circulation are as follows.

1. The **pulmonary trunk** arises from the right ventricle of the heart. After a short course it divides into right and left pulmonary arteries.

2. The right and left **pulmonary arteries** reach the hilum of the corresponding lung. Each artery divides and subdivides into several generations of branches that carry blood to all parts of the lung.

3. After this blood has passed through very rich capillary plexuses present in the walls of alveoli, and has been oxygenated, it passes into venules that drain into larger veins. Ultimately two **pulmonary veins** (upper and lower) emerge from the hilum of each lung, there being four pulmonary veins in all. These veins end by opening into the left atrium of the heart.

THE SYSTEMIC CIRCULATION

The blood vessels of the systemic circulation carry oxygenated blood to all parts of the body. The largest artery of the body is the aorta which arises from the left ventricle of the heart. The aorta and its numerous ramifications carry this blood to all organs and tissues. Blood returns to the heart through the superior and inferior venae

cavae which open into the right atrium of the heart.

THE AORTA

For purposes of description the aorta is divided into the following parts (Fig. 36.2).

1. The **ascending aorta** lies just behind the sternum. It passes upwards from the aortic orifice. At the level of the sternal angle it becomes continuous with the arch of the aorta. The only branches of the ascending aorta are the right and left **coronary arteries** that supply blood to the walls of the heart.

2. The **arch of the aorta** is shaped like a semicircle that is convex upwards. It passes from right to left,

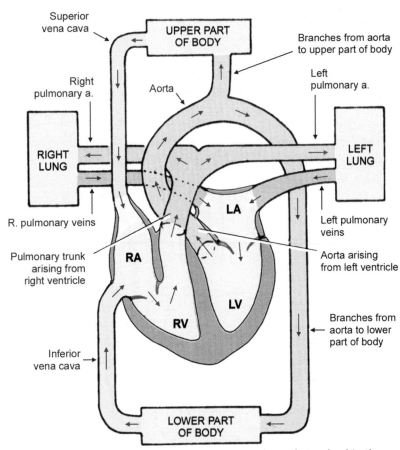

Fig. 36.1. Scheme to illustrate the main channels involved in the circulation of blood

and also from front to back. The summit of the arch reaches the level of the middle of the manubrium sterni. Its posterior end lies on the left side of the body of the fourth thoracic vertebra.

3. The posterior end of the arch of the aorta becomes continuous with the **descending thoracic aorta**. This part runs downwards to reach the aortic opening in the diaphragm, situated at the level of the lower border of the twelfth thoracic vertebra. Here it becomes continuous with the abdominal aorta.

4. The **abdominal aorta** descends in front of the lumbar vertebrae. It terminates in front of the fourth lumbar vertebra by dividing into the right and left common iliac arteries.

BRANCHES ARISING FROM THE AORTA

Branches from ascending aorta
1. **Right coronary artery**
2. **Left coronary artery**

The coronary arteries supply the heart muscle. Narrowing of the arteries takes place with advancing age. It can lead to coronary insufficiency, in which the patient has pain in the region of the sternum on exertion. This is called **angina pectoris**. Blockage of a branch of a coronary artery leads to a heart attack (**coronary thrombosis**).

Branches from arch of aorta
1. **Brachiocephalic artery**. This is the first branch of the arch of the aorta. It ends behind the right

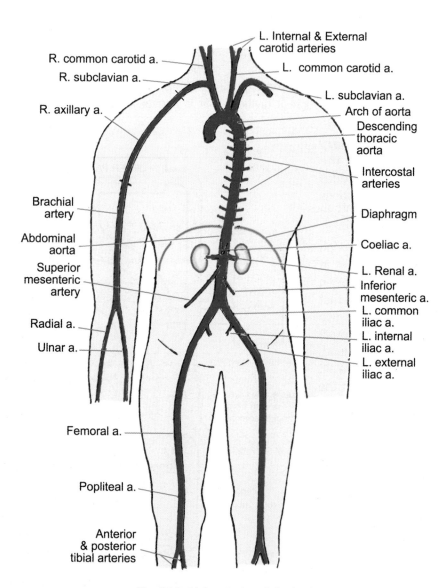

Fig. 36.2. Main arteries of the body

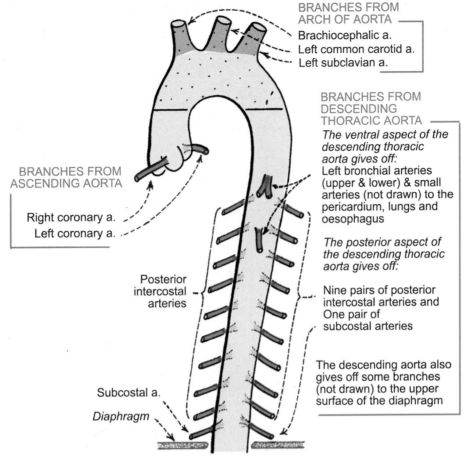

Fig. 36.3. Scheme to show branches arising from the aorta in the thorax.

In the figure:

BRANCHES FROM ARCH OF AORTA
Brachiocephalic a.
Left common carotid a.
Left subclavian a.

BRANCHES FROM ASCENDING AORTA
Right coronary a.
Left coronary a.

Posterior intercostal arteries

Subcostal a.

Diaphragm

BRANCHES FROM DESCENDING THORACIC AORTA

The ventral aspect of the descending thoracic aorta gives off:
Left bronchial arteries (upper & lower) & small arteries (not drawn) to the pericardium, lungs and oesophagus

The posterior aspect of the descending thoracic aorta gives off:

Nine pairs of posterior intercostal arteries and One pair of subcostal arteries

The descending aorta also gives off some branches (not drawn) to the upper surface of the diaphragm

sternoclavicular joint by dividing into the right common carotid and right subclavian arteries.

2. The **left common carotid artery** is the second branch of the arch of the aorta. It runs upwards and enters the neck passing behind the left sternoclavicular joint.

3. The third branch of the arch of the aorta is the **left subclavian artery**. It runs upwards and enters the neck at the level of the left sternoclavicular joint.

The **common carotid arteries** pass upwards in the neck lying lateral to the trachea and oesophagus. They end by dividing into the external carotid and internal carotid arteries.

The right or left **subclavian artery** forms an arch that runs laterally through the lower part of the neck. It then passes behind the clavicle and becomes the axillary artery.

Branches from descending thoracic aorta

These are shown in Fig. 36.3.

1. **Posterior intercostal arteries** for the lower nine intercostal spaces arise from the descending aorta. They supply intercostal muscles, skin of the thoracic wall and parietal pleura. The lowest two intercostal arteries also supply part of the abdominal wall.

2. The **subcostal arteries** lie below the 12th rib. After a short course in the thorax the artery enters the abdominal wall.

3. Some **bronchial arteries** arise from the aorta. In addition to bronchi they supply connective tissue of the lungs.

Branches from abdominal aorta

These are shown in Fig. 36.4. They are classified as follows.

(a) Unpaired **ventral branches** supply the gut. These are:

(1) The **coeliac artery**.
(2) The **superior mesenteric artery**.
(3) The **inferior mesenteric artery**

(b) Paired **lateral branches**.

(1) The most important of these are the right and left **renal arteries**. They supply the kidneys.
(2) **Testicular or ovarian arteries** supply the gonads.
(3) Small branches are given off to the suprarenal gland and the diaphragm.

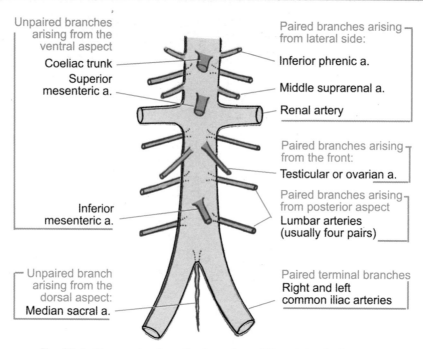

Fig. 36.4. Diagram to show the branches of the abdominal aorta.

(c) **Dorsal branches**. These are:

(1) Right and left **lumbar arteries** (usually four on each side) supply the abdominal wall.

(2) The **median sacral artery** arises from the lower end of the aorta and descends over the sacrum.

(d) **Terminal branches**: The abdominal aorta ends by dividing into the right and left **common iliac arteries**.

Further description of some of the branches of the aorta named above is given below.

RAMIFICATIONS OF BRANCHES ARISING FROM ARCH OF AORTA

BRANCHES OF THE EXTERNAL CAROTID ARTERY

The branches (in order of origin) are as follows (Fig. 36.5).

1. The **superior thyroid artery** takes part in supplying the thyroid ad parathyroid glands.

2. The **ascending pharyngeal artery** supplies the wall of the pharynx and related structures, and gives some branches to the middle ear.

3. The **lingual artery** supplies the tongue.

4. The **facial artery** supplies the face.

5. The **occipital artery** supplies part of the scalp and part of the pinna.

6. The **posterior auricular artery** supplies part of the auricle.

7. The **maxillary artery** supplies structures in relation to the upper and lower jaws (Fig. 36.6). It also supplies parts of the nasal cavity and the orbit.

8. The terminal part of the external carotid artery becomes the **superficial temporal artery**. It supplies the scalp, part of the auricle and part of the face.

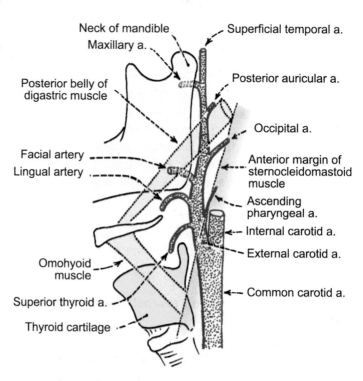

Fig. 36.5. Branches of external carotid artery

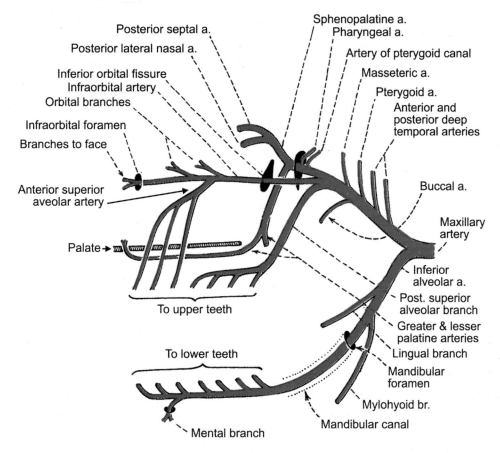

Fig. 36.6. Branches of the maxillary artery.

BRANCHES OF THE INTERNAL CAROTID ARTERY

The internal carotid artery does not give any branch in the neck. After entering the skull the artery gives a number of small branches (shown in Fig. 36.7). The large branches given off are as follows.

1. The *ophthalmic artery* supplies structures in the orbit, including the eyeball. Some of its branches reach the scalp.

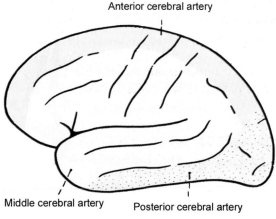

Fig. 36.8. Arteries supplying the superolateral surface of the cerebral hemisphere.

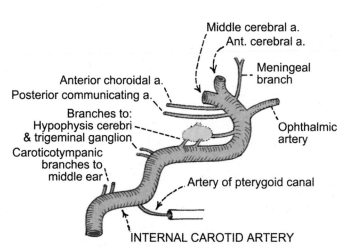

Fig. 36.7. Scheme to show the branches given off by the internal carotid artery.

2, 3. The *anterior cerebral artery* and the *middle cerebral artery* supply part of the cerebral hemisphere. The areas supplied are shown in Figs. 36.8 to 36.10. They take part in forming an arterial circle (*circulus arteriosus*) related to the base of the brain (Fig. 36.11).

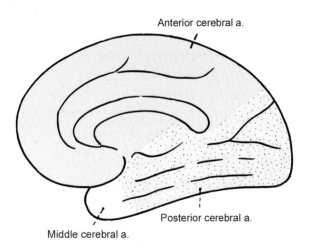

Fig. 36.9. Arteries supplying the medial surface of the cerebral hemisphere.

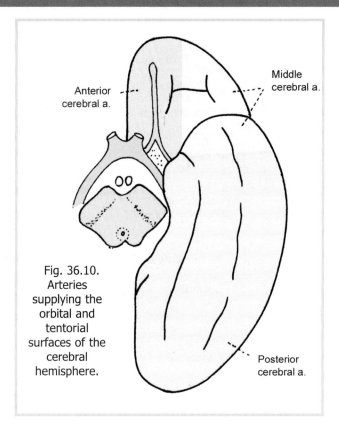

Fig. 36.10. Arteries supplying the orbital and tentorial surfaces of the cerebral hemisphere.

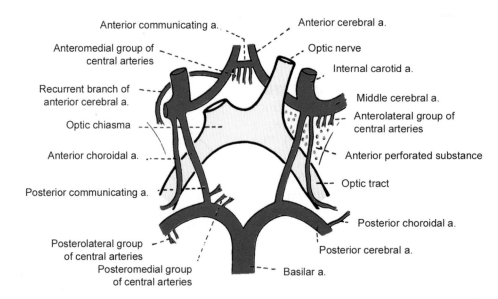

Fig. 36.11. The circulus arteriosus and related structures.

BRANCHES OF SUBCLAVIAN ARTERY

The branches of the subclavian artery are shown in Fig. 36.12.

1. The **vertebral artery** is the first branch. After a short upwards course the artery enters the foramen transversarium of the sixth cervical vertebra (Fig. 36.13). Emerging from the foramen transversarium of the atlas, the artery passes through the suboccipital region. It then passes through the foramen magnum to enter the cranial artery. Here it joins the vertebral artery of the opposite side to form the **basilar artery**. Branches given off by the vertebral artery are shown in Fig. 36.13. Note the **posterior inferior cerebellar artery** to the cerebellum.

The basilar artery is shown in Fig. 36.14. It gives two branches to the cerebellum. These are the **superior cerebellar artery** and the **anterior inferior cerebellar artery**. It terminates by dividing into the

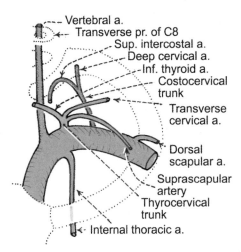

Fig. 36.12. Scheme to show the branches of the subclavian artery.

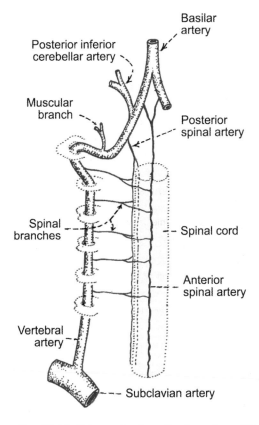

Fig. 36.13. Scheme to show the branches of the vertebral artery.

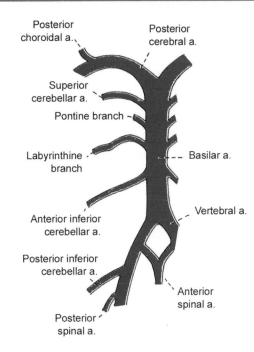

Fig. 36.14. Branches of the basilar artery. Some branches of the vertebral artery are also shown.

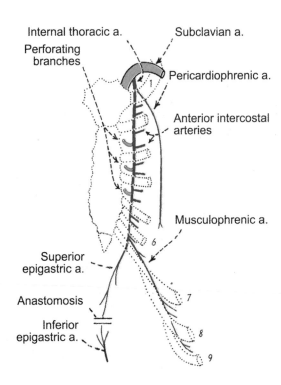

Fig. 36.15. Internal thoracic artery and its branches.

right and left *posterior cerebral arteries* which help to supply the cerebral hemispheres (Figs. 36.8 to 36.10). In Fig. 36.11 note that these arteries take part in forming the circulus arteriosus.

2. The next branch of the subclavian artery (after the vertebral) is the *internal thoracic artery*. It descends into the thorax and gives off a series of *anterior intercostal branches* (Fig. 36.15). It ends by dividing into the *musculophrenic* and *superior epigastric* branches. Other branches are shown in the figure.

3. The third branch of the subclavian artery is the thyrocervical trunk (Fig. 36.12). It ends by dividing into the following.

(a) The *inferior thyroid artery* supplies the thyroid gland.

(b) The *transverse cervical artery* divides into superficial and deep branches. The deep branch

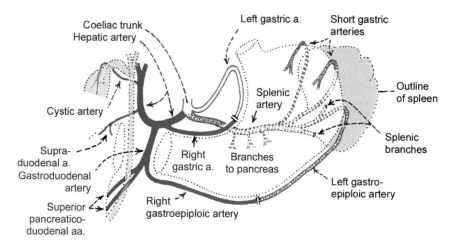

Fig. 36.16. Scheme to show the distribution of the hepatic and splenic arteries.

descends into the scapular region and takes part in the anastomosis around the scapula. (Ch. 26).

(c) the *suprascapular artery* also takes part in the anastomosis around the scapula.

4. The costocervical trunk (Fig. 36.12) divides into the following.

(a) The *superior intercostal artery* supplies the first intercostal space.

(b) The *deep cervical artery* reaches the back of the neck.

5. The *dorsal scapular artery* is not always present. When present it replaces the deep branch of the transverse cervical artery.

We have already seen that the subclavian artery continues into the upper limb as the axillary artery (Chapter 26).

This completes our consideration of the ramifications of branches arising from the arch of the aorta. Branches arising from the descending thoracic aorta do not require further consideration. We will go on to consider the distribution of some branches of the abdominal aorta.

RAMIFICATIONS OF SOME BRANCHES OF ABDOMINAL AORTA

BRANCHES OF COELIAC TRUNK

The coeliac trunk divides into the left gastric, hepatic and splenic arteries (Fig. 36.16). The *left gastric artery* supplies part of the stomach. The *splenic artery* supplies the spleen. It also gives off the *left gastroepiploic artery* to the stomach. The *hepatic artery* supplies the liver. It also gives off the *right gastric artery* to the stomach, and the *gastroduodenal artery*. The *right gastroepiploic artery* is a branch of the gastroduodenal artery. In this way the entire stomach is supplied through branches of the coeliac trunk. Other branches arising

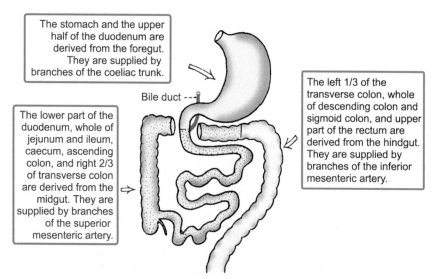

Fig. 36.17. Scheme to show parts of the gut supplied by the coeliac trunk, the superior mesenteric and inferior mesenteric arteries.

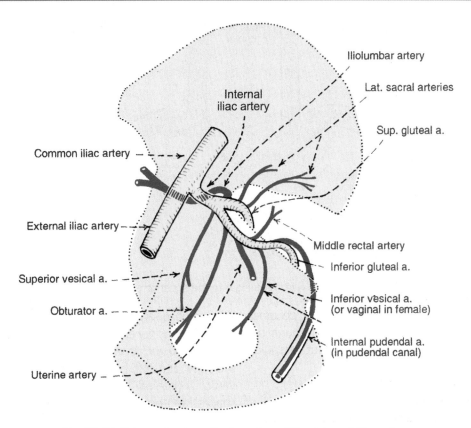

Fig. 36.18. Scheme to show the branches of the internal iliac artery.

from the hepatic artery and the gastroduodenal artery supply part of the duodenum, the gall bladder and the pancreas. The pancreas also receives branches from the splenic artery.

DISTRIBUTION OF SUPERIOR AND INFERIOR MESENTERIC ARTERIES

The superior and inferior mesenteric arteries supply parts of the gut not supplied by the coeliac trunk. Their distribution is summarised in Fig. 36.17.

Further consideration of other branches of the abdominal aorta is not necessary. We will go on to the common iliac arteries.

RAMIFICATIONS OF COMMON ILIAC ARTERIES

The common iliac arteries are terminal branches of the abdominal aorta. Each artery runs downwards and laterally and ends by dividing the external and internal iliac arteries.

The *external iliac artery* continues in the same direction as the common iliac. Reaching the inguinal ligament, it passes deep to it and becomes the femoral artery. The femoral artery has been considered in Chapter 31.

The external iliac artery gives off the *inferior epigastric artery* and the *deep circumflex iliac artery*. Both of them supply the abdominal wall.

The branches of the internal iliac artery are shown in Fig. 36.18. The artery divides into anterior and posterior trunks.

Branches from anterior trunk

1. The *superior vesical artery* supplies the urinary bladder.

2. The *inferior vesical artery* also supplies the urinary bladder. It is present only in the male. In the female its is replaced by the *vaginal artery*.

3. The *middle rectal artery* supplies part of the rectum.

4. The *uterine artery* supplies the uterus and uterine tubes. Some branches reach the vagina and the ovary.

5. The *obturator artery* supplies part of the pelvic wall.

6. The *internal pudendal artery* leaves the pelvis through the greater sciatic foramen. After a short course through the gluteal region the artery passes into the lesser sciatic foramen and comes to lie in the ischiorectal fossa. Finally, it enters the perineum and supplies structures in it.

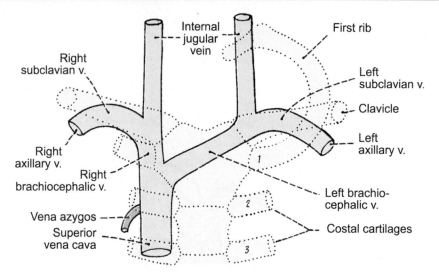

Fig. 36.19. Large veins draining into the superior vena cava.

7. The terminal part of the anterior trunk becomes the **inferior gluteal artery**. It passes through the greater sciatic foramen to reach the gluteal region (Chapter 31).

Branches from the posterior trunk

1. The **iliolumbar artery** supplies the psoas major and the ilacus muscles.

2. The **lateral sacral arteries** supply the sacrum.

3. The **superior gluteal artery** passes through the greater sciatic foramen and supplies structures in the gluteal region.

VEINS OF THE TRUNK

The veins of the trunk are the superior and inferior venae cavae and their tributaries.

TRIBUTARIES OF THE SUPERIOR VENA CAVA

1. The chief vein of the head and neck is the **internal jugular vein** (Fig. 36.20). It begins just below the skull and descends to the sternal end of the clavicle. It ends by joining the corresponding subclavian vein.

2. The **subclavian vein** is a continuation of the axillary vein. It runs transversely through the lower part of the neck and joins the internal jugular vein.

3. On each side the internal jugular vein joins the subclavian vein to form the brachiocephalic vein. The **right brachiocephalic vein** is short and runs vertically in the upper part of the thorax. Note its position in Fig. 36.19. The **left brachiocephalic vein** is much longer.

It runs obliquely behind the manubrium sterni to join the right brachiocephalic vein.

4. The **superior vena cava** is formed by union of the right and left brachiocephalic veins. It descends vertically (behind the first and second right intercostal spaces) and enters the right atrium of the heart. The superior also receives the termination of the vena azygos.

Tributaries of the internal jugular vein

The internal jugular vein receives the facial vein, the lingual vein, and veins from the thyroid gland (Fig. 36.20). The thoracic duct (carrying lymph from a large part of the body) opens into the junction of the left internal jugular and subclavian veins. On the right side the right lymphatic duct has a similar termination.

Some other veins of the head and neck

The **superficial temporal vein** and the **maxillary vein** (which accompany the corresponding arteries) join to form the **retromandibular vein** (Fig. 36.21). After descending for a short distance this vein divides into anterior and posterior divisions. The anterior division joins the facial vein to form the **common facial vein**. The posterior division joins the posterior auricular vein to form the **external jugular vein**. The external jugular vein terminates by joining the subclavian vein. This vein is prominent and can be seen on the side of the neck in living persons. The **anterior jugular vein** runs down the front of the neck and then turns backwards to end in the external jugular vein.

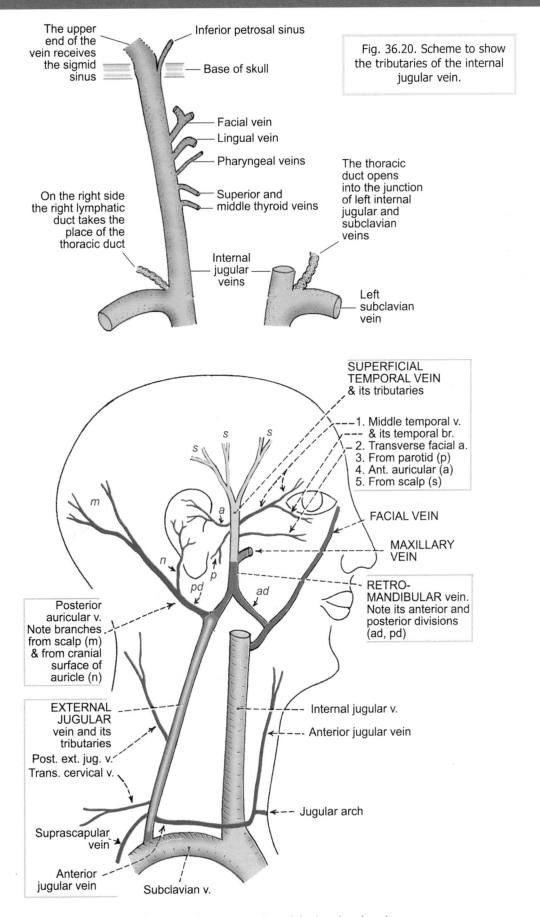

The upper end of the vein receives the sigmid sinus

Inferior petrosal sinus

Base of skull

Fig. 36.20. Scheme to show the tributaries of the internal jugular vein.

Facial vein

Lingual vein

Pharyngeal veins

The thoracic duct opens into the junction of left internal jugular and subclavian veins

On the right side the right lymphatic duct takes the place of the thoracic duct

Superior and middle thyroid veins

Internal jugular veins

Left subclavian vein

SUPERFICIAL TEMPORAL VEIN & its tributaries

1. Middle temporal v. & its temporal br.
2. Transverse facial a.
3. From parotid (p)
4. Ant. auricular (a)
5. From scalp (s)

FACIAL VEIN

MAXILLARY VEIN

RETRO-MANDIBULAR vein. Note its anterior and posterior divisions (ad, pd)

Posterior auricular v. Note branches from scalp (m) & from cranial surface of auricle (n)

EXTERNAL JUGULAR vein and its tributaries

Post. ext. jug. v.
Trans. cervical v.

Internal jugular v.

Anterior jugular vein

Jugular arch

Suprascapular vein

Anterior jugular vein

Subclavian v.

Fig. 36.21. Scheme to show some veins of the head and neck.

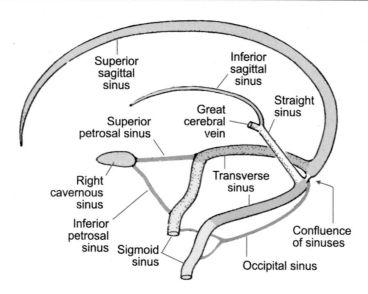

Fig. 36.22. Scheme to show the intracranial venous sinuses. Note that the transverse, sigmoid and cavernous sinus are paired. The petrosal sinuses are also paired. The superior and inferior sagittal sinuses, and the straight sinus are unpaired.

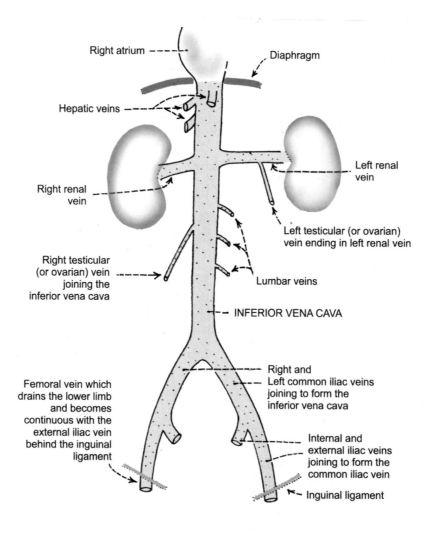

Fig. 36.23. Scheme to show the inferior vena cava and its tributaries.

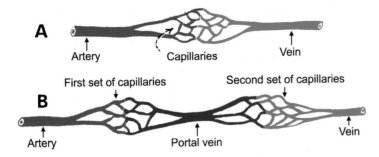

Fig. 36.24. Scheme to compare systemic **(a)** and portal **(b)** circulations.

Intracranial venous sinuses

Within the cranial cavity there are a number of intracranial venous sinuses (Fig. 36.22). Identify the superior and inferior sagittal sinuses, the transverse and sigmoid sinuses, the cavernous sinus, and the straight sinus. Ultimately all the blood from the cranial cavity passes into the sigmoid sinus which becomes continuous with the upper end of the internal jugular vein.

TRIBUTARIES OF INFERIOR VENA CAVA

The **external iliac** and **internal iliac** veins accompany the corresponding arteries. They join to form the **common iliac** veins (Fig. 36.23). The inferior vena cava is formed by union of the right and left common iliac veins. The vena cava runs upwards lying to the right of the abdominal aorta. It ends by piercing the diaphragm to end in the right atrium of the heart. Apart from the common iliac veins that form it, the vena cava receives renal veins from the kidneys, hepatic veins from the liver, and lumbar veins from the body wall. The right testicular (or ovarian) vein joins the vena cava, but on the left side it ends in the renal vein.

THE HEPATIC PORTAL SYSTEM

Normally the arteries supplying an organ end in a set of capillaries from which blood is collected by veins which carry it to the heart (Fig. 36.24A). In some cases,

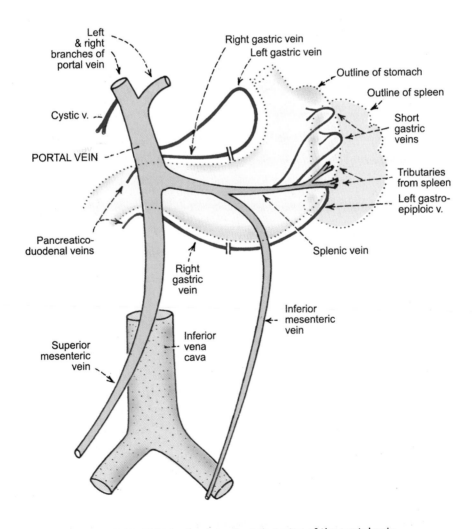

Fig. 36.25. Scheme to show the tributaries of the portal vein.

however, the veins from an organ enter another organ where they divide into another set of capillaries (or sinusoids). Such an arrangement is called a **portal system** (Fig. 36.24B).

The best example of a portal system is the hepatic portal system. The arteries supplying the abdominal part of the gastrointestinal tract (excluding the lower part of the anal canal) break up into capillaries in its wall (first set). Veins draining these capillaries ultimately end in the portal vein which enters the liver. Within the liver the portal vein divides into sinusoids (= 2nd set of capillaries). This blood is returned to the heart through the hepatic veins and the inferior vena cava.

The main veins comprising the hepatic portal system are shown in Fig. 36.25. Observe that the portal vein is formed by the union of the **superior mesenteric** and **splenic** veins. The **inferior mesenteric vein** joins the splenic vein. The right and left **gastric veins** drain directly into the portal vein. The **left gastroepiploic** and **short gastric** veins drain into the splenic vein, while the **right gastroepiploic vein** drains into the superior mesenteric vein.

The splenic vein, the superior and inferior mesenteric veins, and the veins of the stomach accompany the corresponding arteries and have tributaries corresponding to branches of these arteries. Note that veins corresponding to branches of the coeliac trunk end directly in the portal vein.

Index